Encyclopedia of Phytochemicals: Impacts on Health

Volume II

Encyclopedia of Phytochemicals: Impacts on Health

Volume II

Edited by **Vivian Belt**

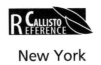

New York

Published by Callisto Reference,
106 Park Avenue, Suite 200,
New York, NY 10016, USA
www.callistoreference.com

Encyclopedia of Phytochemicals: Impacts on Health
Volume II
Edited by Vivian Belt

International Standard Book Number: 978-1-63239-283-1 (Hardback)

Printed in the United States of America.

Contents

Preface

This book on phytochemicals is designed in response to the requirement for more current research on the subject. Phytochemicals are biologically active non-nutritive compounds that occur naturally in plants. They are utilized for food and medicinal purposes. Several topics are encompassed in this book like phytochemicals and their pharmacological aspects, chemical as well as physical aspects and biological activities. This book consists of contributions made by internationally renowned authors. It is intended to satisfy the needs of health professionals, researchers, government regulatory agencies and industries. The aim of this book is to serve as a valuable source of reference for the readers who are related to this significant and rapidly advancing area of phytochemicals, and its impact on human health.

This book is a result of research of several months to collate the most relevant data in the field.

When I was approached with the idea of this book and the proposal to edit it, I was overwhelmed. It gave me an opportunity to reach out to all those who share a common interest with me in this field. I had 3 main parameters for editing this text:

1. Accuracy – The data and information provided in this book should be up-to-date and valuable to the readers.

2. Structure – The data must be presented in a structured format for easy understanding and better grasping of the readers.

3. Universal Approach – This book not only targets students but also experts and innovators in the field, thus my aim was to present topics which are of use to all.

Thus, it took me a couple of months to finish the editing of this book.

I would like to make a special mention of my publisher who considered me worthy of this opportunity and also supported me throughout the editing process. I would also like to thank the editing team at the back-end who extended their help whenever required.

Editor

Phytocannabinoids

Afeef S. Husni and Stephen J. Cutler
University of Mississippi,
USA

1. Introduction

What is marijuana? Marijuana, also known as *Cannabis*, is defined as any preparation of the *Cannabis sativa* plant used to exploit psychoactive effects whether it is recreational or medicinal. According to the 2004 World Drug Report, 3.7% of the population 15-64 years of age consumed marijuana from 2001-2003 (World Drug Report, 2004). The use of marijuana is associated with numerous pharmacological effects; most, but not all may attributed to tetrahydrocannabinol (THC). The combination of THC and other compounds from *Cannabis sativa* may all exhibit specific pharmacological effects. These isolates from *Cannabis* are known as cannabinoids (ElSohly, 2010).

Cannabinoids are a chemical class of C_{21} terpenophenolic compounds that represent a group of compounds found in *Cannabis sativa* (Mechoulam & Gaoni, 1967). Phytocannabinoids are the naturally occurring cannabinoids from *Cannabis* sp (Pate, 1999). It is now known that at least 85 cannabinoids have been derived from *Cannabis sativa* (El-Alfy et al., 2010). It is also known that some of these compounds are of medical importance in today's society.

In order to gain a better understanding of the pharmacological effects of the phytocannabinoids, human and rodent receptors are used to evaluate binding affinity of these compounds to two cannabinoid receptors that have been reported in literature, CB_1 and CB_2. CB_1 receptors are located mainly in the brain, while CB_2 receptors are primarily

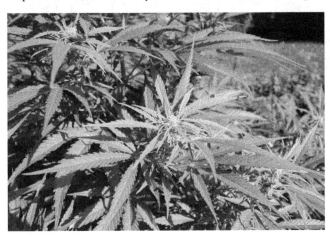

peripheral and found on mature B cells and macrophages within the tonsils and spleen (Raymon & Walls, 2010). When activated, the CB_1 receptors exhibit the psychoactive effects caused by *Cannabis* use. Since CB_1 receptors are not present in the medulla oblongata, part of the brain stem responsible for respiratory and cardiovascular functions, there is not a risk of overdose resulting in respiratory depression or cardiovascular failure that may be seen with abuse of other drugs, such as the opioids. CB_2 receptors are said to be responsible for anti-inflammatory effects.

2. Cannabinoid receptor function

Cannabinoid receptors are G-protein coupled receptors (Figure 1), which are a large family of seven member transmembrane receptors that act in a second messenger fashion. When cannabinoid receptors are activated, they inhibit the enzyme adenylate cyclase. Adenylate cyclase is responsible for breaking ATP to form cyclic AMP (cAMP). When a ligand binds to the extracellular surface of cannabinoid receptors, it causes a conformational change of the receptor. This change activates the second messenger by exchanging guanosine diphosphate (GDP) for guanosine triphosphate (GTP). Then, the G-protein's alpha subunit separates from the beta/gamma subunit to cause intracellular proteins to function properly. In CB_1 and CB_2 receptors, cAMP acts as the second messenger. When these receptors are activated, cAMP levels decrease within the cell. Therefore, the result of activating cannabinoid receptors leads to a decrease in cAMP levels, and in turn leads to an inhibition of function.

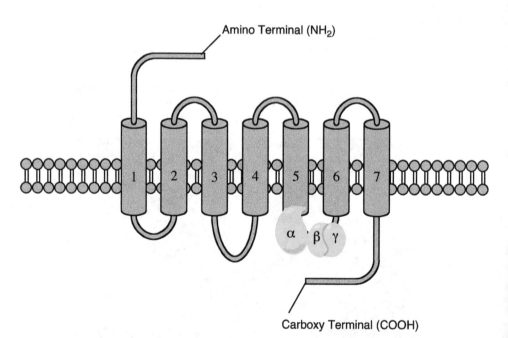

Fig. 1. Example of a G-Protein Coupled Receptor.

3. Endocannabinoids

Endogenous cannabinoids, or endocannabinoids, are substances produced in the body that activate the cannabinoid receptors. Generally, neurotransmitters are released presynaptically and activate the receptors on a postsynaptic cell. However, unlike most neurotransmitters, the endocannabinoids work in a reverse fashion. Endocannabinoids use retrograde signaling to achieve cannabinoid receptor activation. This means that the ligands are being produced postsynaptically, but acting presynaptically (Lambert, 2009). Another critical point in understanding the function of the endocannabinoids is that the endocannabinoid system can produce endocannabinoids "on demand" in response to an increase in intracellular calcium levels (Sugiura et al., 2006).

Shortly after the cloning of the cannabinoid receptors, researchers began searching for endogenous ligands that activate these receptors. The first endocannabinoid discovered was anandamide (Figure 2) in 1992 (Devane et al., 1992). Several years after the discovery of anandamide the second endogenous ligand, 2-arachadonoyl-glycerol (2-AG, Figure 3), was discovered (Sugiura et al., 2006). Anandamide and 2-AG act as a partial agonist and full agonist, respectively, at the CB_1 and CB_2 receptors. Although the structure of anandamide differs significantly from THC, both of these ligands have similar pharmacological profiles (Grotenhermen, 2002). Understanding the mechanism of how cannabinoids produce their effects is in part because of the discovery of the endocannabinoid system.

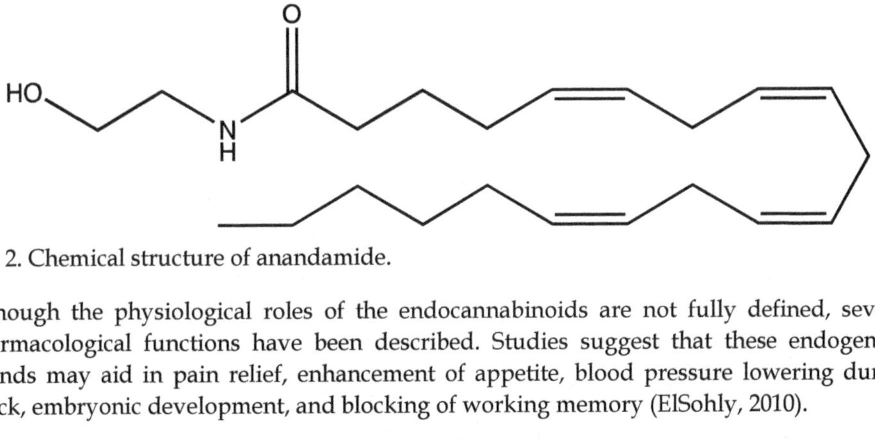

Fig. 2. Chemical structure of anandamide.

Although the physiological roles of the endocannabinoids are not fully defined, several pharmacological functions have been described. Studies suggest that these endogenous ligands may aid in pain relief, enhancement of appetite, blood pressure lowering during shock, embryonic development, and blocking of working memory (ElSohly, 2010).

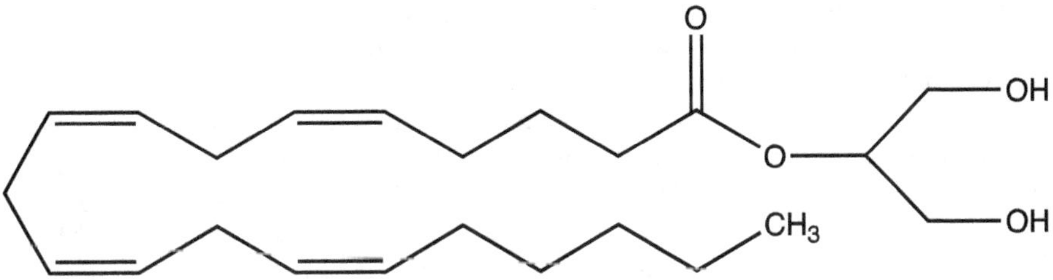

Fig. 3. Chemical structure of 2-AG.

4. Phytocannabinoids

The first cannabinoid identified was cannabigerol, and its precursor cannabigeric acid was shown to be the cannabinoid formed in the plant as well as endogenously (Yamauchi, 1975). Today, the most discussed phytocannabinoid is delta-9-tetrahydrocannabinol. In 1964, Gaoni and Mechoulam isolated and elucidated the chemical structure of THC from the leaves of *Cannabis sativa* (Mechoulam & Gaoni, 1964). THC is pharmacologically and toxicologically the best studied constituent of *Cannabis*, responsible for most of the psychoactive effects of natural *Cannabis* preparations (Grotenhermen, 2002). THC and cannabidiol (CBD) are the two most common naturally occurring cannabinoids.

As mentioned earlier, THC (Figure 4) is the main component of *Cannabis* responsible for the psychoactive effects. Other than *Cannabis* being abused to achieve a state of euphoria, it is now being used medicinally to aid in acquired immunodeficiency syndrome (AIDS) patients with wasting syndrome and for pain management, nausea, and vomiting associated with patients receiving cancer chemotherapy. Since THC is responsible for the psychoactive effects of *Cannabis*, people have learned how to genetically increase the concentration of THC within each plant to produce a stronger "high." Since 1980, the concentration of THC within marijuana has increased from less than 1.5% to approximately 20% (ElSohly et al., 2000). THC acts a partial agonist at the CB_1 and CB_2 receptors, but functions via interaction with the CB_1 receptor.

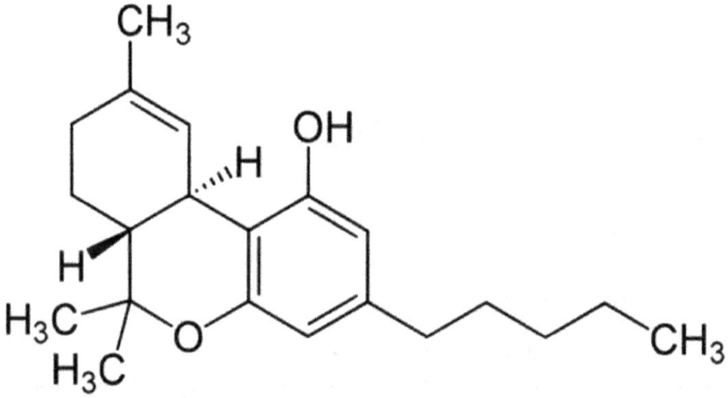

Fig. 4. Chemical structure of delta-9-THC.

The second major constituent of *Cannabis*, cannabidiol (CBD, Figure 5), is responsible for the anti-inflammatory effects due to its interactions with the human CB_2 receptor. CBD was first isolated in 1940 (Adams et al., 1940); however, it was not until 1963 that Mechoulam and Shvo elucidated its correct structure (Mechoulam & Shvo, 1963). At the human CB_2 receptor, CBD's mechanism of action shows inverse agonism activity (Pertwee et al., 2007). In 1995, Benet and colleagues show that cannabidiol is not only responsible for anti-inflammatory effects, but may also aid in reducing unpleasant side effects from THC, including reduced anxiety (Benet et al., 1995). They found that CBD inhibits cytochrome P450 3A11, which causes THC to change into its more potent metabolite 11-hydroxy-THC (Gallily et al., 2002).

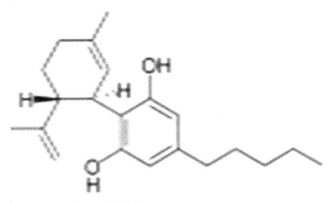

Fig. 5. Chemical structure of cannabidiol.

Tetrahydrocannabinol and cannabidiol are the two most discussed phytocannabinoids, but not the only ones known. ElSohly and co-investigators have divided the phytocannabinoids into ten subclasses: 1) Cannabigerol type – propyl side chains and monomethyl ether derivatives 2) Cannabichromene type – analogs present in the C-5 position 3) Cannabidiol type – analogs varying from C-1 to C-5 positions 4) Delta-9-tetrahydrocannabinol type – double bond in the C-9 position; responsible for psychoactive effects 5) Delta-8-tetrahydrocannabinol type – double bond in the C-8 position; thermodynamically more stable than delta-9-THC , however, 20% less active 6) Cannabicyclol type – five atom ring and C-1 bridge 7) Cannabielsoin type – artifacts formed from CBD 8) Cannabinol and Cannabinodiol types – A ring aromatization 9) Cannabitriol type – additional hydroxyl substitution 10) Miscellaneous types – ex: furano ring, carbonyl function, tetrahydroxy substitution (ElSohly, 2010).

Another phytocannabinoid that shows a significant amount of importance is cannabinol (CBN, Figure 6); it is a metabolite of tetrahydrocannabinol. It was the first cannabinoid identified from *Cannabis sativa*. (Wood et al., 1896). Along with THC, cannabinol is also a psychoactive component of *Cannabis* due to its interaction with CB_1 receptors. Compared to THC, it acts a weak agonist at both the CB_1 and CB_2 receptors.

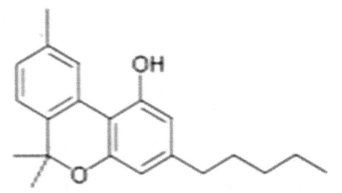

Fig. 6. Chemical structure of cannabinol.

Extracts that have been isolated from marijuana may be tested to see if they have affinity for each of the CB_1- or CB_2- type receptors. THC remains the best phytocannabinoid in terms of affinity for the cannabinoid receptors with a binding Ki of 14nM (Figure 7). Most of the compounds isolated from *Cannabis* show a sufficient amount of binding activity at both of the cannabinoid receptors. However, not all compounds isolated show interactions with either CB_1 or CB_2. For instance, even though cannabidiol is a major constituent of *Cannabis* and shows pharmacological effects, it has little or no activity for CB_1 or CB_2 receptors (Mechoulam & Rodriguez, 2007). To determine binding affinity and functional activity, in vitro assays are performed.

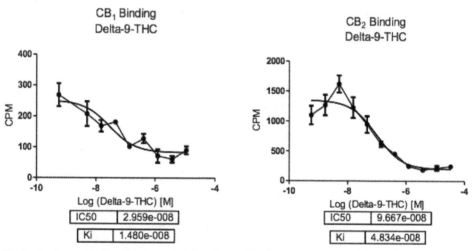

Fig. 7. Binding affinity of delta-9-THC at Cannabinoid Receptor 1 and Cannabinoid Receptor 2.

5. *In vitro* bioassays

In order to have success with in vitro assays, cultured cells containing the specific receptors must be developed. At the University of Mississippi HEK293 cells have been transfected with full length human CB_1 and human CB_2 DNA via electroporation. Once "shocked," the cells open and accept the human CB_1 and CB_2 cDNA with a linked specific antibiotic resistant plasmid. Since not all cells will receive the DNA, a selection process using the specific antibiotic is added to the cultured cells in order to kill off cells without the cDNA. After an allotted time period for growth, a single cell is selected and clonal colonies are grown in cell culture. The replication of a single cell containing either CB_1 or CB_2 DNA allows researchers to guarantee the over expression of cannabinoid receptors on the cell membrane. With this, mass subculture followed by "scraping" of the cells leads to the membrane with the receptors. Once the protein concentration is determined this membrane may be used for in vitro assays.

Phytocannabinoids may be tested for their binding affinity toward each of the cannabinoid receptors. A competitive binding assay is done to determine the binding affinity of each compound. The competition is between the chosen phytocannabinoid and a labeled ligand, such as [3H]- CP-55, 940. It is known that the labeled ligand will tightly bind to each of the cannabinoid receptors; therefore, if a test compound shows affinity for the receptors, the amount of labeled ligand bound to the receptor will be low resulting in high binding affinity of the test compound. A compound showing strong binding affinity for either of the cannabinoid receptors, warrants testing to determine the functional activity.

A functional assay determines whether the compound is acting as an agonist, antagonist, or inverse agonist. As opposed to the binding assay, an in vitro functional assay is not based upon competitive binding, but rather "tracking" the amounts of guanosine triphosphate (GTP). When the membrane is not stimulated, there is a pool of guanosine diphosphate (GDP) associated with it. Upon stimulation, this pool of GDP is converted into GTP. To monitor this response, ^{35}S labeled GTP is added to the assay to bind to the receptors. Therefore, an increase in GTP is directly proportional to stimulation of the receptor by labeled ligand. An agonist compound is indicated by an increase in GTP. Delta-9-THC has a functional Ki of approximately 300nM, which means it is acting as a partial agonist, yet is still responsible for the psychoactive effects associated with *Cannabis* (Figure 8). To detect an antagonist, the compound must be tested in the presence of a known agonist at that specific receptor. The antagonist blocks the ability of the agonist to fully stimulate the receptor, thus resulting in a right shift of the agonist EC$_{50}$.

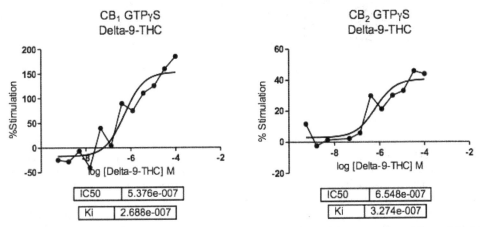

Fig. 8. Functional assay activity of delta-9-THC at Cannabinoid Receptor 1 and Cannabinoid Receptor 2.

6. *In Vivo* bioassays

Cannabinoids that show promising activity in the functional assay, whether acting as an agonist or antagonist, may be tested in vivo using the tetrad assay in mice. In the late 1980s, Little and his colleagues began testing rodents treated with cannabinoids in this tetrad assay. The term tetrad describes a series of four different tests to help evaluate the biological effects of a compound: 1) Locomotor activity 2) Catalepsy 3) Hypothermia and 4) Analgesia. The locomotor activity test allows a researcher to determine if the rodent is acting "lazy." The rodent is placed in a box with perpendicular gridlines, which are beams of light. The test determines the amount of times the beams are broken in an allotted time period, an increase in the number of times broken correlates with a decrease in locomotor activity. To determine if the drug causes cataleptic effects, a rodent is placed on a bar elevated off the ground surface. If the rodent remains immobile, it is considered cataleptic. Hypothermia, also know as a rectal temperature assay, is simply a measure of the rodents rectal temperature after the drug has been administered. For the last part of the tetrad assay, there are two different methods of testing for analgesic effects. One method is the hot plate (Figure 9) assay. In this assay, a rodent is placed upon a hot plate and the time it takes for the rodent to react, usually a small jump, is recorded. The second method is known as the tail-flick assay. In this assay, the rodent is immobilized and a high temperature beam of light is sporadically placed on the tail. If the rodent feels pain, it will move its tail either left or right (Little, 1988).

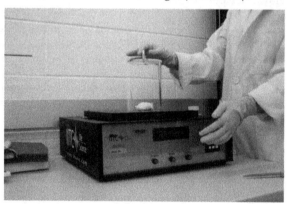

Fig. 9. Analgesic portion of tetrad assay: hot plate test.

7. Medicinal uses of marijuana

According the United Nations, *Cannabis* "is the most widely used illicit substance in the world" (World Drug Report, 2010). There are people who use Cannabis medicinally, and there are others who abuse *Cannabis* in order get "high," or obtain a state of euphoria. Those who use marijuana regularly for medicinal purposes use strict, smaller amounts to control the strength and duration of the "high." However, those who abuse marijuana attempt to smoke or ingest as much as necessary to achieve their own personal state of euphoria. This abuse negatively affects the people who do need *Cannabis* to help with side effects of chemotherapy and AIDS. *Cannabis* is not only used to help those suffering from cancer chemotherapy and AIDS, but it also lowers intraocular eye pressure for those with glaucoma, acts a pain reliever, and more recently has been found to help with symptoms of multiple sclerosis and depression. Therefore, researchers are attempting to formulate a synthetic cannabinoid that resembles the compounds isolated from *Cannabis,* but do not exploit psychotropic properties.

The goal of research in this area is to synthesize a cannabinoid-like compound that warrants a high affinity for either CB_1 or CB_2 receptors, or both, and can help patients without causing some of the unwanted side effects of marijuana, such as the psychotropic effects associated with CB_1. With this said, studies show that *Cannabis* users have fewer psychological side effects than those users administering synthetic THC. There are two synthetic cannabinoid products available on the market in the United States, Nabilone and Dronabinol (Figure 10). Some of these side effects from synthetic cannabinoids include dysphoria, depersonalization, anxiety, and paranoia (Grinsponn & Bakalar, 1997). As previously mentioned, CBD has shown to reduce anxiety and other unpleasant side effects caused by ingestion of pure THC (Zuardi et al., 1982). The preference of whole *Cannabis* over synthetic formulations of THC is due to the lack of extra side effects associated with the whole *Cannabis*. This opens the door for scientists to study what is actually causing all of the side effects associated with synthetic THC. This also shows that some of the compounds associated with *Cannabis sativa* may be working synergistically to alleviate unwanted effects from THC when used alone (McPartland & Russo, 2001). So, the ultimate goal in cannabinoid drug development would be to mimic the non-psychotropic effects associated with CB_1, mimic the beneficial effects associated with CB_2, and not deal with the negative side effects associated with marijuana or synthetic THC.

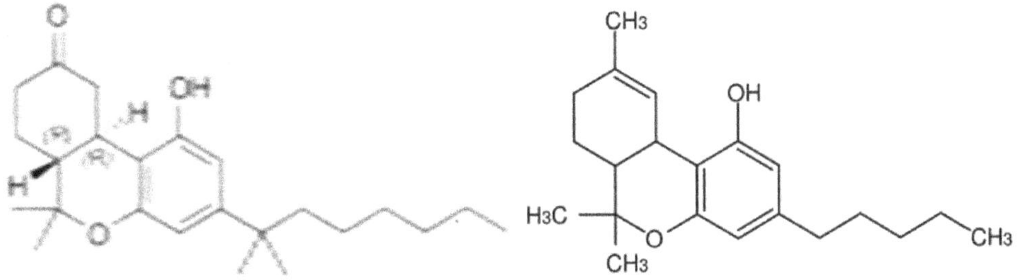

Fig. 10. Chemical structures of Nabilone (left) and Dronabinol (right).

8. Phytocannabinoids and depression

Depression may be described as a mood disorder associated with feeling down, sad, angry, or lost that interferes with everyday life. The most commonly associated drug categories for the treatment of depression include monoamine oxidase inhibitors (MAOIs), tricyclic antidepressants (TCAs), selective-serotonin reuptake inhibitors (SSRIs), and serotonin-norepinephrine reuptake inhibitors (SNRIs). A new field of research involving *Cannabis* may be the link to the treatment of depression. However, studies show conflicting data as to whether *cannabis* is beneficial (Grinsponn & Balkar, 1998) or detrimental for the treatment of depression (Bovassa, 2001). Due to the conflicting results of these studies, Witkin switched the focus to the role of the endocannabinoid system and the treatment of depression from exogenously administered cannabinoids (Witkin et al., 2005). Since 2005, it has been concluded that the endocannabinoid system does play a role in the treatment of depression, but differs from minor depression to major depression.

New research has found that a common characteristic of *Cannabis*, mood elevation, may be the link to the treatment of depression. A study published by El-Alfy and co-investigators in 2010 describes the antidepressant effects associated with administration of phytocannabinoids. The objective of this study was to isolate the major cannabinoids from *Cannabis* and evaluate the antidepressant effects using the mouse forced swim test (FST), followed by the tail suspension test (TST). Typically in mice, when cannabinoids are administered they exert hypothermia and catalepsy, which means that a psychoactive state is being achieved. For these depression studies, only low dosages of these phytocannabinoids were administered so that the test subjects did not demonstrate psychoactive effects. The cannabinoids isolated and tested were cannabigerol (CBG), cannabinol (CBN), cannabichromene (CBC), cannabidiol (CBD), delta-8-THC, and delta-9-THC (THC) (Figure 12).

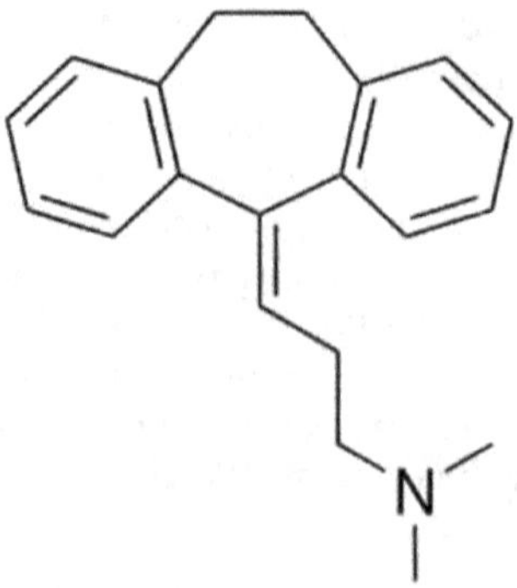

Fig. 11. Chemical structure of the tricyclic antidepressant, Amitriptyline.

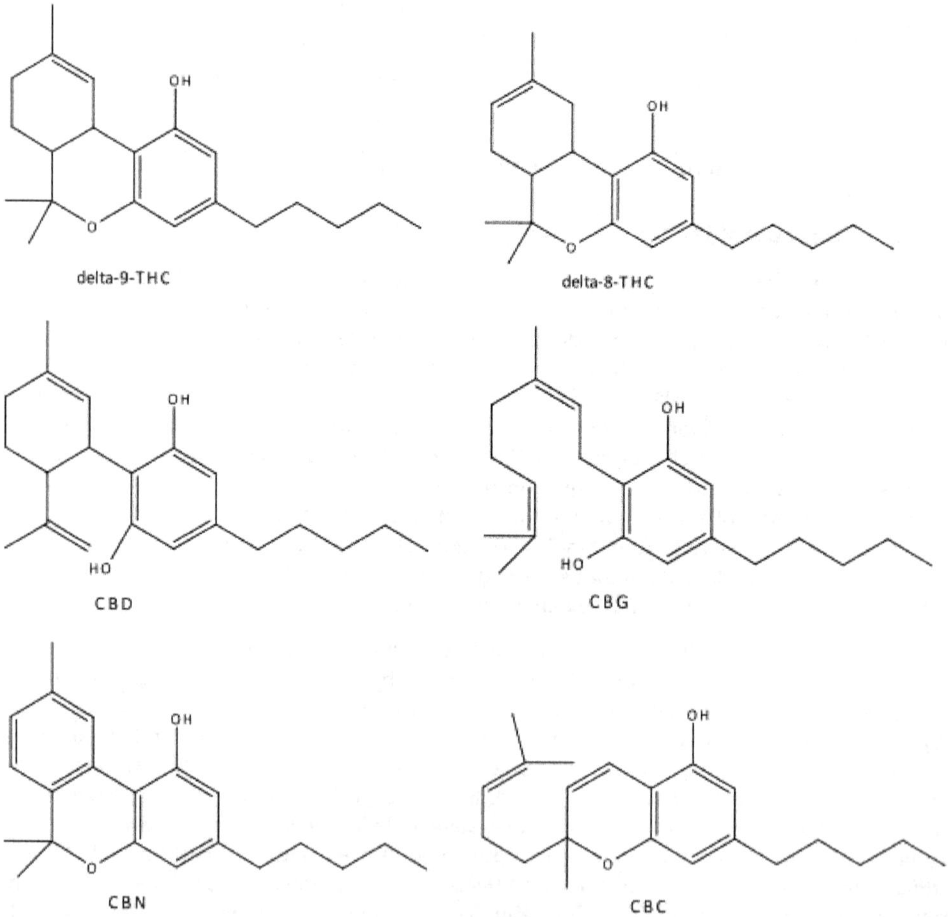

delta-9-THC

delta-8-THC

CBD

CBG

CBN

CBC

Fig. 12. The six phytocannabinoids tested for antidepressant-like effects (El-Alfy et al., 2010).

To assess that hypothermia and catalepsy were not achieved, the tetrad assay was completed after administration of each cannabinoid. Out of the six cannabinoids tested, only delta-8-THC and delta-9-THC showed a U-shaped dose response in the forced swim test. With this, only delta-9-THC showed significant antidepressant-like effects. Administration of the non-psychoactive components revealed that CBC and CBD displayed antidepressant-like effects in the forced swim test. However, a high dose of CBD was used to display these antidepressant-like effects.

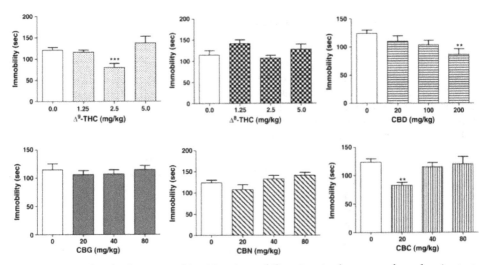

Fig. 13. Effects of each phytocannabinoid on immobility time in the mouse forced swim test (El-Alfy et al., 2010).

To further confirm these tests, delta-9-THC and CBC were evaluated in the tail suspension test. Between these two phytocannabinoids, only delta-9-THC continued to exhibit these antidepressant-like effects at low doses. Therefore, the results of this study show that delta-9-THC and other phytocannabinoids administered exogenously do indeed aid with the treatment of depression (El-Alfy et al., 2010).

9. Phytocannabinoids and appetite stimulation

Patients suffering from AIDS are now becoming the main target for the therapeutic use of *Cannabis*. Those with AIDS tend to lose their desire to eat regularly throughout the day. When this occurs, the patient becomes weak, agitated, tired, and anorexic; this occurrence in known as Wasting Syndrome. Research shows that at least 90% of patients who smoked marijuana had the desire to eat immediately after use (Haines & Green, 1970). With the use of *Cannabis* as a therapeutic drug to stimulate appetite, the suffering patients may be able to eat on a regular basis throughout the day, thus improving their quality of life. Several studies have shown that the use of marijuana does increase appetite, which also increases energy in daily life routines.

In a study conducted by Mattes and colleagues, the appetite stimulating effects of cannabinoids, specifically THC, were examined. A major focus in this study, for a means of clarification from previous research, was the route of administration of THC. The four

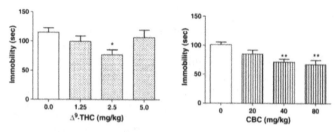

Fig. 14. Effects of THC and CBC on immobility time in the mouse tail suspension test (El-Alfy et al., 2010).

different ways in which THC was administered includes oral, inhaled, sublingual, and suppository. There are high levels of variability in determining if THC does actually stimulate appetite. Factors such as environment, age, gender, tolerance, dosage, and social influences play a role in the effect of THC on appetite. During one study, the suppository route of administration resulted in the highest energy intake when compared to oral, sublingual, and inhaled administration of THC (Figure 15).

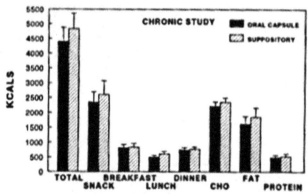

Fig. 15. Mean data from patients dosed orally and via suppository over a 72 hour time period (Mattes et al., 1994).

There is no single outcome on the effect of THC on appetite stimulation no matter the form of administration. The results vary from having no effect to the possibility of having major food cravings. In some circumstances, not only did the food cravings become increased, but during a meal the food seemed to also have an increased taste of delightfulness. The conclusion of this study indicates that THC as an appetite stimulant produces its highest effects on healthy, adult individuals who use low dosage amounts (Mattes et al., 1994).

10. Future directions

The growing population is becoming more aware of *Cannabis* as a medicinal plant, and not only a recreational drug. The first *Cannabis* publications date back to the early 1940's in which there was only one publication from 1940-1949. Today, when a search is performed there are over 7,000 journal articles that discuss anything associated with the words *Cannabis*, cannabinoids, or endocannabinoids. Over the last 50 years, marijuana has become the most widely used illegal drug, along with one of the most widely studied plants. There are still many questions to be answered within the *Cannabis* field of study.

It is possible that the cannabinoid system has several other receptors that may explain the mechanism of action of compounds that exhibit cannabinoid-like effects when there is little or no affinity for CB_1 or CB_2. GPR55 and GPR119, both G-protein coupled receptors, are said to be novel cannabinoid receptors. All cannabinoid receptor antagonists appear to act as inverse agonists instead of neutral antagonists. There are few ligands starting to appear in literature as being neutral antagonists. Interest in this area could is important to help develop pharmacological tools to aid in finding neutral antagonists. These findings may possess unknown therapeutic advantages over receptor antagonists that act as inverse agonists (Pertwee, 2005).

It is now known that phytocannabinoids interact with the CB_1 and CB_2 receptors, and that the human body consists of an endocannabinoid system that activates these two receptors. However, what these receptors look like remains a mystery. A general structure-activity relationship has been determined for the cannabinoids, but there is no limitation to synthesizing new compounds that will interact strongly with these receptors. In *vitro* and in *vivo* bioassays play a crucial role in determining the affinities and functions of compounds associated with the CB_1 and CB_2 receptors. The information determined from these bioassays will continue to help develop novel therapeutic drugs that potentially have pharmacological effects related to *Cannabis* without the deleterious side effects.

11. References

Adams, R., Hunt, M., & Clark, J. (1940). Structure of cannabidiol, a product isolated from the marihuana extract of Minnesota wild hemp. I. *J. Am. Chem. Society.* 62, 196-199.

Bornheim, L., Kim, K., Li, J., Perotti, B., & Benet, L. (1995). Effect of cannabidiol pretreatment on the kinetics of Tetrahydrocannabinol metabolites in mouse brain. *Drug Metab. Dispos.* 23, 825-831.

Bovassa, G. (2001). Cannabis abuse as a risk factor for depressive symptoms. *American Journal Psychiatry.* 158: 2033-2037.

Devane, W., Hanus, L., Breur, A., Pertwee, R., Stevenson, L., Griffin, G., Gibson, D., Mandelbaum, A., Etinger, A., & Mechoulam, R. (1992). Isolation and Structure of a Brain Constituent That Binds to the Cannabinoid Receptor. *Science.* 258, 1946-1949.

El-Alfy, A., Ivey, K., Robinson, K., Ahmed, S., Radwan, M., Slade, D., Khan, I., ElSohly, M., & Ross, S. (2010). Antidepressant-like effect of [Delta]9-tetrahydrocannabinol and other cannabinoids isolated from Cannabis sativa L. *Pharmacology Biochemistry and Behavior*, 95, 4, June 2010, 434-442, ISSN 0091-3057.

ElSohly, M., Ross, S., Mehmedic, Z., Arafat, R., Yi, B., & Banahan, B. (2000). Potency trends of Delta-9-THC and other cannabinoids in confiscated marijuana from 1980-1997. *J. Forens. Sci.* 45, 24-30.

ElSohly, M. (2010). *Marijuana and the Cannabinoids.* Humana Press. ISBN: 978-1-61737-581-1.Totowa, New Jersey.

Gaoni, Y. & Mechoulam, R. (1964). *J. Am. Chem. Soc.* 86, 1646.

Grinsponn, L. & Bakalar, J. (1997). *Marihuana, the forbidden medicine*, revised edition. New Haven, CT: Yale University Press.

Grinsponn, L. & Balkar, J. (1998). The use of cannabis as a mood stabilizer in bipolar disorder: anectodotal evidence and the need for clinical research. *Journal Psychoactive Drugs.* 30, 171-177.

Grotenhermen, F. (2002). Effects of Cannabis and the cannabinoids, in Cannabis and Cannabinoids, In: *Pharmacology, Toxicology, and Therapeutic Potential*, Grotenhermen, F. and Russo, E., pages 55-65, Haworth Press, New York.

Haines, L. & Green, W. (1970). Marijuana use patterns. *British Journal of Addiction*. 65, 347-362.

Lambert, D. (2009). *Cannanbinoids in Nature and Medicine*. Wiley-Verlag Helvetica Chimica Acta. ISBN: 978-3-906390-56-7. Zurich, Switzerland.

Little, P., Compton, D., Johnson, M., Melvin, L., & Martin, B. (1988). Pharmacology and stereoselectivity of structurally novel cannabinoids in mice. *Journal of Pharmacol. Exp. Ther.* 247, 1046-1051.

Mattes, R., Engelman, K., Shaw, L., & ElSohly, M. (1994). Cannabinoids and appetite stimulation. *Pharamcology, Biochemistry, and Behavior*. 49, 187-195

McPartland, J. & Russo, E. (2001). Cannabis and cannabis extracts: greater than the sum of their parts? *J. Cann. Therap.* 1, 103-132.

Mechoulam, R. & Shvo, Y. (1963) Hasish-I. The structure of cannabidiol. *Tetrahedron* 19, 2073-2078.

Mechoulam, R. & Gaoni, Y. (1967). Recent advances in the chemistry of hashish. *Fortschr. Chem. Org. Naturst*, 25, 175-213.

Mechoulam, R., Parker, L., & Gallily, R. (2002) Cannabidiol: an overview of some pharmacological aspects. *J. Clinical Pharmacology*. 42, 11S-19S.

Mechoulam, R. & Peters, M. (2007). Cannabidiol-Recent advances. *Chemistry and Biochemistry* 4, 8, 1678-1692.

Pate, D. (1999) Anandamide structure-activity relationships and mechanisms of action on intraocular pressure in the normotensive rabbit model. *Doctoral dissertation*. Kuopio University Publications, Kuopio.

Pertwee, R. (2005). Pharmacological actions of cannabinoids. *Handbook of Experimental Pharmacology*. 168: 1-51.

Raymon, L. & Walls, H. (2010). Marijuana and the Cannabinoids. *Pharmacology of Cannabinoids*. Page 97-143.

Shoyama, Y., Yagi, M., Nishioka, I., & Yamauchi, T. (1975). Biosynthesis of cannabinoid acids. *Phytochemistry*, 14, 2189-2192.

Sugiura, T., Kishimoto, S., Oka, S., & Gokoh, M. (2006). Biochemistry, pharmacology and physiology of 2-arachadonoylglycerol, and endogenous cannabinoid receptor ligand. *Prog. Lipid Res.* 45, 405-446.

Thomas, A., Baillie, G., Phillips, A., Razdan, R., Ross, R., Pertwee, R. (2007) *British Journal of Pharmacology*. 150, 613.

Witkin, J., Tzavara, E., Davis, R., Li, X., & Nomikos, G. (2005). A therapeutic role for cannabinoid CB1 receptor antagonists in major depressive disorders. *Trends Pharmacol. Sci.* 26, 609-617.

Wood, T., Spivey, W., & Easterfield, T. (1896). *Journal of the Chemical Society*. 69, 539.

Yamauchi, T., Shoyama, Y., Yagi, M., & Nishioka, I. (1975). Biosynthesis of cannabinoid acids. *Phytochemistry*. 14, 10, 2189-2192.

Zuardi, A., Morais, S., Guimaraes, F., & Mechoulam, R. (1995). Antipsychotic effect of cannabidiol. *J. Clinical Psychiatry*. 56, 485-486.

2004 World Drug Report, United Nations, Office of Drugs and Crime. Oxford University Press, Oxford, United Kingdom.

2010 World Drug Report, United Nations, Office of Drugs and Crime. Oxford University Press, Oxford, United Kingdom.

2

Phytochemistry of some Brazilian Plants with Aphrodisiac Activity

Cinara V. da Silva, Fernanda M. Borges and Eudes S. Velozo
Federal University of Bahia,
Brazil

1. Introduction

Since time immemorial man has used various parts of plants in the treatment and prevention of many ailments, including sexual impotence (Ayyanar & Ignacimuthu, 2009 as cited in Chah et al., 2006). Ancient people knew about herbal and animal aphrodisiacs, used in combinations like potions to mystical rites to infertility, to increase sexual performance, desire and pleasure (Malviya et al., 2011).

One of the first mentions of aphrodisiacs is in the Egyptian papyruses from 2300 to 1700 B.C. In the papyrus of Ebers, mandragora, garlic, onion and blue lotus were found as plants with aphrodisiac activity (Zanolari, 2003).

The tomb of Tutankhamon contain a gold plated shrine decorated with a bas-relief of a pharaoh holding a blue lotus and two mandragoras in his left hand, since the Egyptians believed in sexual life after death (Bertol et al., 2004).

Hindu poems dating from 2000 to 1000 B.C. and the Kama Sutra had already reported to the use of some products to enhance the sex (Zanolari, 2003). The traditional Chinese Medicine uses with aphrodisiac purpose, among others, ginseng, Chinese chive and parts of animals for example: dogs, rhino, bear and tiger penis and testicles (Still, 2003).

On this basis, the legendary love potions, such as Spanish fly, glandular products from musk deer and civet cats, varieties of natural oats (*Avena sativa*), ginseng, belladonna, and erotic foods like fish and oysters, are known aphrodisiacs (Drewes et al., 2003 as cited in Choudhary & Ur-Rahman, 1997).

The word aphrodisiac has its origin in Greek Mythology, most precisely from the goddess of love, Aphrodite. It has been used to define the products applied with proposal of increasing desire and drive associated with sexual instinct. Besides they have represented a passion of man, since historically, in all cultures, the sexual potency is considered as a significant part of the male ego and the anxiety and humiliation is frequently associated with a declining sexual ability (Malviya et al., 2011; Zanolari, 2003).

An aphrodisiac includes any food or drug that arouses the sexual instinct, induces venereal desire and increases pleasure and performance. There are two main types of aphrodisiacs: psychophysiological stimuli (visual, tactile, olfactory and aural) preparations and internal preparations (food, alcoholic drinks and love potion) (Malviya et al., 2011).

Currently, the increase in life expectancy of human beings has increased the demand for substances capable of improving quality of this longevity. Among these are products that enhance sexual performance, treat impotence or erectile dysfunction.

Brazil is the country with around 55,000 species of higher plants about a quarter of all known and greatest biodiversity in the world (Velozo et al., 2002). Many of these plants are used in folk medicine to aphrodisiac purposes in the form of teas, mixed with alcohol and other beverages. Some of them are belonging to the families like Anacardiaceae, Fabaceae, Sapindaceae, Amarantaceae, Amaryllidaceae, Aristolochiaceae, Bignoniaceae, Erythroxylaceae, Oleaceae, Asteraceae, Sapindaceae, Annonaceae and Dilleniaceae.

Several phytochemical studies, with species from these families above cited, have enabled the isolation of secondary metabolites possibly related to its pharmacological activity, such as alkaloids, flavonoids and saponins.

This chapter is a review on the chemical composition of Brazilian plants most used by the population for aphrodisiac purpose, searching rationalization between the chemical structure and biological activity (SAR).

2. Erectile dysfunction and aphrodisiac products

Erectile dysfunction (ED) is experienced at least some of the time by the most of men who have reached 45 years of age, and it is projected to affect 322 million men worldwide by 2025. This prevalence is high in men of all ages but increases greatly in the elderly (Seftel et al., 2002).

Sexual dysfunction, erectile dysfunction or male impotence is characterized by the inability to develop or maintain an erection of the penis and can be caused by psychological disorders like anxiety, stress and depression, physical disorders like chronic diseases: diabetes and hypertension; hormonal problems or sedentary life-style, alcohol and smoking abuses (Malviya et al., 2011; Sumalatha et al., 2010).

Drugs play a significant role in the pathogenesis of ED, altering hormonal or vascular mechanics needed for erection. Alterations in penile vessels can be observed in the elderly and in particular, lack of androgens may lead to a reduction of smooth muscle cells content in the penis and an increase in the caliber of vascular spaces (Vignera et al., 2011 as cited in Galiano et al., 2010).

An erection is a hemodynamic balance between inflow and outflow of blood within two chambers named corpus cavernosum and it starts with sensory and mental stimulation. There is a relaxation of the smooth muscles and arterioles which allows blood supply to flow in the sinusoidal space. The increased flow of blood, compress venules between sinusoids and the tunica albuginea of the corpus cavernosum. The lack of the distension of tunica albuginea results in venous occlusion, which increases the intracavernosal pressure, generating and sustaining a full erection (Zanolari, 2003).

The erection ends when the muscles of penis contract, opening outflow channels. The relaxation of cavernous smooth muscle is mediated by Nitric Oxide (NO) via cyclic guanosine monophosphate (cGMP). After sexual stimulation, nitric oxide is released by nerve endings and endothelial cells. Nitric oxide (NO) stimulates GMP cyclase to produce cGMP, which leads to relaxation of smooth muscle. The erection ceases after a while because cGMP is hydrolysed by phosphodiesterase enzime into inactive GMP. Five types of phosphodiesterases are known to cause hydrolysis in cGMP. In the penis, phosphodiesterase is type V. Thus, a drug that inhibits the phosphodiesterase type V (cGMP-specific) should accelerate the action of nitric oxide and cGMP in erection (Drewes et al., 2003).

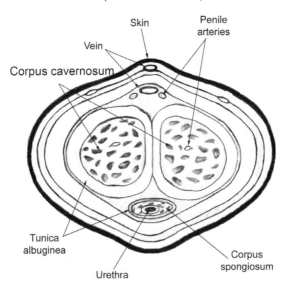

Fig. 1. Penis anatomy diagram

2.1 Male dysfunction therapies

The treatment with a psychotherapeutic approach is indicated to patients with psychological disorders. To patients with physical disorders, current treatments include oral medication, intracavernosal injection, vacuum pumps and penile prosthesis.

Some oral medications are available and well-established for ED treatment, among of them, two natural products: Cantharidin (Spanish fly) and Yohimbine, besides synthetic selective inhibitors, such as sildenafil (Viagra®), vardenafil (Levitra®), tadalafil (Cialis®), lodenafil (Helleva®) and udenafil (Zydena®) (see fig.2). The PDE-5 inhibitors have shown efficacy compared to placebo, in addition to present similar form of action and side effects like headache, flushing, dyspepsia and nasal congestion (Matheus et al., 2009; Wang et al., 2008).

The cantharidin is a lactone found in Spanish flies (also called Cantharides), beetles that have been cited in most of Asian and European Pharmacopoeias and have been used in dried form in internal preparations to impotence. Cantharides acts causing irritation of the urethra with vascular congestion, and inflammation of the erectile tissue. The Spanish flies are fallen into disuse due to their toxic effects (Zanolari, 2003).

Yohimbine is an indole alkaloid with a 2-adrenergic blocking activity. It comes from the bark of the African tree *Corynanthe yohimbe*, its first isolation was in the early 1930s and remained on the African market until 1973 like a drug marketed Aphrodex. Renewed interest in yohimbine for ED has prompted several new investigative trials; however, there are indications of side-effects such as hypertension, anxiety, manic symptoms and interactions with used medications (Drewes et al., 2003).

Some natural products act like non-selective PDE inhibitors as the methylxanthines caffeine and theophylline, but others show similar effects to PDE-5 inhibitors, for example: flavonoids and derivatives (quercetin from *Allium cepa*, pyrano-isoflavones from *Eriosema kraussianum* - Kraussianone 1 and 2); alkaloids (Neferin from *Nelumbo nucifera*, Berberine from *Berberis aristata*, Papaverine from *Papaver somniferum* - used in association with Prostaglandin-E1 to injections intracavernosal), saponins (Steroidal saponins from *Allium tuberosum*), coumarins (Osthole from *Angelica pubescens*) and terpenes (Forskolin from *Coleus forskohlii*) (Drewes et al., 2003; Guohua et al., 2009; Rahimi et al., 2009; Sumalatha et al., 2010; Zanolari, 2003).

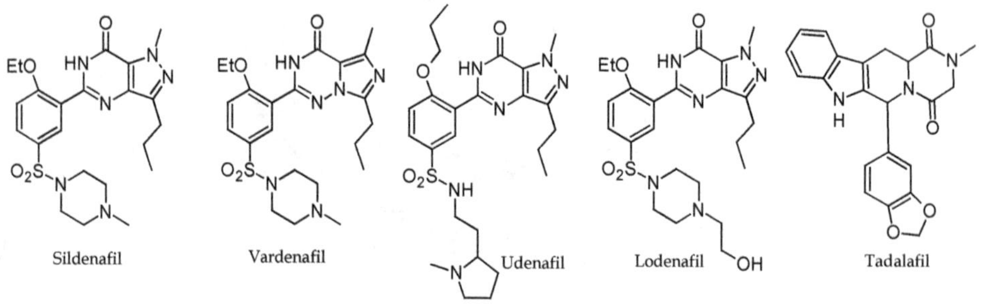

Sildenafil   Vardenafil   Udenafil   Lodenafil   Tadalafil

Fig. 2. Selective inhibitors of PDE-5

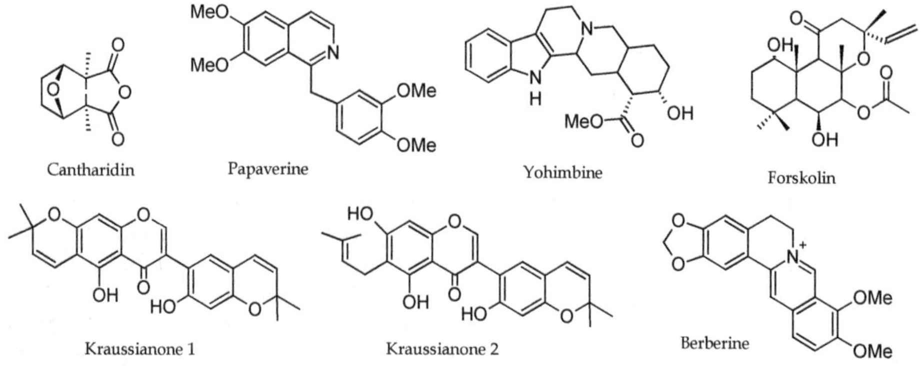

Cantharidin   Papaverine   Yohimbine   Forskolin

Kraussianone 1   Kraussianone 2   Berberine

Fig. 3. Examples of natural products with aphrodisiac effect

2.2 Chemical of some Brazilian aphrodisiacs species and rationalization between structure and activity

The success of PDE-5 inhibitors, particularly of Viagra, the first inhibitor that has been marketed, the aging of the population and the quest for improved quality of life led to the search for new drugs with fewer side effects. As sources of research, plants used as aphrodisiacs have turned to folk medicine in whole world.

There are many herbal drugs that have been used by men with ED with varying degrees of success. Most potent aphrodisiacs herbal are available and have few side effects (Malviya et al., 2011).

Some of the genera and species listed in this work in *in vitro* tests showed satisfactory answers to such an aphrodisiac effect like *Turnera diffusa* (Estrada-Reyes et al., 2009), *Pfaffia paniculata* (Arletti et al., 1999), *Passiflora* (Patel et al. 2009), *Mucuna pruriens* (Suresh et al., 2009), *Mimosa pudica* (Pande & Pathak, 2009), *Mimosa tenuiflora* (Souza et al., 2008), *Achyrocline satureioides* (Hnatyszyn et al, 2004; Simões et al., 1986) and *Anemopaegma arvense* (Chieregatto, 2005).

The effects of the Brazilian herbal medicine Catuama® and each of its plant constituents (*Paullinia cupana, Trichilia catigua, Zingiber officinalis and Ptychopetalum olacoides*) were investigated on rabbit corpus cavernosum. Catuama® induced relaxations, but P. *cupana* was the most effective, increased the cAMP levels by 200% indicating that it is the main extract responsible for the relaxing effect (Antunes et al., 2001).

Specie (Family)	Part used	Popular Name
Achyrocline satureioides (Asteraceae)	Inflorescence	Macela do campo Macela
Anacardium Ocidentale (Anacardiaceae)	Nut Pseudo-fruit	Caju
Anemopaegma arvense (Bignoniaceae)	Stem bark Roots	Catuaba verdadeira Marapuama Alecrim do campo
Aristolochia cymbifera (Aristolochiaceae)	Stem	Cipó mil homens
Arrabidaea chica (Bignoniaceae)	Leaves	Cipó cruz Carajiru
Artocarpus integrifolia (Moraceae)	Seeds	Jaca
Davilla rugosa (Dilleniaceae)	Stem , Leaves	Cipó caboclo
Erythroxylum viceniifolium (Erythroxylaceae)	Stem bark	Catuaba
Hippeastrum psittacinum (Amaryllidaceae)	Bulbs	Alho-bravo Alho-do-mato Açucena-do-campo
Mimosa pudica (Fabaceae)	Stem bark	Dormideira
Mimosa tenuiflora (Fabaceae)	Stem bark	Jurema preta
Mucuna pruriensis (Fabaceae)	Seeds	Pó-de-mico Mucuna preta
Nymphaea ampla (Nymphaeaceae)	Whole plant	Ninfa branca
Passiflora sp. (P. edulis, P. alata and P. caerulea) (Passifloraceae)	Leaves	Maracujá
Paulinia cupana (Sapindaceae)	Seeds	Guaraná
Pfaffia paniculata (Amarantaceae)	Roots	Ginseng brasileiro
Ptychopetalum olacoides (Oleaceae)	Bark	Marapuama
Schinus terebinthifolius (Anarcadiaceae)	Bark	Aroeira vermelha
Trichilia catigua (Meliaceae)	Bark , Leaves	Catuaba
Turnera diffusa (Turneraceae)	Leaves	Damiana

Table 1. Main Brazilian species with aphrodisiac activity

2.2.1 Aphrodisiacs chemical classes

The classes of substances discussed were those with proven aphrodisiac activity or with this possible action. The compounds were separated in three main groups, according to structures similarities: flavonoids and others phenolics compounds; alkaloids, xanthins and others amines; and saponins.

2.2.1.1 Flavonoids and other phenolic compounds

Flavonoids are polyphenols with a diphenylpropane core. According to the chemical and biosynthetic routes, flavonoids are separated into different classes: chalcones, flavonols, flavones, dihydroflavonoids, anthocyanidins, isoflavones, aurones, pterocarpanes, neoflavonoids, bioflavonoids and are presents in all flowering plants.

The major classes are flavones, flavonols, anthocyanins, isoflavones and the flavan-3-ol derivatives (catechin and tannins) (Miean & Mohamed, 2001).

The flavonoids are widely distributed in gymnosperms and angiosperms with therapeutic potential because of their antioxidant, anti-inflammatory, hepatoprotective, cardio protective, antiulcer, anticancer, antimutagenic, antispasmodic, anti-allergic and antiviral activities, besides to show inhibit xanthine oxidase, protein kinase C and PDE (Rahimi et al., 2009; Ko et al., 2004).

Miean & Mohamed (2001) studied 62 tropical species to presence of flavonoids and observed that flavonol quercetin and derivatives, mainly quercetin glycosides, had major occurrence, however glycosides of kaempferol, luteolin and apigenin were also present. In fruits contained almost exclusively quercetin glycosides.

In plants surveyed, in addition to flavonoids, other phenols were found such as caffeic and chlorogenic acid in *Achyrocline satureioides* (Desmarchelier et al., 2000) and chlorogenic acid in *Trichilia catigua* (Lagos, 2006), besides anacardic acid in *Anacardium ocidentale* (Kubo et al., 1994).

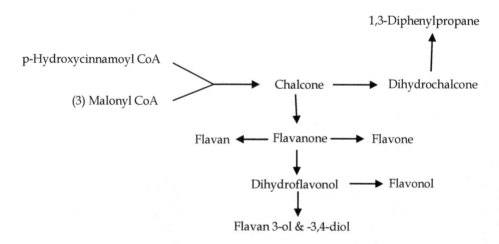

Fig. 4. Biosynthetic relationship among classes of flavonoids (Barron & Ibrahim, 1996)

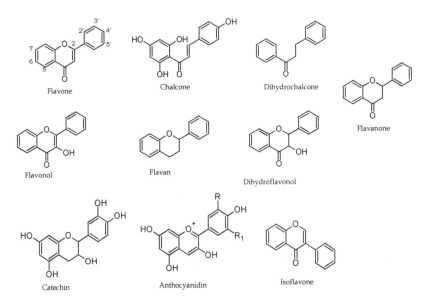

Fig. 5. Basic Structures of Flavonoids

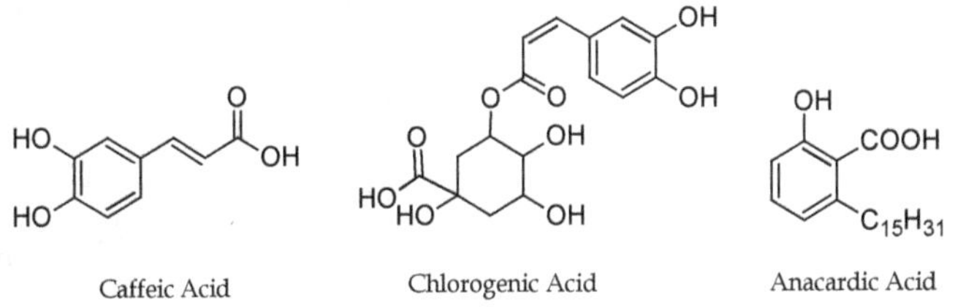

Fig. 6. Phenolic substances

Studies conducted by Ko and colleagues (2004) in flavonoids as inhibitors of PDE have suggested that C-4' and C-5' hydroxyl groups is not important for PDE-5 inhibition. The replacement of the hydroxyl by a methoxyl did not alter its inhibitory effect and it deletion resulted in no effect on PDE-5 inhibition. However, the C-7 hydroxyl group is very important for PDE-5 inhibition. C-7-glucoside showed no inhibition of the enzyme, being possible that the bulky glycosyl residues may hinder its binding to active site. Also, the C-3-hydroxyl group of flavonols seems difficult the binding with the PDE-5.

The luteolin showed more potent than other flavonoids, indicating that the presence of a double bond between C-2 and C-3 is important for PDE-5 inhibition. Between a flavon and an isoflavone, it may be easier for isoflavones than flavones to bind to the moiety of PDE-5. The removal of the C-5 hydroxyl group promoted the loss of inhibition of PDE, proposing that the hydroxyl group is vital for PDE-5 inhibition (Ko et al., 2004).

Specie (Family)	Flavonoids and phenols
Achyrocline satureioides (Asteraceae)	Quercetin 3-O-Metil Quercetin Luteolin And Caffeic, chlorogenic and isochlorogenic acids (Desmarchelier et al., 2000).
Anacardium Ocidentale (Anacardiaceae)	Myricetin And Quercetin, Anacardic Acids and derivatives (Kubo et al., 1994; Miean & Mohamed, 2001).
Anemopaegma arvense (Bignoniaceae)	Catuabine A Cinchonain Ia R= —OH Cinchonain IIa R= ''''OH KandelinAl (Tabanca et al.,2007)
Arrabidaea chica (Bignoniaceae)	Vicenin-A (Barbosa et al., 2008) Carajuruflavone (Takemura et al., 1995) Acacetin (Zorn et al., 2001) R₁= H; R = CH₃ - Carajurin 4'-hydroxi-3,7-dimethoxiflavone (Barbosa et al., 2008) Kaempferol (Barbosa et al., 2008) R₁= OH; R= H - 6,7,3',4'-tetrahydroxy-5-methoxyflavylium R₁= H; R= H - 6,7,4'-trihydroxy-5- methoxyflavylium (Zorn et al., 2001)

Specie (Family)	Flavonoids and phenols
Davilla rugosa (Dilleniaceae)	Narigenin 4'-O-methyltaxifolin Quercetin (David et al, 2006)
Mimosa tenuiflora (Fabaceae)	 R= O Me; R₁= OH; R₂= Me - Tenuiflorin A R= R₁= OMe; R₂= H - Tenuiflorin B R= H; R₁= OH; R₂= Me - Tenuiflorin C R= H; R₁= H; R₂= H - 6-Dimethoxycapilarisin R= H; R₁= H; R₂= Me - 6-Dimethoxy-4'-O-methylcapilarisin R= O Me - Kukulkan A R= OH - Kukulkan B (Souza et al., 2008)
Nymphaea ampla (Nymphaeaceae)	Quercetin derivatives (glycosides) (Marquina et al., 2005)
Passiflora sp. (Passifloraceae)	Vitexin Scoparin Isoorientin Orientin Isovitexin Chrysin (*P. Caeruleae*) Dhwan et al., 2002) Apigenin and luteolin derivatives (*P. edulis*) (Ferreres et al., 2007) Flavonoids above (*P. alata*)(Doyama et al, 2005)
Paulinia cupana (Sapindaceae)	Epicathechins, Cathechins (Ushirobira et al., 2007)
Schinus terebinthifolius (Anarcadiaceae)	Quercetin, myricetin, Kaempferol and derivatives (Ceruks et al., 2007; Johann et al., 2010)
Trichilia catigua (Meliaceae)	Chlorogenic acid, catechin and epicatechin (Lagos, 2006)

Specie (Family)	Flavonoids and phenols
Turnera diffusa (Turneraceae)	Luteolin, apigenin, quercetin, orientin and vitexin derivatives (Zhao et al., 2007)

Table 2. Aphrodisiacs plants, their flavonoids and phenols

2.2.1.2 Alkaloids, xanthines and others amines

In broad sense, the alkaloids are natural nitrogen-containing secondary metabolites mostly derived from amino acids and found in about 20% of flowering plants. They are not limited to plants but also occur in marine organisms, insects, microorganisms and some animals (Rahimi et al., 2009).

Until 2005, 150,000 compounds were known and 14% these have been alkaloids. They are special interesting due to the heterogeneity of the group and the great bioactive potential particularly as inhibitors of PDE (Silva, 2006). Many of them have been used as a basis for design and development of new and more selective drugs with reduced side effects.

The methylxanthines are purine bases and have structural similarity with the cAMP and cGMP, therefore bind competitively to the sites of the various PDEs. They are considered non-selective inhibitors, such as caffeine found in *Paullinia cupana* seeds, theobromine and adenine from *Ptychopetalum olacoides*, which validate its aphrodisiac effect.

Introducing achiral cyclopenthyl and hexylamines moiety in xanthines analogues enhanced inhibitory activity. The ethyl group at the N-1 and N-3 positions showed the highest effect in PDE-5 (Wang et al., 2002).

Aporphines alkaloids act as dopamine agonists, due to their structural similarity. They improve central pro-erectile mechanisms by binding to receptors in the paraventricular nucleus of the hypothalamus. In clinical trials, apomorphine was found to be effective in patients with ED of various aetiologies and levels of severity, albeit with substantially less efficacy than any of the PDE-5 inhibitors (Seftel, 2002).

Other plants that seem to act this way are: *Mimosa tenuiflora, Mimosa pudica and Mucuna pruriens*, but they need more studies to investigation their aphrodisiac activities.

While many β-carbolines have effect as a selective inhibitor of PDE-5, the alkaloids of *Passiflora* seems to have effect as serotonin uptake inhibitors and therefore act with antidepressants. Recently, harmine and numerous related β-carboline derivatives were found as potent and specific inhibitors of cyclin-dependent kinases (CDKs), and the structure activity relationships (SARs) analysis demonstrated that the degree of aromaticity

Specie (Family)	Alkaloids, xanthines and others amines
Aristolochia cymbifera (Aristolochiaceae)	Magnoflorine (Wu et al.,2005)
Erythroxylum viceniifolium (Erythroxylaceae)	Catuabin A Catuabin B Catuabin C Catuabin D Catuabin E Catuabin F Catuabin G Catuabin H Catuabin I Vaccinine A Vaccinine B And derivatives (Zanolari, 2003)
Hippeastrum psittacinum (Amaryllidaceae)	Galanthamine Montanine Hippeastrine Pretazettine Lycorine Lycosinine (Jin, 2011; Pagliosa et al., 2010)

Specie (Family)	Alkaloids, xanthines and others amines
Mimosa pudica (Fabaceae)	Mimopudine Mimosiine Pheniletylamine (Muthumani et al., 2010; Ueda & Yamamura, 1999a, 1999b)
Mimosa tenuiflora (Fabaceae)	1) R=R₁= H 2) R=H; R₁=Me 3) R=R₁= Me 4) R=R₁= Me L-dopa Yuremamine 5 Hydroxytryptamine N,N-dimethyltryptamine (Souza et al., 2008)
Mucuna pruriensis (Fabaceae)	1) R=R₁= H 2) R=H; R₁=Me 3) R=R₁= Me 4) R=R₁= Me L-dopa (Misra & Wagner, 2004; Siddhuraju &Becker, 2001)
Passiflora sp. (Passifloraceae)	R=H- Harman R=OH - Harmol R=OCH₃ - Harmin R=OH - Harmalol R=OCH₃ - Harmalin (Ingale & Hivrale, 2010)

Specie (Family)	Alkaloids, xanthines and others amines
Paulinia cupana (Sapindaceae)	Caffeine (Ushirobira et al., 2007)
Ptychopetalum olacoides (Oleaceae)	Adenine Theobromine And caffeine, muirapuamine (Montrucchio, 2005)

Table 3. Aphrodisiacs plants and their alkaloids, xanthines and others amines

of the tricyclic ring and the positioning of substituents were crucial for inhibitory activity. In addition, N-2-furoyl and N-2- pyrimidinyl β-carbolines were found to strongly inhibit activity against phosphodiesterases (PDEs) (Cao et al., 2007).

Tropane alkaloids present in *Erytroxylum* species have a structure similar to cocaine and seem to have the same action in the transport of dopamine (Singh, 2000).

2.2.1.3 Saponins

Saponins are a vast group of non-nitrogenous compounds, in general glycosides of steroids or polycyclic terpenes and widely distributed in higher plants. Their surfactant properties are what distinguish these compounds from others. They are soluble in water and form colloidal solutions that foam upon shaking (Schenkel et al., 2007; Sparg et al. 2004).

They have a diverse range of biological activities including hemolytic, hepatoprotective, antimutagenic, antiviral, antileishmanial and antiinflammatory (Rahimi et al., 2009).

Saponins are high molecular weight substances and occur in complex mixtures due to the concomitant presence of structures with varying number of sugars or because of the presence of various aglycones. As a result of structural complexity, isolation and structural elucidation of these compounds can be very difficult and has developed only recently (Schenkel et al., 2007).

Although some saponins inhibit PDE-5, like those present in *Allium tuberosum*, those found in plants studied did not have any reports for this activity (Guohua et al., 2009; Rahimi et al, 2009), except *Pfaffia paniculata* (Brazilian ginseng) presented saponins as the main active components due to its similarity with those saponins from *Panax ginseng*, known as ginsenosides (Rates & Gosmann, 2002). The ginsenosides are adaptogens substances or anti-stress agents, but their action mechanisms are not clear (Schenkel et al., 2007).

The term adaptogen, or resistogen, as it is called to classify a group of substances that can improve nonspecific resistance of body after being exposed to various stressing factors, promoting a state of adaptation to the exceptional situation. Some plants like *Pfaffia paniculata, Paulinia cupana, Turnera diffusa, Anemopaegma arvense, Ptychopetalum olacoides* and *Trichilia catigua* are considered adaptogens (Mendes, 2011).

Specie (Family)	Saponins
Mimosa tenuiflora (Fabaceae)	(Souza et al., 2008)
Passiflora sp. (Passifloraceae)	3-sophorosil oleanolic acid (R=sophorose) Quadrangoloside (R= gentibiose) (*P. alata*) (Doyama et al., 2005)
Pfaffia paniculata (Amarantaceae)	R= H - Pfaffic acid R= β-D-glucoronic acid(2-1)-β-D-xilose (Rates & Gosmann, 2002)

Table 4. Saponins and derivatives found in some Brazilian plants

Pharmacological studies of *P. paniculata* extracts indicate that they might act mainly by increasing central noradrenergic and dopaminergic tone, and possibly (indirectly) oxytocinergic transmission (Arletti et al., 1999).

It is possible to speculate that the activity is related to the distance between the groups at C-3 and groups at C-17 and the architecture of the molecule must be important.

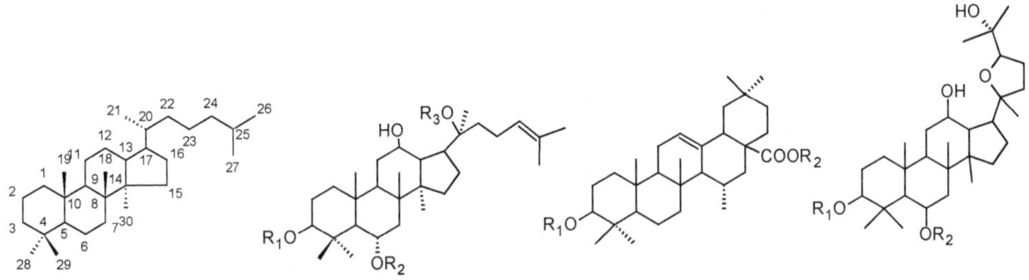

Fig. 7. Saponins basic strutures from *Panax Ginseng* (Jia & Zhao, 2009)

3. Conclusion

Despite the search promoted by pharmaceutical companies for analogues of sildenafil, the use and interest in herbal products based on folk and traditional medicine is growing globally, aiming to increase access to treatment for erectile dysfunction and to reduce the adverse effects and costs, improving the quality of life.

The investigation of classes of metabolites present in plants can indicate a possible rationalization of relations between the structure - aphrodisiac activity of substances, contributing to the development and generation of new drugs more effective and secure derivatives from regional floras.

4. References

Antunes, E.; Gordo, W. M.; Oliveira, J. F. de; Teixeira, C.E. ; Hyslop, S. & Nucci, G. de. (2001). The relaxation of isolated rabbit corpus cavernosum by the herbal medicine Catuama® and its constituents. *Phytotherapy Research*, Vol. 15, n.d., pp. 416-421. ISSN: 1099-1573.

Arletti, R.; Benelli, A; Cavazzuti, E.; Scarpetta, G. & Bertolini, A. (1999). Stimulating property of *Turnera diffusa* and *Pfaffia paniculata* extracts on the sexual-behavior of male rats. *Psychopharmacology*, Vol. 143, No. 1, n.d., pp. 15-19. ISSN: 0033-3158.

Ayyanar, M. & Ignacimuthu, S. (2009). Herbal medicines for wound healing among tribal people in Southern India: Ethnobotanical and Scientific evidences. *International Journal Of Applied Research in Natural Products*, Vol. 2, No. 3, n.d., pp. 29-42. ISSN: 1940-6223.

Barbosa, W. L. R.; Pinto, L. Do N.; Quignard, E.; Vieira, J.M. dos S. ; Silva Jr., J.O.C. & Albuquerque, S. (2008). *Arrabidaea chica* (HBK) Verlot: phytochemical approach, antifungal and trypanocidal activities. *Revista Brasileira de Farmacognosia*, Vol. 18, No. 4, (October/December 2008), pp. 544-548. ISSN: 0102-695X.

Barron, D.& Ibrahim, R. K. (1996). Isoprenylated flavonoids—a survey. *Phytochemistry*, Vol. 43, No. 5, n.d., pp. 921-982. ISSN: 0031-9422.

Bertol, E.; Fineschi, V.; Karch, S. B.; Mari, F. & Riezzo, I. (2004). *Nymphaea* cults in ancient Egypt and the New World: a lesson in empirical pharmacology. *Journal of the Royal Society of Medicine*, Vol. 97, No. 2, (February 2004), pp. 84-85. ISSN: 0141-0768.

Cao, R.; Peng, W.; Wang, Z. & Xu, A. (2007). β-Carboline alkaloids: biochemical and pharmacological functions. *Current Medicinal Chemistry*, Vol. 14, No. 4, n.d., pp. 479-500. ISSN: 0929-8673.

Ceruks, M.; Romoff, P.; Fávero, O. A. & Lago, J. H. G. (2007). Constituíntes fenólicos polares de *Schinus Terebinthifolius* Raddi (Anacardiaceae). *Química Nova*, Vol. 30, No. 3, n.d., pp. 597-599. ISSN: 0100-4042.

Chieregatto, L. C. (2005). *Efeito do tratamento crônico com extratos de Heteropterys aphrodisiaca O. Mach. e Anemopaegma Arvense (Vell.) Stellf. no testículo de ratos wistar adultos.* Thesis of Master Degrees. Universidade Federal de Viçosa.

David, J. M.; Souza, J. C.; Guedes, M. L. S. & David, J. P.(2006). Estudo fitoquímico de *Davilla rugosa*: flavonóides e terpenóides. *Revista Brasileira de Farmacognosia*, v. 16, No. 1, (January/March 2006), pp. 105-108. ISSN: 0102-695X.

Desmarchelier, C.; Ciccia, G. & Coussio, J. (2000). Recent advances in the search for antioxidant activity in South American plants. In : *Studies in Natural Products Chemistry.* Rahman, A. Vol. 22, n.d., pp. 343-367. Elsevier. ISBN: 9780444531810. Amsterdam, Netherlands.

Dhawan, K.; Kumar, S. & Sharma, A. (2002). Beneficial Effects of Chrysin and Benzoflavone on Virility in 2-Year-Old Male Rats. *Journal Of Medicinal Food*, Vol. 5, No. 1, n.d., pp. 43-48. ISSN: 1096-620X.

Doyama, J. T.; Rodrigues, H. G.; Novelli, E. L. B.; Cereda, E. & Vilegas, W. (2005). Chemical investigation and effects of the tea of *Passiflora alata* on biochemical parameters in rats. *Journal of Ethnopharmacology*, Vol. 96, No. 3, n.d., pp. 371-374. ISSN: 0378-8741.

Drewes, S. E.; George, J. & Khan, F. (2003). Recent findings on natural products with erectile-dysfunction activity. *Phytochemistry*, Vol. 62, No. 7, n.d., pp. 1019-1025. ISSN: 0031-9422.

Estrada-Reyes, R.; Ortiz-López, P.; Gutiérrez-Ortíz, J. & Martínez-Mota, L. (2009). *Turnera diffusa* Wild (Turneraceae) recovers sexual behavior in sexually exhausted males. *Journal of Ethnopharmacology*, Vol. 123, No. 3, n.d., pp. 423-429. ISSN: 0378-8741.

Ferreres, F.; Sousa, C.; Valentão, P.; Andrade, P. B. ; Seabra, R. M. & Gil-Izquierdo, A. (2007). New C-deoxyhexosyl flavones and antioxidant properties of *Passiflora edulis* leaf extract. *Journal of Agricultural and Food Chemistry*, Vol. 55, No. 25, (November 2007), pp. 10187-10193. ISSN: 0021-8561

Guohua, H.; Yanhua, L.; Rengang, M.; Dongzhi, W.; Zhengzhi, M. & Hua, Z. 2009. Aphrodisiacs properties of *Allium tuberosum* seeds extract. *Journal of Ethnopharmacology*, Vol. 122, n.d., pp. 579-582. ISSN: 0378-8741.

Hnatyszyn, O.; Moscatelli, V.; Garcia, J.; Rondina, R ; Costa, M. ; Arranz, C.; Balaszczuk, A. ; Ferraro, G. & Coussio, J.D. (2003). Argentinian plant extracts with relaxant effect on the smooth muscle of the corpus cavernosum of guinea pig. *Phytomedicine: International Journal of Phytotherapy and Phytopharmacology*, Vol. 10, No. 8, n.d., pp. 669-674. ISSNČ 0944-7113.

Ingale, A. G. & Hivrale, A. U. (2010). Pharmacological studies of *Passiflora sp.* and their bioactive compounds. *African Journal of Plant Science*, Vol. 4, No. 10, (October 2010), pp. 417-426. ISSN: 1996-0824.

Jia, L. & Zhao, Y. (2009). Current Evaluation of the Millennium Phytomedicine-Ginseng (I): Etymology, Pharmacognosy, Phytochemistry, Market and Regulations. *Current Medicinal Chemistry*, Vol. 16, No. 19, (January 2010), pp. 2475-2484. ISSN: 0929-8673.

Jin, Z. (2011). *Amaryllidaceae* and *Sceletium* alkaloids. *Natural Product Reports*, Vol. 28, No. 6, n.d., pp. 1126-42. ISSN : 1460-4752.

Johann, S.; Sá, N. P.; Lima, L. A. R. S.; Cisalpino, P. S.; Cota, B. B.; Alves, T. M.A.; Siqueira, E. P. & Zani, C. L. (2010). Antifungal activity of schinol and a new biphenyl compound isolated from *Schinus terebinthifolius* against the pathogenic fungus *Paracoccidioides brasiliensis*. *Annals of Clinical Microbiology and Antimicrobials*, Vol. 9, No. 1, n.d., pp. 09-30. ISSN: 1476-0711.

Ko, W-C.; Shih, C-M.; Lai, Y-H.; Chen, J-H. & Huang, H-L. (2004). Inhibitory effects of flavonoids on phosphodiesterase isozymes from guinea pig and their structure-activity relationships. *Biochemical Pharmacology*, Vol. 68, No. 10, n.d., pp. 2087-2094. ISSN: 0006-2952.

Kubo, I.; Kinst-Hori, I. & Yokokawa, Y. (1994). Tyrosinase inhibitors from *Anacardium Occidentale* fruits. *Journal of Natural Products*, Vol. 57, No. 4, n.d., pp. 545-551. ISSN: 0163-3864.

Lagos, J. B. (2006). *Estudo comparativo da composição química das folhas e cascas da Trichilia catigua A. Juss., Meliaceae*. Thesis of Master Degrees. Universidade Federal da Paraná.

Malviya, N.; Jain, S.; Gupta, V. B. & Vyas, S. (2011). Recent studies on aphrodisiac herbs for the management of male sexual dysfunction - a review. *Acta Poloniae Pharmaceutica*, Vol. 68, No. 1, n.d., pp. 3-8. ISSN 0001-6837.

Marquina, S.; Bonilla-Barbosa, J. & Alvarez, L. (2005). Comparative phytochemical analysis of four Mexican *Nymphaea* species. *Phytochemistry*, Vol. 66, No. 8, n.d., pp. 921-927. ISSN: 0031-9422.

Matheus, W. E.; Fregonesi, A. & Ferreira, U. (2009). Disfunção erétil. *Revista Brasileira de Medicina*, Vol. 66, No. 12, (October 2009), pp. 85-89. ISSN: 0034-7264.

Mendes, F. R. (2011). Tonic, fortifier and aphrodisiac: adaptogens in the Brazilian folk medicine. *Revista Brasileira de Farmacognosia*, Vol. 21, No. 3, in print. ISSN: 0102-695X.

Miean, K. H. & Mohamed, S. (2001). Flavonoid (Myrcetin, Quercetin, Kaempferol, Luteolin, and Apigenin) content of edible tropical plants. *Journal of Agricultural and Food Chemistry*, Vol. 49, n.d., pp. 3106-3112. ISSN: 0021-8561.

Misra, L. & Wagner, H. (2004). Alkaloidal constituents of *Mucuna pruriens* seeds. *Phytochemistry*, Vol. 65, No. 18, n.d., pp. 2565-2567. ISSN: 0031-9422.

Montrucchio, D. P.; Miguel, O. G.; Miguel, M. D.; Monache, F. D. & Carvalho, J. L. S. Componentes Químicos e Atividade Antimicrobiana de *Ptychopetalum Olacoides* Bentham. *Visão Acadêmica*, Vol. 6, No. 2, (July-December 2005), pp. 48-52. ISSN: 1518-5192.

Muthumani, P.; Meera, R.; Devi, P.; Koduri, L.V.S.K. ; Manavarthi, S. & Badmanaban, R. (2010). Phytochemical investigation and enzyme inhibitory activity of *Mimosa pudica* Linn. *Journal of Chemical and Pharmaceutical Research*, Vol. 2, No. 5, n.d., pp. 108-114. ISSN: 0975-7384

Pagliosa, L.B.; Monteiro, S. C.; Silva, K. B.; de Andrade, J. P.; Dutilh, J. Bastida, J.; Cammarota, M & Zuanazzi, J. A. S. (2010). Effect of isoquinoline alkaloids from two *Hippeastrum* species on in vitro acetylcholinesterase activity. *Phytomedicine: International Journal of Phytotherapy and Phytopharmacology*, Vol. 17, No. 8-9, n.d., pp. 698-701. ISSN: 0944-7113.

Pande, M. & Pathak, A. (2009). Aphrodisiac Activity of Roots of *Mimosa pudica* Linn. ethanolic extract in mice. *International Journal of Sciences and Nanotechnology Pharmaceutical*, Vol. 2, No. 1, (April-June 2009), pp. 477-486. ISSN: 0974-3278.

Patel, S. S.; Verma, N. K. & Gauthaman, K. (2009). *Passiflora Incarnata* Linn: A Review on Morphology, Phytochemistry and Pharmacological Aspects. *Pharmacognosy Reviews*, Vol. 3, No. 5, n.d., pp. 186-192. ISSN: 0973-7847.

Rahimi, R.; Ghiasi, S.; Azimi, H.; Fakhari, S. & Abdollahi, M. (2009). A review of the herbal phosphodiesterase inhibitors; future perspective of new drugs. *Cytokine*, Vol. 49, No. 2, (November 2009), pp. 123-129. ISSN: 1043-4666.

Rates, S. M. K. & Gosmann, G. Gênero *Pfaffia*: aspectos químicos, farmacológicos e implicações para o seu emprego terapêutico. *Revista Brasileira de Farmacognosia*, Vol. 12, No. 2, (July-December 2002), pp. 85-93. ISSN: 0102-695X.

Schenkel, E. P.; Gosmann, G. & Athayde, M. L. (2007). Saponinas. In : *Farmacognosia: da planta ao medicamento*. Simões, C.M.O. ; Schenkel, E. P.; Gosmann, G. Mello, J. C. P.; Mentz, L.A & Petrovick, P.R. pp. 711-740. UFRGS : Universidade Federal do Rio Grande do Sul. ISBN : 9788570259271, Porto Alegre-RS, Brazil.

Seftel, A. D. (2002). Challenges in oral therapy for erectile dysfunction. *Journal of Andrology*, Vol. 23, No. 6, (November/December 2002), pp. 729-736. ISSN: 0196-3635.

Siddhuraju, P. & Becker, K. (2001). Rapid reversed-phase high performance liquid chromatographic method for the quantification of L-Dopa tetrahydroisoquinoline compounds from *Mucuna* beans. *Food Chemistry*, Vol. 72, n.d., pp. 389-394. ISSN: 0308-8146.

Silva, C. V. da. (2006) *Alcalóides benzofenantridínicos e outros metabólitos do caule e frutos de Zanthoxylum tingoassuiba St. Hil*. Thesis of Master Degrees. Universidade Federal da Bahia.

Simões, C. M. O.; Rech, N. & Lapa, A. J. (1986). Investigação farmacológica do extrato aquoso de folhas/caules de *Achyrocline satureioides* (Lam.) Dc., Compositae (Marcela). *Caderno de Farmácia*, Vol. 2, No. 1, n.d., pp. 37-54. ISSN: 0102-6593.

Singh, S. (2000). Chemistry, design, and structure-activity relationship of cocaine antagonists. *Chemical Reviews*, Vol. 100, No. 3, n.d., pp. 925-1024. ISSN: 0009-2665.

Souza, R. S. O. D.; Albuquerque, U. P. D.; Monteiro, J. M. & Amorim, E. L. C. D. (2008). Jurema-Preta (*Mimosa tenuiflora* [Willd.] Poir.): a review of its traditional use, phytochemistry and pharmacology. *Brazilian Archives of Biology and Technology*, Vol. 51, No. 5, (September-October 2008), pp. 937-947. ISSN: 1516-8913.

Sparg, S. G.; Light, M. E. & Staden, J. Van. (2004). Biological activities and distribution of plant saponins. *Journal of Ethnopharmacology*, Vol. 94, No. 2-3, n.d., pp. 219-243. ISSN: 0378-8741.

Still, J. (2003). Use of animal products in traditional Chinese medicine: environmental impact and health hazards. *Complementary Therapies in Medicine*, Vol. 11, No. 2, n.d., pp. 118-122. ISSN: 0965-2299.

Sumalatha, K. & Kumar, A. (2010). Review on natural aphrodisiac potentials to treat sexual dysfunction. *International Journal of Pharmacy & Therapeutics*, Vol. 1, No. 1, n.d., pp. 6-14. ISSN: 0976 – 0342.

Suresh, S.; Prithiviraj, E. & Prakash, S. (2009). Dose-and time-dependent effects of ethanolic extracts of *Mucuna pruriens* Linn. seed on sexual behaviour of normal male rats. *Journal of Ethnopharmacology*, Vol. 122, n.d., pp. 497-501. ISSN: 0378-8741.

Tabanca, N.; Pawar, R. S.; Ferreira, D.; Marais, J.P.J. ; Khan, S. I. ; Vaishali, J. ; Wedge, D. E. & Khan, I. A. (2007). Flavan-3-ol-Phenylpropanoid Conjugates from *Anemopaegma arvense* and their antioxidant activities. *Planta Medica*, Vol. 73, n.d., pp. 1107-1111, ISSN: 0032-0943.

Takemura, O. (1995). A flavone from leaves of *Arrabidaea chica* f. cuprea. *Phytochemistry*, Vol. 38, No. 5, n.d., pp. 1299-1300. ISSN: 0031-9422.

Ueda, M. & Yamamura, S. (1999a). Leaf-opening substance of *Mimosa pudica* L.; chemical studies on the other leaf movement of mimosa. *Tetrahedron Letters*, v. 40, No. 2, (January 1999), pp. 353-356. ISSN: 0040-4039

Ueda, M. & Yamamura, S. (1999b) Leaf-closing Substance of *Mimosa pudica* L.; Chemical Studies on Another Leaf-movement of Mimosa II. *Tetrahedron Letters*, v. 40, No. 15, (April 1999), pp. 2981-2984. ISSN: 0040-4039

Ushirobira, T. M. A.; Yamaguti, E.; Uemura, L. M.; Nakamura, C.V. ; Dias Filho, B.P. & Palazzo de Mello, J.C. (2007). Chemical and Microbiological Study of Extract from Seeds of Guaraná (*Paullinia cupana* var. *sorbilis*). *Acta Farmacéutica Bonaerense*, Vol. 26, No. 1, n.d., pp. 5-9. ISSN: 0326-2383.

Velozo, E. da S.; Barreto, M. M.; Jesus, E. L. de & Silva, C. V. da. (2002). A Etnofarmacologia dos terreiros nagôs-baianos. In : *O Mundo das folhas*. Serra, O.; Velozo, E. da S. ; Bandeira, F. ; Pacheco, L. pp.143-175. UEFS/EDUFBA. ISBN: 8573950862, Salvador – BA, Brazil.

Vignera, S. L.; Condorelli, R.; Vicari, E.; Agata, R. D. & Calogero, A. E.(2011). Physical activity and erectile dysfunction in middle-aged men : a brief review. *Journal of Andrology*, Vol. 32, No. 3, (May/June 2011), pp. 1-17, ISSN: 0196-3635.

Wang, Y.; Chackalamannil, S.; Hu, Z.; Boyle, C. D. ; Lankin, C. M. ; Xia, Y. ; Xu, R. ; Asberom, T. ; Pissarnitski, D. ; Stamford, A. W. ; Greenlee, W. J.; Skell, J. ; Kurowski, S. ; Vemulapalli, S. ; Palamanda, J. ; Chintala, M. ; Wu, P.; Myers, J. & Wang, P. (2002). Design and synthesis of xanthine analogues as potent and selective PDE5 inhibitors. *Bioorganic & Medicinal Chemistry Letters*, Vol. 12, No. 21, n.d., pp. 3149-3152. ISSN: 0960-894X

Wang, H.; Ye, M.; Robinson, H.; Francis, S. H. & Ke, H. (2008). Conformational Variations of Both Phosphodiesterase-5 and Inhibitors Provide the Structural Basis for the Physiological Effects of Vardenafil and Sildenafil. *Molecular Pharmacology*, Vol. 73, No. 1, n.d., pp. 104-110. ISSN: 0026-895X.

Wu, T-S.; Damu, A. G.; Su, C-R. & Kuo, P-C. (2005). Chemical constituents and pharmacology of *Aristolochia* species. In : *Studies in Natural Products Chemistry*. Rahman, A. Vol. 32, n.d., pp. 855-1018. Elsevier. ISBN: 9780444531810. Amsterdam, Netherlands.

Zanolari, B. (2003). *Natural Aphrodisiacs. Studies of comercially-available herbal recipes, and phytochemical investigation of Erythroxylum vacciniifolium Mart. from Brazil.* Thesis of Doctor Degrees. University of Lausanne.

Zhao, J.; Pawar, R. S.; Ali, Z.; Khan, I. A. (2007). Phytochemical investigation of *Turnera diffusa. Journal of Natural Products.* Vol. 70, No. 2, n.d., pp. 289-292. ISSN 0163-3864.

Zorn, B.; Garcia-Piñeres, A. J.; Castro, V.; Murillo, R. ; Mora, G. & Merfort, I. (2001). 3-Desoxyanthocyanidins from *Arrabidaea chica. Phytochemistry*, Vol. 56, No. 8, n.d., pp. 831-835. ISSN: 0031-9422.

3

A Phytochemical and Ethnopharmacological Review of the Genus *Erythrina*

João X. de Araújo-Júnior, Mariana S.G. de Oliveira, Pedro G.V. Aquino,
Magna S. Alexandre-Moreira and Antônio E.G. Sant'Ana
Universidade Federal de Alagoas
Brazil

1. Introduction

Considered in acient times as a connection to the divine, the use of this medicinal plant is as old as human civilization itself. Whole nations dominated its secrets, often associated with magic and religious rites, searching in nature's resources to improve life conditions, and increase chances of survival (Herbarium, 2008).

In 1978, the World Health Organization (WHO) recognized folk medicine and its beneficial effects to health, during the *Alma Ata* conference, which published in 1985 that approximatly 80% of the global population, resorted to traditional medicine as their primary health treatment (Herbarium, 2008). Medicinal plants have been used as a means of curing or preventing diseases, now called phytotherapy, in all regions of the world, with regional variations due to the influence of cultural characteristics of the population, as well as its flora, soil and climate (Lewinsohn, 2003).

Since the nineteenth century, humanity discovered the endless and diverse therapeutic arsenal present in medicinal plants, due to the discovery of active substances that in their natural state or after chemical transformation showed biological activity, and often already confirmed by popular use and/or proven scientifically (Miguel & Miguel, 2004).

According to Yamada (1998) it is necessary to carry out more studies and to propagate medicinal plant utilization as a way to diminish the costs of public health programs since the utilization of these plants may constitute a very useful therapeutic value due their efficacy coupled with low operating costs and the relative ease of obtaining the plants (Matos, 1994).

According to Brazilian legislation, a new herbal medicine can be introduced to the market in two forms: as a finished product – industrially produced, or as an official product – manufactured in pharmacies. Both forms should ensure quality, safety and efficacy of the herbal medicines supplied to the consumer. On the other hand, medicinal plants sold at popular markets or obtained directly from farmers at an informal market, have no guarantee provided by law, especially with regards to safety and efficacy (Herbarium, 2008). However we cannot rule out the cultural importance that popular knowledge inputs, being transmitted from generation to generation.

The WHO strategy on traditional medicine for the period of 2002-2005 has brought as one of its objectives, the strengthening of traditional remedies by placing them in the National Health Systems through policies and programs determined by their respective governments. The National Policy on Integrative and Complementary Practices of the Brazilian Unified Health System (SUS, *Sistema Único de Saúde*) (2006), for example, fulfills these requests by proposing the inclusion of medicinal plants, phytotherapy, homeopathy, traditional Chinese medicine, acupuncture, hydrotherapy and crenotherapy as therapeutic options for the SUS. Another example is the Brazilian National Policy on Medicinal Plants and Herbal Medicines, which includes as one of its guidelines the promotion and recognition of popular practices in the use of herbal and home remedies. Therefore, a strategy that can be used to meet this demand proposed by the federal government is to conduct a survey of plants used by communities in order to strengthen with the establishment a list of Medicinal Plants of Interest to SUS (RENISUS), which aims to give priority to the naturally occurring species of regions or to those easily cultivated. In this context, the Brazilian Ministry of Health released the RENISUS list, containing 71 species of medicinal plants for therapeutic use (http://portal.saude.gov.br/portal/ arquivos/pdf/RENISUS.pdf).

2. The Fabaceae family

Also known as a sub-family of Leguminosae, the Fabaceae family is one of the largest botanical families and widely distributed around the world, spread out over temperate, tropical and cold regions. Thus family is composed of 32 tribes, whose genera are chemically represented by a variety of flavonoid skeletons, notably pterocarpans and isoflavones. There are about 650 genera comprising about 18,000 species (Polhil & Raven, 1981). The genus *Erythrina* is represented by about 290 species (Cronquist, 1981; http://www.tropicos.org/Name/40005932). The Fabaceae family produces valuable medicinal drugs, ornamental species, fodders plants, oil producing plants, inseticides and species with various other functions (Salinas, 1992).

3. The *Erythrina* Genus

The genus *Erythrina* is one among several genera from the Fabaceae family. The origin of the name *Erythrina* comes from the Greek word "erythros" which means red, alluding to the bright red flowers of the trees of the genus (Krukoff & Barneby, 1974). Over 130 species of "coral tree" belong to the genus *Erythrina*, which has been widely studied and are distributed in tropical and subtropical regions of the world. In South America, these species are present in Argentina, Bolivia, Paraguay, French Guiana, Colombia and Peru (Hickey & King, 1981). In Brazil the genus is spread throughout all of the Brazilian biomes, like the Atlantic forest, *cerrado*, Amazon rainforest and Brazilian northeast *caatinga* (Corrêa, 1984). In Brazil, there are eight species found: *E. mulungu, E. velutina, E. cista-galli, E. poeppigiana, E. fusca, E. falcata, E. speciosa* and *E. verna* (Lourenzi, 1992).

Phytochemical analysis has demonstrated the presence of terpenes in plants from the *Erythrina* genus (Serragiotto et al., 1981; Nkengfack et al., 1997), that are also recognized as bioactive alkaloid-rich plants (Ghosal et al., 1971; Barakat et al., 1977) and flavonoids, especially, isoflavones, pterocarpanes, flavanones and isoflavanones (Chacha et al., 2005). Some of these flavonoids have demonstrated a wide variety of biological activities (Table 2).

Studies have demonstrated the presence of analgesic and anti-inflammatory effects in extracts obtained from *E. senegalensis*, *E. velutina* and *E. mulungu* (Vasconcelos et al., 2003). In folk medicine, various species are utilized as a tranquilizer, against insomnia and to treat inflammation (Garcia-Mateos et al., 2001).

3.1 Bibliographic review

We conducted a literature review using the database SciFinder Scholar®, and from the results obtained, we prepared two tables of data showing the correlation between popular use and the plant part utilized, as well as the form of utilization (Table 1), and the biological activities of the extracts obtained from *Erythrina* species (Table 2). Due to the large amount of data for phytochemicals isolated from the *Erythrina* species, we organized them in a simplified table (Table 3).

Uses	Part Utilized	Kind of Extract/ Way of Use and Administration	Species	Locality	Reference
Trachoma Malaria Syphilis Elephantiasis	Bark Roots Roots Bark	Unspecified, oral Unspecified,oral Unspecified Unspecified, external	*Erythrina abyssinica*	Kenya	Ichimaru et al. (1996) Kamat et al. (1981) Moriyasu et al. (1998)
Colic	Roots	Decoction, oral	*Erythrina abyssinica*	Tanzania	Chhabra et al. (1984)
Syphilis	Flowers	Infusion, oral	*Erythrina abyssinica*	Uganda	Kamusiime et al. (1996)
Fever Leprosy Dysentery Gonorrhea Hepatitis	Leaves Stalk Stalk	Unspecified, oral	*Erythrina abyssinica*	Rwanda	Chagnon (1984) Boily & Van Puyvelde (1986) Maikere-Faniyo et al. (1989) Vlietinck et al. (1995)
Schistosomiasis of the urinary tract	Unspecified	Decoction, oral	*Erythrina abyssinica*	Zimbabwe	Ndamba et al. (1994)
Poison antidote	Roots	Unspecified	*Erythrina abyssinica*	India	Selvanayahgam et al. (1994)
Anthelmintic	Green bark stem	Unspecified, oral	*Erythrina abyssinica*	East Africa	Kokwaro (1976)
Contraception Parturition Malaria Insomnia	Bark Bark Whole plant Flowers	Unspecified, oral Unspecified, oral Unspecified, oral Unspecified, oral	*Erythrina americana*	Mexico	Hastings (1990) Dominguez & Alcorn (1985)

Uses	Part Utilized	Kind of Extract/ Way of Use and Administration	Species	Locality	Reference
Hypnotic Inflammation of the arms, legs, hair and eyes. Abscesses Insect bites Ulcers Curare-like effect	Flowers Fruits Leaves Leaves Leaves Seeds	Unspecified, oral Unspecified, External Unspecified, external Unspecified, oral Unspecified, external Unspecified, external			
Anthelmintic Earache	Bark Leaves	Decoction, oral Juice of leaves, aural	*Erythrina arborescens*	Nepal	Manandhar (1995) Bhattarai (1991)
Pork skin disease	Leaves	Unspecified, external	*Erythrina arborescens*	India	Rao (1981)
Snakebite Abscesses Boils Infections of skin and mucous Dermatitis and inflammation	Bark Leaves Leaves Leaves Leaves	Infusion, oral Unspecified, external Unspecified, external Unspecified, external Unspecified, external	*Erythrina berteroana*	Guatemala	Giron et al. (1991) Caceres et al. (1987)
Poison antidote	Bark	Infusion, oral	*Erythrina berteroana*	India	Selvanayahgam et al. (1994)
Fish poison Female diseases Sedative Bleeding Dysentery Poison Narcotic	Branches Whole plant Flowers Flowers Flowers Seeds Unspecified	Unspecified Unspecified, oral Decoction, oral Decoction, oral Decoction, oral Unspecified, oral Decoction, Unspecified	*Erythrina berteroana*	Mexico	Hastings (1990)
Sedative Bleeding Dysentery	Levaes and flowers Flowers Flowers	Infusion, oral Unspecified, oral Unspecified, oral	*Erythrina berteroana*	Central America	Morton (1994)
Female diseases	Unspecified	Unspecified, oral	*Erythrina berteroana*	Panama	Duke & Ayensu (1994)
Antiasthmatic Expel placenta	Bark Leaves	Unspecified Unspecified, oral	*Erythrina corallodendron*	Antilles	Ayensu (1978)
Measles	Seeds	Unspecified, external	*Erythrina coralloides*	Mexico	Hastings (1990)

Uses	Part Utilized	Kind of Extract/ Way of Use and Administration	Species	Locality	Reference
Urinary Tract Infection Respiratory Tract Infection Diarrhea Anti- hemorrhoids Narcotic Antiseptic	Bark Bark Bark Leaves Stalk Stalk	Decoction, oral Decoction, oral Decoction, oral Unspecified, external Unspecified, oral Unspecified, external	*Erythrina crista-galli*	Argentina	Perez & Anesini (1994) Bandoni et al. (1976)
Antimicrobial Throat infections Astringent in wound healing	Stalk+leaves Stalk+leaves Stalk+leaves	Unspecified, external Unspecified, oral Unspecified, external	*Erythrina crista-galli*	Brazil	Simões et al. (1999)
Swelling Healing	Bark Bark	Suspension in water, oral	*Erythrina dominguezii*	Argentina	Filipoy (1994)
Diarrhea Toothache Erotic dreams Toxic Purgative Contraceptive	Leaves Seeds Seeds Seeds Seeds Seeds	Infusion, oral Unspecified, oral Unspecified, oral Unspecified, oral Unspecified, oral Unspecified, oral	*Erythrina flabelliformis*	Mexico	Hastings (1990) Diaz (1977) Pennington (1973) Bye (1986)
Inflammation of uterus Appendicitis Diuretic	Bark Whole plant Seeds	Decocction, oral Unspecified, oral Unspecified	*Erythrina folkersii*	Mexico	Zamora- Martinez & Pola (1992) Hastings (1990)
Migraine Infected wounds Fungal dermatosis Antitussive	Bark Bark Bark Flowers	Infusion, external Decoction, external Decoction, external Decoction, oral	*Erythrina fusca*	Peru	Duke (1994)
Anti- inflammatory	Bark and leaves	Unspecified, oral	*Erythrina fusca*	Thailand	Wasuwat (1967)
Skin infections Itch	Seeds Seeds	Unspecified Unspecified	*Erythrina fusca*	Indonesia	Widianto (1980)
Headache Narcotic Kidney	Bark and leaves Bark and	Infusion, oral Infusion, oral Infusion, oral	*Erythrina glauca*	Peru	Jovel et al.(1996) Duke (1994)

Uses	Part Utilized	Kind of Extract/ Way of Use and Administration	Species	Locality	Reference
inflammation Purgative Antimalarial	leaves Bark and leaves Bark and leaves Unspecified	Infusion, oral Decocction, oral			
Rats and dogs poison	Seeds	Unspecified, oral	*Erythrina herbacea*	Mexico	Hastings (1990)
Tuberculosis	Bark	Infusion, oral	*Erythrina humeana*	South Africa	Pillay et al. (2001)
Antipyretic Anthelmintic Astringent Expectorant Eye drops Antibilious Stomach upset Menstrual regulator Aphrodisiac Laxative Diuretic Stimulation of milk production	Bark Bark and leaves Bark Bark Bark Bark Bark+roots Leaves Leaves Leaves Leaves	Unspecified, oral Unspecified, oral Unspecified, external Unspecified, oral Unspecified, ophthalmic Unspecified, oral Juice, oral With milk, oral Unspecified, oral Unspecified, oral Unspecified, oral Unspecified, oral	*Erythrina indica*	India	Khan et al. (1994) John (1984) Chopra & Ghosh (1935) Pushpangadan & Atal (1984)
Poison	Whole plant	Unspecified	*Erythrina lanata*	Mexico	Hastings (1990)
Aphrodisiac	Bark	Unspecified, oral	*Erythrina mildbraedii*	Guinea	Vasileva (1969)
Antipyretic	Bark	Decoction, oral	*Erythrina mulungu*	Brazil	Brandão (1985)
Antimalarial	Leaves an roots	Decoction/ infusion, oral	*Erythrina sacleuxii*	Tanzania	Gessler et al.(1995)
Postpartum (women) Treatment of female sterility	Bark Bark+leaves	Unspecified, oral Unspecified, oral	*Erythrina senegalensis*	Guinea	Vasileva (1969)
Serious injury Yellow fever Bronchial diseases Eye disorders Injuries	Bark Bark Bark Bark Twigs and leaves	Unspecified, oral, external Unspecified, oral Unspecified, oral Unspecified, oral Unspecified, external	*Erythrina senegalensis*	Senegal	Le Grand & Wondergem (1987) Le Grand (1989)

Uses	Part Utilized	Kind of Extract/ Way of Use and Administration	Species	Locality	Reference
Ulcers Venereal diseases	Twigs and leaves Twigs and leaves	Unspecified, oral Unspecified, oral			
Antimalarial	Roots	Unspecified	*Erythrina senegalensis*	Nigeria	Etkin (1997)
Broken bones Antipyretic	Bark Leaves	Decoction, external Unspecified, oral	*Erythrina species*	Thailand	Anderson (1986) Mokkhasmit et al. (1971)
Analgesic	Leaves	Unspecified, oral	*Erythrina species*	Solomon Islands	Blackwood (1935)
Parturition induction Toothache Nosebleed	Bark and leaves Roots Roots	Infusion, oral Unspecified, oral Unspecified, external	*Erythrina standleyana*	Mexico	Hastings (1990) Dominguez & Alcorn (1985)
Epilepsy Leprosy	Bark Bark	Unspecified, oral Unspecified	*Erythrina stricta*	India	Chopra (1933)
Menorrhagia	Leaves	Unspecified, oral	*Erythrina subumbrans*	East Indias	Burkill (1966)
Antiseptic	Bark	Unspecified, external	*Erythrina ulei*	Peru	Desmarcheilier et al. (1997) Desmarcheilier et al. (1996)
Antiseptic	Stem Bark	Unspecified, external	*Erythrina ulei*	Argentina	Desmarcheilier et al. (1996)
Antipyretic	Bark	Decoction, oral	*Erythrina variegata*	Adaman Islands	Awasth (1991)
Epilepsy Stomach ache	Bark Bark	Unspecified, oral Juice, oral	*Erythrina variegata*	India	Pushpangadan & Atal (1984) John (1984)
Swelling	Bark	Unspecified, external	*Erythrina variegata*	New Guinea	Holdsworth (1984)
Amenorrhea Conception Dysmenorrhea	Bark Bark Bark	Infusion, oral Infusion, oral Infusion, oral	*Erythrina variegata*	Rotuma	Mc Clatchey (1996)
Antipyretic Sedative Antiasthmatic	Flowers Flowers Flowers	Unspecified, oral Unspecified, oral Unspecified, oral	*Erythrina variegata*	Brazil	Sarragiotto et al. (1981)
Induce menstruation	Leaves	Juice, oral	*Erythrina variegata*	India	Das (1955)

Table 1. Popular uses of *Erythrina* species

3.1.1 Ethnopharmacological data

Plants of the *Eryhtrina* genus are utilized for a wide array of human diseases (Table 1). With regards the parts of the plants that are utilized, the most used is the bark, being 40.8% of the total of citations, as shown in Graphic 1.

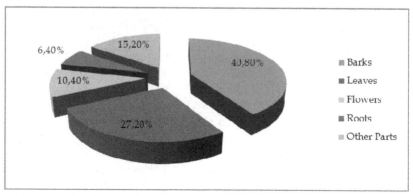

Graphic 1. Parts of the plants utilized in folk medicine.

3.1.2 Biological activity data

Analysis of the biological activity data (Table 2) shows the wide variety of biological activity of plants from the *Erythrina* genus, and shows too that most of this corroborates with popular knowledge and uses.

It is noteworthy to point out that most of these activities, mainly the antibacterial and analgesic properties, confirm the different popular applications of extracts obtained from plants of this genus. We would like also to draw attention to the fact that in the Brazilian market there is the availability of a phytotherapeutic product from *Erythrina mulungu* widely used for anxiolytic purposes and as a sedative, activities confirmed by popular knowledge, but that, to our knowledge, have not yet been confirmed in pharmacological tests, showing that, despite the wide array of available data related to plants of this genus, there is still a need for more research about some of them.

It is important to note that some of the activities shown in the biological tests were not cited in the ethnopharmacological studies, which indicates yet another importance for plants of the *Erythrina* genus, which have the potential to provide new compounds for the development of drugs for the treatment of diseases such as cancer, diabetes and hypertension.

3.1.3 Phytochemical data

The phytochemical data (Table 3) analysis allowed for the verificationof a predominance of alkaloids and flavonoids in the *Erythrina* genus. It is important to note that alkaloids are recognized as markers for plants of this genus in addition to showing a wide array of biological activities, and being important candidates in the development of new drugs.

Species	Part of the Plant	Biological Activities	Location	Reference
Erythrina abyssinica	Bark Leaves Roots Roots Root Bark Root Bark	Mitogenic activity Cell Culture Molluscicidal (*Biomphalaria pfeifferi*) Anti-bacterial Anti-bacterial (Gram-positive species, *Escherichia coli*) Anti-yeast (*Saccharomyces cerevisiae*) Antimalárico	Kenya	Tachibana et al (1993) Kloos et al (1987) Kamat et al. (1981) Taniguchi et al. (1978) Yenesew et al. (2003a)
Erythrina abyssinica	Bark	Anti-bacterial (*Escherichia coli, Pseudomonas aeruginosa, Bacillus subtilis e Staphylococcus aureus*)	Sudan	Omer et al. (1998)
Erythrina abyssinica	Leaves Trunk	Uterine relaxing and stimulant Muscle Relaxing and stimulant Periferic muscle relaxing and stimulant Toxic effect in rats Antidiarrheal Anti-bacterial (*Salmonella typhi, Shigella flexnerishigella dysenteriae, Shigella boyd, Shigella sonnei*) Antiviral	Rwanda	Chagnon (1984) Maikere-faniyo et al. (1989) Vlietinck et al. (1995)
Erythrina abyssinica	Root bark	Anti-bacterial Anti-fungal	East Africa	Taniguchi & Kubo (1993)
Erythrina addisoniae	Stem Bark	Anti-inflammatory	Cameroon	Talla et al. (2003)
Erythrina americana	Bark	Plant germination inhibition Molluscicidal	Unspecified	Dominguez & Alcorn (1985)
Erythrina americana	Seeds	Central Nervous System depressor	Mexico	Garin-Aguilar et al. (2000)
Erythrina arborescens	Leaves Leaves, stem Stem Stem	Hypotensive Cytotoxic Antispasmodic Uterine stimulant	India	Dhar et al. (1968)
Erythrina berteroana	Leaves	Anti-yeast Anti-bacterial	Guatemala	Caceres et al. (1987)
Erythrina	Leaves+Twigs	Cytotoxic	Panamá	Chapuis et al.

Species	Part of the Plant	Biological Activities	Location	Reference
berteroana	Root bark	Anti-fungal		(1988) Maillard et al. (1987)
Erythrina berteroana	Stem	Pherormone	Puerto Rico	Keiser et al. (1975)
Erythrina bidwillii hybrid	Root bark	Anti-fungal Anti-bacterial Anticoagulant	Okinawa	Iinuma & Tanaka (1994) Iinuma et al. (1994)
Erythrina breviflora	Leaves+stem	Cancer induction	USA	Caldwell & Brewer (1983)
Erythrina caffra	Bark, leaves	COX1 inhibitor Anti-bacterial	South Africa	Pillay et al. (2001)
Erythrina corallodendron	Dry fruit + leaves + stem	Antiphagocytic	Greece	Yannitsaros (1996)
Erythrina corallodendron	Seeds	Trypsin inhibition	Israel	Joubert & Sharon (1985)
Erythrina coromandelianum	Whole plant	Molluscicidal	Puerto Rico	Medina& Woodbury (1979)
Erythrina crista-galli	Aerial parts Bark	Analgesic Anti-inflammatory Anti-bacterial Anti-fungal	Argentina	Mino et al. (2002) Perez & Anesini (1994)
Erythrina crista-galli	Flowers	Anti-mutagenic	Unspecified	Ishii et al. (1984)
Erythrina crista-galli	Fresh fruit + leaves + stem	Anti-phagocytic	Greece	Yannitsaros (1996)
Erythrina crista-galli	Leaves	Anti-fungal Anti-bacterial	Egypti	Ross et al. (1980)
Erythrina crista-galli	Leaves + stem	Cytotoxic Antiviral	Brazil	Simoes et al. (1999)
Erythrina crista-galli	Leaves + stem	Animal repellent	Germany	Wink (1984)
Erythrina crista-galli	Root and stem bark	Anti-bacterial Anti-mycobacterial	Bolivia	Mitscher et al. (1984) Mitscher et al. (1988)
Erythrina crista-galli	Seeds	Trypsin inhibition	Uruguay	Joubert & Sharon (1985)
Erythrina eriotricha	Root bark	Anti-bacterial	Cameroon	Nkengfack et al. (1995)
Erythrina excelsa	Root bark	Anti-bacterial/anti-fungal	East Africa	Taniguchi et al. (1993)
Erythrina	Seeds	Larvicidal	Unspecified	Janzen et al.

Species	Part of the Plant	Biological Activities	Location	Reference
flabelliformis				(1977)
Erythrina fusca	Leaves	Hypotensive Uterine stimulant Diuretic	Thailand	Unakul (1950)
Erythrina fusca	Seeds	Central Nervous System depressor	Indonesia	Widianto et al. (1980)
Erythrina glauca	Bark	Antiviral	Guatemala	Mc Kee et al. (1997)
Erythrina humeana	Bark, leaves	Anti-bacterial COX1 inhibitor	South Africa	Pillay et al. (2001)
Erythrina indica	Leaves	Anti-fungal Anti-bacterial	Egypt	Ross et al. (1980)
Erythrina indica	Leaves	Central Nervous System depressor	Sri Lanka	Ratnasooriya & Dharmasiri (1999)
Erythrina indica	Unspecified	Stimulant and inhibitor of lymphocyte blastogenesis	India	Singh & Chatterjee (1979)
Erythrina indica	Root bark Stem bark	Anti-mycobacterial Anti-bacterial Cytotoxic	Nigeria	Waffo et al. (2000) Nkengfack et al. (2001)
Erythrina indica	Seeds	Anti-fungal Anti-bacterial	Egypt	Ross et al. (1980)
Erythrina indica	Seeds	Immunosuppressor	India	Singh (1979)
Erythrina latissima	Bark, leaves	COX1 inhibitor Anti-bacterial	South Africa	Pillay et al. (2001)
Erythrina lysistemon	Bark, leaves	COX1 inhibitor Anti-bacterial Anti-yeast	South Africa	Pillay et al. (2001) Rabe & Van Staden (1997) Motsei et al. (2003)
Erythrina lysistemon	Root	Antiviral	Tanzania	Mc Kee et al. (1997)
Erythrina lysistemon	Stem bark	Estrogenic Bone formation stimulant Antidiabetic Rises seric LDL	Cameroon	Njamen et al. (2007)
Erythrina mildbraedii	Whole plant	Anti-tumoral Toxic effect Cytotoxic	Unspecified	Suffness et al (1988)
Erythrina mildbraedii	Root	Anti-mycobacterial Anti-bacterial	Nigeria	Mitscher et al. (1988)

Species	Part of the Plant	Biological Activities	Location	Reference
Erythrina poeppigiana	Unspecified	Cytotoxic	Colombia	De Cerain et al. (1996)
Erythrina resupinata	Roots	Fetal anti-implantation Anti-tumoral Uterine stimulant Abortive Toxicity evaluation	India	Aswal et al. (1984)
Erythrina rubrinervia	Twigs	"DNA linker" Cytotoxic	Unspecified	Pezzuto et al. (1991)
Erythrina sacleuxii	Leavess, root bark	Antimalarial Cytotoxic	Tanzania	Gessler et al. (1994) Gessler et al. (1995)
Erythrina senegalensis	Bark, root, stem bark

Flowers | Antimalarial Analgesic Anti-inflammatory Anti-bacterial Molluscicidal | Nigeria | Saidu et al. (2000) Etkin (1997) Ajaiyeoba et al. (2004) Hussain & Deeni (1991) Okunji & Iwu (1988) |
| Erythrina senegalensis | Bark | Anti-bacterial Anti-fungal | Senegal | Le Grand & Wondergem (1988) |
| Erythrina senegalensis | Raiz | Antiviral | Guinea-Bissau | Silva et al. (1997) |
| Erythrina sigmoidea | Bark Bark, root bark

Stem bark | Anti-yeast Anti-bacterial Anti-fungal Skeletal muscle relaxing Antispasmodic Spasmolytic | Cameroon | Biyiti et al. (1988) Nkengfack et al. (1994) Benedicta et al. (1993) Nkeh et al. (1996) |
Erythrina species	Bark	Anti-bacterial	China	Gaw & Wang (1949)
Erythrina species	Leaves	Pherormone	Puerto Rico	Keiser et al. (1975)
Erythrina species	Leaves	Anti tumoral	Indonesia	Itokawa et al. (1990)
Erythrina species	Leaves	Antipyretic	Thailand	Mokkhasmit et al. (1971)
Erythrina species	Stem bark	Anti-leishmaniasis Anti-trypanossomiasis	Bolivia	Fournet et al. (1994)

Species	Part of the Plant	Biological Activities	Location	Reference
Erythrina standleyana	Bark	Molluscicidal Inhibition of plant germination	Unspecified	Dominguez & Alcorn (1985)
Erythrina stricta	Stem Leaves	Spasmolytic Hypotermic Diuretic Anticonvulsant Analgesic Antiviral Anti-fungal Anti-yeast Anti-protozoan Toxicity evaluation Cytotoxic	India	Bhakuni et al. (1988) Dhar et al. (1968)
Erythrina suberosa	Leaves Stem bark	Hypotensive Anti-spermatogenic Anti-androgen Anti-gonadotropin Anti tumoral Toxicity evaluation Hypoglicemic Cytotoxic Antispasmodic	India	Dhar et al. (1968)
Erythrina suberosa	Leaves, seed oil	Anti-bacterial Anti-fungal	Thailand	Silpasuwon (1979) Joshi et al. (1981)
Erythrina subumbrans	Aerial parts	Fetal anti-implantation Uterine stimulant Anti tumoral Abortive effect Toxicity evaluation	India	Aswal et al. (1984)
Erythrina ulei	Bark	Anti-crustacean "DNA linker" Antioxidant	Peru	Desmarcheilier et al. (1996) Desmarcheilier et al. (1997)
Erythrina variegata	Bark	Anti gastric ulcer	Japan	Muto et al. (1994)
Erythrina variegata	Bark, leaves Seeds oil Stem	Inhibition of plant germination and growing Anti-bacterial Anti-fungal Juvenile hormone activity	India	Chauhan et al. (1989) Bhale et al. (1979) Tripathi & Rizvi (1984) Prabhu & John (1975)

Species	Part of the Plant	Biological Activities	Location	Reference
Erythrina variegata	Bark Stem bark	Phospholipase A2 inhibitor Prostaglandin synthesis inhibidor Central Nervous System effects Spasmolytic	Samoa	Hegde et al. (1997) Dunstan et al. (1997) Cox et al. (1989)
Erythrina variegata	Flowers	Anti-yeast Anti-bacterial	Thailand	Avirutnant & Pongpan (1983)
Erythrina variegata	Fresh flowers	Anxiolytic	Brazil	Flausino et al. (2007)
Erythrina variegata	Leaves Unspecified	Anti-inflammatory Skeletal muscle relaxing Barbiturates potentiator	Vietnam	Nguyen et al. (1991) Nguyen et al. (1992)
Erythrina variegata	Roots	Inhibitor of glutamate-pyruvate-transaminase	Taiwan	Yanfg et al. (1987)
Erythrina variegate var. orientalis	Leaves Roots Stem bark	Antispasmodic Cytotoxic Toxicity evaluation Anti-yeast Anti-bacterial Anti-mycobacterial Cytotoxic Antispasmodic	India	Dhar et al. (1968) Telikepalli et al. (1990) Dhar et al. (1968)
Erythrina variegate var. orientalis	Leaves	Anti tumoral	Philippines	Masilungan et al. (1971)
Erythrina velutina	Leaves Stem bark Trunk bark	Analgesic Anti-inflammatory Uterine stimulant Molluscicidal	Brazil	Marchioro et al. (2005) Barros et al. (1970) Pinheiro de Sousa & Rouquayrol (1974)
Erythrina vespertilio	Bark	Inhibition of platelet aggregation Serotonin release inhibition	Australia	Rogers et al. (2001)
Erythrina vogelii	Root bark	Anti-fungal	Ivory Coast	Queiroz et al. (2002)
Erythrina zeyheri	Leaves	Anti-bacterial COX1 Inhibitor	South Africa	Pillay et al. (2001)

Table 2. Biological activity of *Erythrina* extracts.

Classes of Compounds	Occurrence	Percentage
Alkaloids	461	41.57
Coumarins	1	0.09
Steroids	29	2.62
Flavonoids	330	29.76
Lipids	32	2.88
Proteins	112	10.10
Triterpenes	31	2.80
Other compounds	113	10.19
Total	1109	100

Table 3. Occurrence of the different classes of compounds in the *Erythrina* genus

Some important alkaloids that are distributed within plants from the *Erythrina* genus are erytharbine, erythartine, erysotramidine and erysotrine, shown in figure 1. It is noteworthy that a characteristic feature of these alkaloids is the spiro structure in the rings bearing the nitrogen atom.

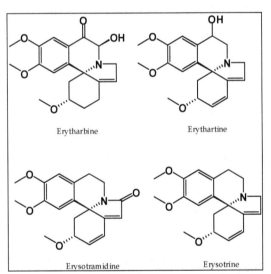

Fig. 1. Common alkaloids found in the *Erythrina* genus.

4. Conclusion

This review showed that *Erythrina* species are commonly utilized for numerous diseases and that many ethnopharmacological studies have been performed in order to confirm the activities attributed to these species. Moreover, several classes of substances have been isolated from the *Erythrina* genus, mainly alkaloids (41.57%) and flavonoids (29.76%).

Despite the large amount of available data, some of the plants of this genus remain to be studied. An example is *Erythrina mulungu*, largely used in Brazil, yet a significant number of studies regarding its pharmacological properties and chemical composition were unable to be found. A recent contribution to the knowledge about this plant is given by our group, regarding the anti-inflammatory and antinociceptive activities of a hydroalcoholic extract obtained from *E. mulungu* (Oliveira et al., *in press*).

5. Acknowledgments

The authors aknowledge the Brazilian National Research Council (CNPq), FAPEAL and CAPES for their financial support in the form of grants and fellowship awards.

6. References

Ajaiyeoba, E., Ashidi, J., Abiodun, O., Okpako, L., Ogbole, O., Akinboye, D., Falade, C., Bolaji, O., Gbotosho, G., Falade, M., Itiola, O., Houghton, P.,Wright, C., & Oduola, A. (2004). Antimalarial ethnobotany: in vitro antiplasmodial activity of seven plants indentified in the Nigerian middle belt. Pharmaceutical Biology, Vol.42, No.8, pp. 588-591, ISSN 1744-5116

Anderson, E. F. (1986). Ethnobotany of hill tribes of northern Thailand. II. Lahu medicinal plants. Economic Botany, Vol.40, No.4, pp. 442-450, ISSN 0013-0001

Aswal, B. S., Bhakuni, D. S., Goel, A. K., Kar, K., Mehrotra, B. N., & Mukherjee, K. C. (1984). Screening of indian plants for biological activity: part X. Indian Journal of Experimental Biology, Vol.22, No.6, pp. 312-332, ISSN 0019-5189

Avirutnant, W. & Pongpan, A. (1983). The antimicrobial activity of some thai flowers and plants. Mahidol University Journal of Pharmaceutical Sciences, Vol.10, No.3, pp. 81-86, ISSN 0125-1570

Awasth, A. K. (1991). Ethnobotanical studies on the negrito islanders of andaman islands, India - the great andamanese. Economic Botany, Vol.45, No.2, pp. 274-280, ISSN 0013-0001

Ayensu, E. S. (1978). Medicinal plants of the West Indies, Unpublished Manuscript, p. 110

Bandoni, A. L., Mendiondo, M. E., Rondina, R. V. D., & Coussio, J. D. (1976). Survey of Argentine medicinal plants. Economic Botany, Vol.30, pp. 161-185, ISSN 0013-0001

Barakat, I., Jackson, A. H., & Abdulla, M. I. (1977). Further studies of *Erythrina* alkaloids. Lloydia, Vol.40, No.5, pp. 471-475, ISSN 0024-5461

Barros, G. S. G., Matos, F. J. A., Vieira, J. E. V., Sousa, M. P., & Medeiros, M. C. (1970). Pharmacological screening of some brazilian plants. Journal of Pharmacy and Pharmacology, Vol.22, p. 116, ISSN 0022-3573

Benedicta, N. N., Kamanyi, & A. Bopelet, M. (1993). Anticholinergic effects of the methanol stembark extract of *Erythrina sigmoidea* on isolated rat ileal preparations. Phytotherapy Research, Vol.7, No.2, pp. 120-123, ISSN 0951-418X

Bhakuni, D. S., Goel, A. K., Jain, S., Mehrotra, B. N., Patnaik, G. K., & Prakash, V. (1988). Screening of indian plants for biological activity: part XIII. Indian Journal of Experimental Biology, Vol.26, No.11, pp. 883RY-904, ISSN 0019-5189

Bhale, B., Jain, P. K., & Bokadia, M. M. (1979). The in vitro antimicrobial activity of the fixed oil of *Erythrina indica*. Indian Drugs Pharm Ind, Vol.14, No.3, pp. 39-40

Bhattarai, N. K. (1991). Folk herbal medicines of Makawanpur district, Nepal. International Journal of Pharmacognosy, Vol.29, No.4, pp. 284-295, ISSN 0925-1618

Biyiti, L., Pesando, D., & Puiseux-Dao, S. (1988). Antimicrobial activity of two flavanones isolated from the cameroonian plant *Erythrina sigmoidea*. Planta Medica, Vol.54, No.2, pp. 126-128, ISSN 0032-0943

Blackwood, B. (1935). Both sides of buka passage, Clarendon Press, ISBN 0404159079, Oxford, United Kingdom

Boily, Y. & Van Puyvelde, L. (1986). Screening of medicinal plants of Rwanda (central Africa) for antimicrobial activity. Journal of Ethnopharmacology, Vol.16, No.1, pp. 1-13, ISSN 0378-8741

Brandão, M., Botelho, M., & Krettli, E. (1985). Antimalarial experimental chemotherapy using natural products. Ciência e Cultura, Vol.37, No.7, pp. 1152-1163, ISSN 1980-0029

Burkill, I. H. (1966). Dictionary of the economic products of the Malay Peninsula. Ministry of agriculture and cooperatives, Volume I, Kuala Lumpur, Malaysia

Bye, J. R. (1986). Medicinal plants of the Sierra Madre: comparative study of Tarahumara and Mexican market plants. Economic Botany, Vol.40, No.1, pp. 103-124, ISSN 0013-0001

Caceres, A., Giron, L. M., Alvarado, S. R., & Torres, M. F. (1987). Screening of antimicrobial activity of plants popularly used in Guatemala for the treatment of dermatomucosal diseases. Journal of Ethnopharmacology, Vol.20, No.3, pp. 223-237, ISSN 0378-8741

Caldwell, M. E. & Brewer, W. R. (1983). Plants with potential to enhance significant tumor growth. Cancer Research, Vol.43, No.12, pp. 5775-5777, ISSN 0008-5472

Chacha, M., Bojase-Moleta, G., & Majinda, R. R. T. (2005). Antimicrobial and radical scavenging flavonoids from the stem wood of *Erythrina latissima*. Phytochemistry, Vol.66, pp. 99-104, ISSN 0031-9422

Chagnon, M. (1984). General pharmacologic inventory of medicinal plants of Rwanda. Journal of Ethnopharmacology, Vol.12, No.3, pp. 239-251, ISSN 0378-8741

Chapuis, J. C., Sordat, B., & Hostettmann, K. (1988). Screening for cytotoxic activity of plants used in traditional medicine. Journal of Ethnopharmacology, Vol.23, No.2/3, pp. 273-284, ISSN 0378-8741

Chauhan, J. S. (1989). Screening of higher plants for specific herbicidal principle active against dodder, *Cuscuta reflexa* roxb. Indian Journal of Experimental Biology, Vol.27, No.10, pp. 877-884, ISSN 0019-5189

Chhabra, S. C., Uiso, F. C., & Mshiu, E. N. (1984). Phytochemical screening of tanzanian medicinal plants. Journal of Ethnopharmacology, Vol.11, No.2, pp. 157-179, ISSN 0378-8741

Chopra, R. N. (1933). Indigenous drugs of india. Their medical and economic aspects, The Art Press, ASIN B003E2YJ6W, Calcutta, India

Chopra, R. N. & Ghosh, S. (1935). Some common indigenous remedies. Indian Medical Record, Vol.55, p. 77, ISSN 0019-5898

Corrêa, M. P. (1984). Dicionário das plantas úteis do Brasil e das exóticas cultivadas, Vol. 5, Ministério da Agricultura, Rio de Janeiro, Brazil

Cox, P. A., Sperry, L. B., Tuominen, M., & Bohlin, L. (1989). Pharmacological activity of the Samoan ethnopharmacopoeia. Economic Botany, Vol.43, No.4, pp. 487-497, ISSN 0013-0001

Cronquist, A. (1981). An integrated system of classification of flowering plants, Columbia University Press, ISBN 0231038801, 9780231038805, New York, United States of America

Das, S. K. (1955). Medicinal, economic and useful plants of India, West Bengal, ISBN B00117DIX2, India

De Cerain A. L. (1996). Cytotoxic activities of colombian plant extracts on chinense hamster lung fibroblasts. Phytotherapy Research, Vol.10, No.5, pp. 431-432, ISSN 0951-418X

Desmarchelier, C., Gurni, A., Ciccia, G., & Giulietti, A. M. (1996). Ritual and medicinal plants of the ese'ejas of the amazonian rainforest (Madre de Dios, Peru). Journal of Ethnopharmacology, Vol.52, No.1, pp. 45-51, ISSN 0378-8741

Desmarchelier C., Repetto, M., Coussio, J., Llesuy, S., & Ciccia, G. (1997). Total reactive antioxidant potential (TRAP) and total antioxidant reactivity (TAR) of medicinal plants used in southwest Amazonas (Bolivia and Peru). International Journal of Pharmacognosy, Vol.35, No.4, pp. 288-296, ISSN 1388-0209

Dhar, M. L., Dhar, M. M., Dhawan, B. N., Mehrotra, B. N., & Ray, C. (1968). Screening of indian plants for biological activity: part I. Indian Journal of Experimental Biology, Vol.6, pp. 232-247, ISSN 0019-5189

Diaz, J. L. (1977). Ethnopharmacology of sacred psychoactive plants used by the Indians of Mexico. Annual Review of Pharmacology and Toxicology, Vol.17, pp. 647-75, ISSN:0362-1642

Dominguez, X. A. & Alcorn, J. B. (1985). Screening of medicinal plants used by huastec mayans of northeastern Mexico. Journal of Ethnopharmacology, Vol.13, No.2, pp. 139-156, ISSN 0378-8741

Duke, J. A. (1994). Amazonian ethnobotanical dictionary, CRC Press, ISBN 0849336643, USA

Dunstan, C. A., Noreen, Y., Serrano, G., Cox, P. A., Perera, P., & Bohlin, L. (1997). Evaluation of some Samoan and Peruvian medicinal plants by prostaglandin biosynthesis and rat ear edema assays. Journal of Ethnopharmacology, Vol.57, pp. 35-56, ISSN 0378-8741

Etkin, N. L. (1997). Antimalarial plants used by Hausa in northern Nigeria. Tropical Doctor, Vol.27, No.1, pp. 12-16, ISSN 0049-4755

Filipoy, A. (1994). Medicinal plants of the pilaga of central chaco. Journal of Ethnopharmacology, Vol.44, No.3, pp. 181-193, ISSN 0378-8741

Flausino, O., Santos, L. S.,Verli, H., Pereira, A. M., Bolzani, S., & Nunes-De-Souza, R. L. (2007). Anxiolytic effects of erythrinian alkaloids from Erythrina mulungu. Journal of Natural Products, Vol.70, pp. 48-53, ISSN 0163-3864

Fournet, A. Barrios, A. A., & Munoz, V. (1994). Leishmanicidal and trypanocidal activities of bolivian medicinal plants. Journal of Ethnopharmacology, Vol.41, No.1/2, pp. 19-37, ISSN 0378-8741

García-Mateos, R., Soto-Hernández, M., & Vibrans, H. (2001). Erythrina americana Miller ('Colorín'; Fabaceae), a versatile resource from Mexico: a review. Economic Botany, Vol.55, pp. 391–400, ISSN 0013-0001

Garin-Aguilar, M. E., Luna, J. E. R., Soto-Hernandez, M., Del Toro, G. V., & Vazquez, M. M. (2000). Effect of crude extracts of Erythrina americana Mill. on aggressive behavior in rats. Journal of Ethnopharmacology, Vol.69, No.2, pp. 189-196, ISSN 0378-8741

Gaw, H. Z. & Wang, H. P. (1949). Survey of chinese drugs for presence of antibacterial substances. Science, Vol.110, pp. 11-12, ISSN 1095-9203

Gessler, M. C., Nkunyak, M. H. H., Mwasumbi, L. B., Heinrich, M., & Tanner, M. (1994). Screening tanzanian medicinal plants for antimalarial activity. Acta Tropica, Vol.56, No.1, pp. 65-77, ISSN 0001-706X

Gessler, M. C., Tanner, M., Chollet, J., Nkunya, N. H. H., & Heinrich, M. (1995). Tanzanian medicinal plants used traditionally for the treatment of malaria: in vivo antimalarial and *in vitro* cytotoxic activities. Phytotherapy Research, Vol.9, No.7, pp. 504-508, ISSN 0951-418X

Ghosal, S., Singh, S., & Bhattacharya, S. K. (1971). Alkaloids of Mucuna pruriens, Chemistry and Pharmacology, Planta Medica, Vol.19, p. 279, ISSN 0032-0943

Giron, L. M., Freire, V., Alonzo, A., & Caceres, A. (1991). Ethnobotanical survey of the medicinal flora used by the caribs of Guatemala. Journal of Ethnopharmacology, Vol.34, No.2/3, pp. 173-187, ISSN 0378-8741

Hastings, R. B. (1990). Medicinal legumes of mexico: Fabaceae, Papilionoidea, part one. Economic Botany, Vol.44, No.3, pp. 336-348, ISSN 0013-0001

Hegde, V. R., Dai, P., Patel, M. G., Puar, M. S., Das, P., Pai, J., Bryant, R., & Cox, P. A. (1997). Phospholipase A 2 inhibitors from an *Erythrina* species from Samoa. Journal of Natural Products, Vol.60, No.6, pp. 537-539, ISSN 0163-3864

Herbarium (2008). Introdução à fitoterapia: utilizando adequadamente as plantas medicinais, Colombo: Herbarium Lab. Bot. Ltda

Hickey, M. & King, C. (1981). 100 families of flowering plants, Cambridge University Press, ISBN 0521337003, 9780521337007, Cambridge, United Kingdom

Holdsworth, D. (1984). Phytomedicine of the Madang province, Papua New Guinea part I. Karkar island. International Journal of Crude Drug Research, Vol.22, No.3, pp. 111-119, ISSN 0167-7314

Hussain, H. S. & Deeni, Y. Y. (1991). Plants in kano ethomedicine; screening for antimicrobial activity and alkaloids. International Journal of Pharmacognosy, Vol.29, No.1, pp. 51-56, ISSN 0976-8858

Ichimaru, M., Moriyasu, M., Nishiyama, Y., Kato, A., Mathenge, S. G., Juma, F. D., & Nganga, J. N. (1996). Structural elucidation of new flavanones isolated from *Erythrina abyssinica*. Journal of Natural Products, Vol.59, No.12, pp. 1113-1116, ISSN 1520-6025

Iinuma, M. & Tanaka, T. (1994). Isoflavanone derivatives with antibacterial activity from *Erythrina bidwilli* and antibacterial agents for mouth. Patent-Japan Kokai Tokkyo Koho-1994. 6,312,983.

Iinuma, M., Okawa,Y., Tanaka, T., Kobayashi, Y., & Miyauchi, K. I. (1994). Phenolic compounds in *Erythrina bidwillii* and their activity against oral microbial organisms. Heterocycles, Vol.39, No.2, pp. 687-692, ISSN 1881-0942

Ishii, R., Yoshikawa, K., Minakata, H., Komura, H., & Kada, T. (1984). Specificities of bio-antimutagens in plant kingdom. Agricultural and Biological Chemistry, Vol.48, No.10, pp. 2587-2591, ISSN 0002-136

Itokawa, H., Furukawa, H., & Tanaka, H. (1990). Screening test for antitumor activity of crude drugs (III). Studies on antitumor activity of indonesian medicinal plants. Shoyakugaku Zasshi. Vol.44, No.1, pp. 58-62, ISSN 0037-4377

Janzen,D. H., Juster, H. B., & Bell, E. A. (1977). Toxicity of secondary compounds to the seed-eating larvae of the bruchid beetle *callosobruchus maculatus*. Phytochemistry, Vol.16, pp. 223-227, ISSN 0031-9422

John, D. (1984). One hundred useful raw drugs of the kani tribes of trivandrum forest division, Kerala, India. International Journal of Crude Drug Research, Vol.22, No.1, pp. 17-39, ISSN 0167-7314

Joshi, R., Jain, N. K., & Garg, B. D. (1981). Antimicrobial activity of the oil and its unsaponifiable matter from the seeds of *Erythrina suberosa* roxb. Indian Drugs, Vol.18, p. 411, ISSN 0019-462X

Joubert, F. J. & Sharon, N. (1985). Proteinase inhibitors from Erythrina corallodendron and *Erythrina cristagalli* seeds. Phytochemistry, Vol.24, No.6, pp. 1169-1179, ISSN 0031-9422

Jovel, E. M., Cabanillas, J., & Towers, G. H. H. (1996).An ethnobotanical study of the traditonal medicine of the mestizo people of suni mirano, Loreto, Peru. Journal of Ethnopharmacology, Vol.53, pp. 149-156, ISSN 0378-8741

Kamat, V. S., Chuo, F. Y., Kubo, I., & Nakanishi, K. (1981). Antimicrobial agents from an east african medicinal plant *Erythrina abyssinica*. Heterocycles, Vol.15, pp. 1163-1170, ISSN 1881-0942

Kamusiime, H., Pedersen, A. T., Andersen, O. M., & Kiremire, B. (1996). Kaempferol 3-o-(2-o-beta-d-glucopyranosyl-6-o-alpha-l-rhamnopyranosyl-beta-d-glucopyranoside) from the african plant *Erythrina abyssinica*. International Journal of Pharmacognosy, Vol.34, No.5, pp. 370-373, ISSN 0975-4873

Keiser, I., Harris, E. J., Miyashita, D. H., Jacobson, M., & Perdue, R. E. (1975). Attraction of ethyl ether extracts of 232 botanicals to oriental fruit flies, melon flies, and mediterranean fruit flies. Lloydia, Vol.38, No.2, pp. 141-152, ISSN 0024-5461

Khan, M. A., Khan, T., & Ahmad, Z. (1994). Barks used as source of medicine in madhya pradesh, India. Fitoterapia, Vol.65, No.5, pp. 444-446, ISSN 0367-326X

Kloos, H., Thiongo, F. W., Ouma, J. H., & Butterworth, A. E. (1987). Preliminary evaluation of some wild and cultivated plants for snail control in machakos district, Kenya. Journal of Tropical Medicine & Hygiene, Vol.90, No.4, pp. 197-204, ISSN 0022-5304

Kokwaro, J. O. (1976). Medicinal Plants of East Africa, East Africa Literature Bureau, ISBN 9789966846846 Nairobi, Kenya

Krukoff, B. A. & Barneby, R. C. (1974). Conspectus of species of the genus *Erythrina*. Lloydia, Vol.37, No.3, pp. 332-459, ISSN 0024-5461

Le Grand, A. & Wondergem, P. A. (1987). Antiinfective phytotherapy of the savannah forests of Senegal (east Africa). I. An inventory. Journal of Ethnopharmacology, Vol.21, No.2, pp. 109-125, ISSN 0378-8741

Le Grand, A. & Wondergem, P. A. (1988). Anti-infectious phytotherapies of the tree-savannah of senegal (west-africa). II. Antimicrobial activity of 33 species. Journal of Ethnopharmacology, Vol.22, No.1, pp. 25-31, ISSN 0378-8741

Le Grand, A. (1989). Anti-infectious phytotherapy of the tree-savannah, Senegal (western Africa) III: a review of the phytochemical substances and anti-microbial activity of

43 species. Journal of Ethnopharmacology, Vol.25, No.3, pp. 315-338, ISSN 0378-8741

Lewinsohn, R. (2003). Três Epidemias. Lições do Passado, p. 81-85, Editora Unicamp, ISBN 8526805827, Campinas, Brazil

Lourenzi, H. (1992). Árvores brasileiras: manual de identificação e cultivo de plantas, Plantarum, ISBN 9788586714320, São Paulo, Brazil

Maikere-Faniyo, R., Van Puyvelde, L., Mutwewingabo, A., & Habiyaremye, F. X. (1989). Study of rwandese medicinal plants used in the treatment of diarrhea. Journal of Ethnopharmacology, Vol. 26, No.2, pp. 101-109, ISSN 0378-8741

Maillard, M., Gupta, M. P., & Hostettmann, K. (1987). A new antifungal prenylated flavanone from Erythrina berteroana. Planta Medica, Vol.53, No.6, pp. 563-564, ISSN 0032-0943

Manandhar, N. P. (1995). Medicinal Folk-Lore about the plants used as anthelmintic agents in Nepal. Fitoterapia, Vol.66, No. 2, pp. 149-155, ISSN 0367-326X

Marchioro, M., Blank, M. D. F. A., Mourao, R. H. V., & Antoniolli, A. R. (2005). Antinociceptive activity of the aqueous extract of Erythrina velutina leaves. Fitoterapia, Vol.76, No.7-8, pp. 637-642, ISSN 0367-326X

Masilungan, V. A., Vadlamudi, S., & Goldin, A. (1971). Screening of philippine medicinal plants for anticancer agents using CCNSC protocols. Cancer Chemother Reports Part 2, Vol.2, pp. 135-140, ISSN 0069-0120

Matos, F. J. (1994). Farmácias vivas: sistema de utilização de plantas medicinais projetado para pequenas comunidades, 2nd Ed, EUFC, ISBN 10 8572820086, Fortaleza, Brazil

Mc Clatchey, W. (1996). The ethnopharmacopoeia of Rotuma. Journal of Ethnopharmacology, Vol.50, No.3, pp. 147-156, ISSN 0378-8741

Mc Kee T. C., Bokesch, H. R., Mc Cormick, J. L., Rashid, A., Spielvogel, D., Gustafson, K. R., Alavanja, M. M., Cardelina I. I. J. H., & Boyd, M. R. (1997). Isolation and characterization of new anti-HIV and cytotoxic leads from plants, marine, and microbial organisms. Journal of Natural Products, Vol.60, No.5, pp. 431-438, ISSN 0163-3864

Medina, F. R. & Woodbury, R. Terrestrial plants molluscicidal to lymnaeid hosts of Fasciliasis hepatica in Puerto Rico. Journal of Agriculture of the University of Puerto Rico, Vol.63, pp. 366-376, ISSN 0041-994X

Miguel, M. D. & Miguel, O. G. (2004). Desenvolvimento de fitoterápicos, 2nd Ed., Robe Editorial, ISBN 9788586652196, São Paulo, Brazil

Mino, J., Gorzalczany, S., Moscatelli, V., Ferraro, G., Acevedo, C., & Hnatyszyn, O. (2002). Actividad antinociceptiva y antiinflammatoria de Erythrina crista-galli. Acta Farmaceutica Bonaerense, Vol.21, No.2, pp. 93-98, ISSN 0326-2383

Mitscher,L. A., Ward, J. A., Drake, S., & Rao, G. S. (1984). Antimicrobial agents from higher plants. Erycristagalin, a new pterocarpene from the roots of the bolivian coral tree, Erythrina crista-galli. Heterocycles, Vol.22, No.8, pp. 1673-1675, ISSN 1881-0942

Mitscher, L. A., Okwute, S. K., Gollapudi, S. R., Drake, S., & Avona, E. (1988). Antimicrobial pterocarpans of nigerian Erythrina mildbraedii. Phytochemistry, Vol.27, No.11, pp. 3449-3452, ISSN 0031-9422

Mokkhasmit, M., Ngarmwathana, W., Sawasdimongkol, K., & Permphiphat, U. (1971). Pharmacological evaluation of Thai medicinal plants. Journal of the Medical Association of Thailand, Vol.54, No.7, pp. 490-504, ISSN 0125-2208

Moriyasu, M., Ichimaru, M., Nishiyama, Y., Kato, A., Mathenge, S. G., Juma, F. D., & Nganga, J. N. (1998). Minor flavanones from *Erythrina abyssinica*. Journal of Natural Products, Vol.61, No.2, pp. 185-188, ISSN 1520-6025

Morton, J. F. (1994). Pito (*Erythrina berteroana*) and chipilin (*Crotalaria longirostrata*), (Fabaceae), two soporific vegetables of central america. Economic Botany, Vol.48, No.2, pp. 130-138, ISSN 0013-0001

Motsei, M. L., Lindsey, K. L., Van Staden, J., & Jager, A. K. (2003). Screening of traditionally used south african plants for antifungal activity aganist Candida albicans. Journal of Ethnopharmacology, Vol.76, No.2/3, pp. 235-241, ISSN 0378-8741

Muto, Y., Ichikawa, H., Kitagawa, O., Kumagai, K., Watanabe, M., Ogawa, E., Seiki, M., Shirataki, Y., Yokoe, I., & Komatsu, M. (1994). Studies on antiulcer agents. I. The effects of various methanol and aqueous extracts of crude drugs on antiucler activity. Yakugaku Zasshi, Vol.114, No.2, pp. 980-994, ISSN 1347-5231

National Policy on Integrative and Complementary Practices (2006). Avaiable at: http://www.telessaudebrasil.org.br/lildbi/docsonline/3/1/113-Politica_Nacional_de_Praticas_Integrativas_e_Complementares_SUS.pdf

Ndamba, J., Nyazema, N., Makaza, N., Anderson, C., & Kaondera, K. C. (1994). Traditional herbal remedies used for the treatment of urinary schistosomiasis in Zimbabwe. Journal of Ethnopharmacology, Vol.42, No.2, pp. 125-132, ISSN 0378-8741

Nguyen, V. T., Pham, T. K., Pho, D. T., & Do, C. H. (1991). The pharmacological action of total alkaloids extracted from *Erythrina orientalis* (L.) Murr. Tap Chi Duoc Hoc, Vol.6, pp. 13-17, ISSN 0258-6967

Nguyen, V. T., Pham, T. K., Pho, D. T., & Do, C. H. (1992). The anti-inflammatory effect of the total alkaloids extracted from the leaves of Erythrina orientalis Murr. Tap Chi Duoc Hoc, Vol.1, pp. 25-27, ISSN 0258-6967

Njamen, D., Nde, C. B. M., Fomum, Z. T., & Mbanya, J. C. (2007). Preventive effects of an extract of *Erythrina lysistemon* (Fabaceae) on some menopausal problems: studies on the rat. Journal of Complementary and Integrative Medicine, Vol.4, No.1, pp. 1-17

Nkeh, B., Kamany, A., Bopelet, M., Ayafor, J. F., & Mbfor, J. T. (1996). Inhibition of histamine-induced contraction of rat ileum by promethazine and the methanol stembark extract of *Erythrina sigmoidea*. Phytotherapy Research, Vol.10, No.5, pp. 444-446, ISSN 0951-418X

Nkengfack, A. E., Vouffo, T. W., Formum, Z. T., Meyer, M., Bergendorff, O., & Sterner, O. (1994). Prenylated isoflavanone from the roots of *Erythrina sigmoidea*. Phytochemistry, Vol.36, No.4, pp. 1047-1051, ISSN 0031-9422

Nkengfack, A. E., Vardamides, J. C., Fomum, Z. T., & Meyer, M. (1995). Prenylated isoflavanone from *Erythrina eriotricha*. Phytochemistry, Vol.40, No.6, pp. 1803-1808, ISSN 0031-9422

Nkengfack, A. E., Vouffo, W., Vardamides, J. C., Kouam, J., Fomum, Z. T., Meyer, M., & Sterner, O. (1997). Phenolic metabolites from *Erythrina* species. Phytochemistry, Vol.46, No.3, pp. 573-578, ISSN 0031-9422

Nkengfack, A. E., Azebaze, A. G. B., Waffo, A. K., Fomum, Z. T., Meyer, M., & Van Heerden, F. R. (2001). Cytotoxic isoflavones from *Erythrina indica*. Phytochemistry, Vol.58, No.7, pp. 1113-1120, ISSN 0031-9422

Okunji, C. O. & Iwu, M. M. (1988). Control of schistosomiasis using nigerian medicinal plants as molluscicides. International Journal of Crude Drug Research, Vol.26, No.4, pp. 246-252, ISSN 0167-7314

Oliveira, M. S. G., Aquino, A. B., Silva, D. L., Aquino, P. G. V., Santos, M. S., Porfírio, A. P. R., Sant'Ana, A. E. G., Santos, B. V. O. Alexandre-Moreira, M. S., & Araújo-Júnior, J. X. (*Article in Press*) Antinociceptive and anti-inflammatory activity of hydroalcoholic extracts and phases from *Erythrina mulungu*. Revista Brasileira de Farmacognosia, ISSN 0102-695X

Omer, M. E. A., Al Magboul, A. Z., & El Egami, A. A. (1998). Sudanese plants used in folkloric medicine: screening for antibacterial activity. Part IX. Fitoterapia, Vol.69, No.6, pp. 542-545, ISSN 0367-326X

Pennington, C. W. (1973). Medicinal plants utilized by the pima montanes of chihuahua. America Indigena, Vol.33, pp. 213-232, ISSN 0185-1179

Pérez, C. & Anesini C. (1994). In vitro antibacterial activity of Argentine folk medicinal plants against *Salmonella typhi*. Journal of Ethnopharmacology, Vol.44, No.1, pp. 41-46, ISSN 0378-8741

Pezzuto, J. M., Che, C. T., Mc Pherson, D. D., Zhu, J. P., Topcu, G., Erdelmeier, C. A. J., & Cordell, G. A. (1991). DNA as an affinity probe useful in the detection and isolation of biologically active natural products. Journal of Natural Products, Vol.54, No.6, pp. 1522-1530, ISSN 0163-3864

Pillay C. C. N., Jager, A. K., Mulholland, D. A., & Van Staden, J. (2001). Cyclooxygenase inhibiting and anti-bacterial activities of South African *Erythrina* species. Journal of Ethnopharmacology, Vol.74, No.3, pp. 231-237, ISSN 0378-8741

Pinheiro de Sousa, M. & Rouquayrol, M. Z. (1974). Molluscicidal activity of plants from northeast Brazil. Revista Brasileira de Pesquisa Medica e Biológica, Vol.7, No.4, pp. 389-394

Polhill, R. M. & Raven P. H. (E.d.) (1981). Advances in legume systematic I and II, Kew Publishing, ISBN 9780855212247, United Kingdom

Prabhu, V. K. K. & John, M. (1975). Juvenomimetic activity in some plants. Univ Kerala Dept Zoology Trivandrum Kerala India. Experientia, Vol. 31, p. 913, ISSN 0014-4754

Pushpangadan, P. & Atal, C. K. (1984). Ethno-medico-botanical investigations in kerala i. Some primitive tribals of western ghats and their herbal medicine. Journal of Ethnopharmacology, Vol.11, No.1, pp. 59-77, ISSN 0378-8741

Queiroz, E. F., Atindehou, K. K., Terreaux, C., Antus, S., & Hostettmann, K. (2002). Prenylated isoflavonoids from the root bark of *Erythrina vogelii*. Journal of Natural Products, Vol.65, No.3, pp. 403-406, ISSN 0163-3864

Rabe, T. & Van Staden, J. (1997). Antibacterial activity of south african plants used for medicinal purposes. Journal of Ethnopharmacology, Vol.56, pp. 81-87, ISSN 0378-8741

Rao, R. R. (1981). Ethnobotany of Meghalaya: medicinal plants used by khasi and garo tribes. Economic Botany, Vol.35, No.1, pp. 4-9, ISSN 0013-0001

Ratnasooriya, W. D. & Dharmasiri, M. G. (1999). Aqueous extract of sri lankan *Erythrina indica* leaves had sedative but not analgesic activity. Fitoterapia, Vol.70, No.3, pp. 311-313, ISSN 0367-326X

Rogers, K. L., Grice, I. D., & Griffiths, L. R. (2001). Modulation of in vitro platelet 5-ht release by species of *Erythrina* and *Cymbopogon*. Life Sciences, Vol.69, No.15, pp. 1817-1829, ISSN 0024-3205

Ross, S. A., Megalla, S. E., Bishay, D. W., & Awad, A. H. (1980). Studies for determining antibiotic substances in some egyptian plants. Part I. Screening for antimicrobial activity. Fitoterapia, Vol.51, pp. 303-308, ISSN 0367-326X

Saidu, K., Onah, J., Orisadipe, A., Olusola, A., Wambebe, C., & Gamaniel, K. (2000). Antiplasmodial, anaglesic, and anti-inflammatory activities of the aqueous extract of the stem bark of *Erythrina senegalensis*. Journal of Ethnopharmacology, Vol.71, No.1/2, pp. 275-280, ISSN 0378-8741

Selvanayahgam, Z. E., Gnanevendhan, S. G., Balakrishna, K., & Rao, R. B. (1994). Antisnake venom botanicals from ethnomedicine. Journal of Herbs, Spices and Medicinal Plants, Vol.2, No.4, pp. 45-100, ISSN 1540-3580

Serragiotto, M. H., Leitão Filho, H., & Marsaioli, A. (1981). Erysotrine-N-oxide and erythartine-N-oxide, two novel alkaloids from *Erythrina mulungu*. Canadian Journal of Chemistry, Vol.59, No.18, pp. 2771-2775, ISSN 1480-3291

Silpasuwon, S. (1979). Studies of the effects of some medicinal plants on growth of some bacteria in the family enterobacteriaceae. Ms.Thesis Res Chiangmai University, p. 2522

Silva, O., Barbosa, S., Diniz, A., Valdeira, M. L., & Gomes, E. (1997). Plant extracts antiviral activity against herpes simplex virus type 1 and african swine fever virus. International Journal of Pharmacognosy, Vol.35, No.1, pp. 12-16, ISSN 0976-8858

Simões, C. M. O., Falkenberg, M., Auler Mentz, L., Schenkel, E. P., Amoros, M., & Girre, L. (1999). Antiviral activity of south Brazilian medicinal plant extracts. Phytomedicine, Vol.6, No.3, pp. 205-214, ISSN 0975-0185

Singh, L. M. & Chatterjee, S. (1979). Effect of amoora rohituka on in vitro blastogenesis of lymphocytes. Journal of Research in Indian Medicine, Yoga and Homeopathy, Vol.14, No.1, pp. 45-48

Suffness, M., Abbott, B., Statz, D. W., Wonilowicz, E., & Spjut, R. (1988). The utility of p388 leukemia compared to b16 melanoma and colon carcinoma 38 for in vivo screening of plant extracts. Phytotherapy Research, Vol.2, No.2, pp. 89-97, ISSN 0951-418X

Tachibana, Y., Kato, A., Nishiyama, Y., Kawanishi, K., Tobe, H., Juma, F. D., Ogeto, J. O., & Mathenge, S. G. (1993). Mitogenic activities in african traditional herbal medicines. Planta Medica, Vol.59, No.4, pp. 354-358, ISSN 0032-0943

Talla, E., Njamen, D., Mbafor, J. T., Fomum, Z. T., Kamanyi, A., Mbanya, J. C., Giner, R. M., Recio, M. C., Manez, S., & Rios, J. L. (2003). Warangalone, the isoflavonoid anti-inflammatory principle of *Erythrina addisoniae* stem bark. Journal of Natural Products, Vol.66, No.6, pp. 891-893, ISSN 0163-3864

Taniguchi, M., Chapya, A., Kubo, I., & Nakanishi, K. (1978). Screening of east African plants for antimicrobial activity. Chemical and Pharmaceutical Bulletin, Vol.26, pp. 2910-2913, ISSN 1347-5223

Taniguchi, M. & Kubo, I. (1993). Ethnobotanical drug discovery based on medicine men's trials in the african savanna: screening of east african plants for antimicrobial activity II. Journal of Natural Products, Vol. 56, No.9, pp. 1539-1546, ISSN 0163-3864

Telikepalli, H., Gollapudi, S. R., Keshavarz-Shokri, A., Velazquez, L., Sandmann, R. A., Veliz, E. A., Rao, K. V. J., Madhavi, A. S., & Mitscher, L. A. (1990). Isoflavonoids and a cinnamyl phenol from root extracts of Erythrina variegata. Phytochemistry, Vol.29, No.6, pp. 2005-2007, ISSN 0031-9422

Tripathi, A. K. & Rizvi, S. M. A. (1984).Antifeedant activity of indigenous plants against diacrisia obliqua walker. Curr Science, Vol.54, No.13, pp. 630-631, ISSN 0011-3891

Unakul, S. (1950). Pharmacological studies. 2. Study of the leaves of Erythrina fusca lour. Siriraj Hospital Gazette, Vol.2, No.4, pp. 177-189, ISSN 0125-152X

Vasconcelos, S. M. M., Oliveira, G. R., Carvalho, M. M., Rodrigues, A. C. P., Silveira, E. R., Fonteles, M. M. F., Sousa, F. C. L., & Viana, G. S. B. (2003). Antinociceptive activities of the hydroalcoholic extracts from Erythrina velutina and Erythrina mulungu in mice. Biological and Pharmaceutical Bulletin, Vol. 26, pp. 946-949, ISSN 1347-5215

Vasileva, B. (1969). Plantes medicinales de Guinee. Univ Moscow, Russia

Vlietinck, A. J., Van Hoof, L., Totte, J., Lasure, A., Vanden Berghe, D., Rwangabo, P. C., & Mvukiyumwami, J. (1995). Screening of hundred rwandese medicinal plants for antimicrobial and antiviral properties. Journal of Ethnopharmacology, Vol.46, No.1, pp. 31-47, ISSN 0378-8741

Waffo, A. K., Azebaze, G. A., Nkengfack, A. E., Fomum, Z. T., Meyer, M., Bodo, B., & Van Heerden, F. R. Indicanines B and C, two isoflavonoid derivatives from the root bark of Erythrina indica. Phytochemistry, Vol.53, No.8, pp. 981-985, ISSN 0031-9422

Wasuwat, S. (1967). A list of thai medicinal plants, ASRCT, Bangkok report project. 17 Research report, A.S.R.C.T., N°.1 on Research Project, Vol. 17, p. 22

Widianto, M. B., Padmawinata, K., & Suhalim, H. (1980). An evaluation of the sedative effect of the seeds of Erythrina fusca lour, 4th Asian Symposium on Medicinal Plants and Spices, p. 147, Bangkok, Thailand, 1980

Wink, M. (1984). Chemical Defense of lupins. Mollusc-repellent properties of quinolizidine alkaloids. Zeitschrift für Naturforschung C., Vol.39, No.6, pp. 553-558, ISSN 0939-5075

Yamada, C. S. B. (1998). Fitoterapia sua história e importância. Revista Racine, Vol.43, pp. 50-51, ISSN 1807-166X

Yanfg, L. L., Yen, K. Y., Kiso, Y., & Kikino, H. (1987). Antihepatotoxic actions of formosan plant drugs. Journal of Ethnopharmacology, Vol.19, No.1, pp. 103-110, ISSN 0378-8741

Yannitsaros, A. (1996). Screening for antiphage activity of plants growing in greece. Fitoterapia, Vol.67, No.3, pp. 205-214, ISSN 0367-326X

Yenesew, A., Derses, S., Irungu, B., Midiwo, J. O., Waters, N. C., Liyala, P., Akala, H., Heydenreich, M., & Peter, M. G. (2003a). Flavonoids and isoflavonoids with antiplasmodial activites from the root bark of Erythrina abyssinica. Planta Medica, Vol.69, No.7, pp. 658-661, ISSN 0032-0943

Zamora-Martinez, M. C. & Pola, C. N. P. (1992). Medicinal plants used in some rural
      populations of Oaxaca, Puebla and Veracruz, Mexico. Journal of
      Ethnopharmacology, Vol. 35, No.3, pp. 229-257, ISSN 0378-8741
http://portal.saude.gov.br/portal/arquivos/pdf/RENISUS.pdf
http://www.tropicos.org/Name/40005932

4

Phytochemistry, Pharmacology and Agronomy of Medicinal Plants: *Amburana cearensis*, an Interdisciplinary Study

Kirley M. Canuto, Edilberto R. Silveira, Antonio Marcos E. Bezerra,
Luzia Kalyne A. M. Leal and Glauce Socorro B. Viana
Empresa Brasileira de Pesquisa Agropecuária, Universidade Federal do Ceará,
Brazil

1. Introduction

Plants are an important source of biologically active substances, therefore they have been used for medicinal purposes, since ancient times. Plant materials are used as home remedies, in over-the-counter drug products, dietary supplements and as raw material for obtention of phytochemicals. The use of medicinal plants is usually based on traditional knowledge, from which their therapeutic properties are oftenly ratified in pharmacological studies.

Nowadays, a considerable amount of prescribed drug is still originated from botanical sources and they are associated with several pharmacological activities, such as morphine (I) (analgesic), scopolamine (II) atropine (III) (anticholinergics), galantamine (IV) (Alzheimer's disease), quinine (V) (antimalarial), paclitaxel (VI), vincristine (VII) and vinblastine (VIII) (anticancer drugs), as well as with digitalis glycosides (IX) (heart failure) (Fig. 1). The versatility of biological actions can be attributed to the huge amount and wide variety of secondary metabolites in plant organisms, belonging to several chemical classes as alkaloids, coumarins, flavonoids, tannins, terpenoids, xanthones, etc.

The large consumption of herbal drugs, in spite of the efficiency of synthetic drugs, is due to the belief that natural products are not toxic and/or have fewer side effects, the preference/need for alternative therapies, and their associated lower costs. In developing countries, herbal medicine is the main form of health care. In Brazil, where there is one of greatest biodiversity of plants in the world, pharmaceutical assistance programs, such as "Living Pharmacies", have a prominent role in spreading the rational use of medicinal plants mainly for poor people, under recognition by World Health Organization (WHO). Furthermore, herbal medicines also represent a significant pharmaceutical market share in some industrialized countries like Germany.

On the flip side, herbal drugs are discredited by most of the health related professionals, owing to a lack of scientific research supporting its efficacy and safety. In general, physicians feel insecure in prescribing herbal medicines, as most of them do not undergo through clinical trials, phytochemical analysis, and their active principles not being determined. Therefore, herbal medicines do not have a defined dosage, information on the chemical composition and warnings about possible risks. Additionally, the poor quality control of herbal drugs, which are subject to adulteration and intrinsic factors related to used raw material, do produce variables and inconsistent effects. Furthermore, most herbal drugs are produced from wild source, limiting the production at industrial level and putting the species used under threat of extinction.

Due to these aforesaid limitations, disadvantages and drawbacks of herbal medicine, we would like to present an updated review of chemical, pharmacological and agronomic studies of *Amburana cearensis* as a well succeeded example of a scientific research on wild plants and a model of a sustainable economic utilization of medicinal plants.

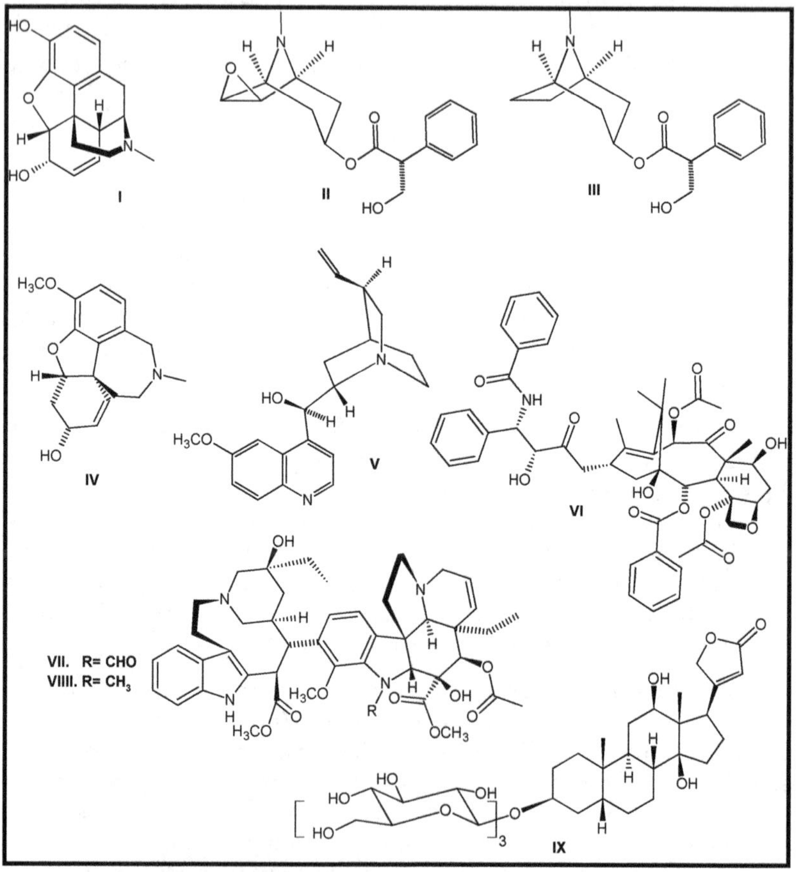

Fig. 1. Chemical structures of plant-derived drugs

2. Herbal drugs and phytopharmaceuticals

According to the WHO definition, herbal drugs are preparations containing plant parts (leaves, roots, seeds, stem bark, etc.) or whole plant materials in the crude or processed form, as active ingredients, besides some excipients. Herbal preparations can be found under different forms: oral tablets, capsules, gel caps, syrup, extracts and infusions. In general, combinations with chemically defined active substances or isolated constituents, are not considered to be herbal medicines. (Calixto, 2000).

The information about the therapeutical properties and usage of medicinal plants are commonly based on the empirical knowledge of ancient people, which was passed over several generations and originated the traditional medicine systems, utilized all over the world (Traditional Chinese Medicine, Ayurvedic system, Western and African Herbalisms). An estimated quantity of 50 000 plant species are used for medicinal purposes, from which the stand out species of the following families, such as Apocynaceae, Araliaceae, Apiaceae, Asclepiadaceae, Canellaceae, Clusiaceae and Menispermaceae (Schippmann et al., 2002). From the total of 252 drugs in the WHO's essential medicine list, 11% are exclusively derived from plant origins (Sahoo et al., 2010)

Herbal drugs are consumed by three-quarters of the world's population in the treatment of mainly chronic diseases, particularly headache, rheumatological disorders and asthma (Inamdar et al., 2010). In the developing countries, the population relies basically on medicinal plants for primary health care, since modern medicine is expensive and not easily accessible. However, the consumption of herbal drugs is also large in developed countries. Phytotherapy is popular in many countries of Western Europe (Germany, France, Italy, etc.), since people believe that either herbal drugs are devoid of side-effects or seek a healthier life style. Americans usually buy herbal products as a dietary supplement in the United States, aiming at preventing aging and diseases like cancer, as well as diabetes (Calixto, 2000).

Herbal drugs have some features which distinguish themselves considerably from synthetic drugs. Herbal medicines are always formed from a complex mixture of chemical compounds (eg. *Scutellaria baicalensis* has over 2000 components), and they may be constituted by many plants, therefore herbal drugs show an ample therapeutic usage. It is quite common to find a medicinal plant with several therapeutic properties (Sahoo et al., 2010; Calixto, 2000). The combination of either many plants, containing diverse bioactive substances or a pool of structural analogs, can produce a synergistic action that results in a stronger effect, therefore, permitting a reduction of dosage, which implies in lower risks of intoxication and undesirable side effects. As some diseases (e.g. AIDS or various types of cancer) possess a multi-causal etiology and a complex pathophysiology, a medical treatment may be more effective through well-chosen drug combinations than a single drug. Ginkgolides A and B, isolated from *Ginkgo biloba*, duly demonstrated a greater effect on the thrombocyte aggregation inhibition, when used as a mixture as opposed to what would be expected from the sum of the two compounds separately (Wagner, 2011).

On the other hand, plant-based products do not possess a well-defined chemical composition, due partially to chemical complexity stated above. Hence, the active principles of herbal drugs are frequently unknown, in addition to their standardization and quality control, being hardly achieved (Calixto, 2000) owing to mainly chemical variability in raw material. Secondary metabolites are the bioactive components from herbal drugs and their contents are strongly influenced by several factors: genetic (genotypes, chemotypes), physiologic (circadian rhythm, phenology, age), environmental (climate, sunlight exposure, water availability, soil, agronomic conditions) and manufacturing conditions (harvesting, storage and processing) (Tab. 1), (Sahoo et al., 2010; Gobbo-Beto & Lopes, 2007).

Evaluated Effect	Plant	Compound (s)	Result
Seasonality	*Hypericum perforatum*	Hypericin	300x content larger in summer than winter. (Southwell & Bourke, 2001)
Harvesting time	*Ocimum gratissimum*	Eugenol	98 % at 17h, but it is 11 % at midday (Silva et al. 1999)
Age	*Papaver somniferum*	Morphine	6x content larger on the 75th day after germination than on the 50th day (Williams & Ellis, 1989)
Phenology	*Gentiana lutea*	Mangiferin/ isoorientin	Before flowering-↑ [Mangiferin] ; during flowering- ↑ [Isoorientin] (Menković et al., 2000)
Temperature	*Nicotiana tabacum*	Scopolamine	[Scopolamine] 4x larger after freezing (Koeppe et al, 1970)
Water availability	*H. perforatum*	Hyperforin/ Hypericin	Under water stress: ↑ 2x [Hyperforin] and ↓ [Hypericin] (Zobayed et al, 2007)

Table 1. Effects on the production of secondary metabolites

Furthermore, most herbal drugs are utilized and commercialized without having a proven efficacy and safety through well-controlled double-blind clinical and toxicological trials, as pharmaceuticals are usually tested prior to being marketed. The safety and efficacy of herbal drugs are supported by their long historical use. Nevertheless, it is known that various herbal drugs fail, after testing in clinical trials and there are numerous reports on intoxication cases associated with their consumption. The WHO database has over sixteen thousand suspected case reports, related to intoxication by herbal drugs. The most frequent adverse reactions are hypertension, hepatitis, convulsions, thrombocytopenia and allergic reactions. Cardiovascular problems with the use of ephedra, hepatotoxicity caused by the consumption of kava-kava and comfrey, as well as licorice-related water retention, are some side effects claimed by the pharmacovigilance authorities. In addition to intrinsic factors mentioned above, the herbal drugs efficacy and safety, may also be seriously affected due to botanical misidentification or intentional usage of fake plants, contamination with pesticide residue, toxic heavy metals, pathogens and mycotoxins, as well as adulterants added to increase potency (synthetic substances) or the weight of herbal products in order to reduce costs (Sahoo et al., 2010; Calixto, 2000).

For the purpose of overcoming or mitigating the aforesaid inconvenient issues, WHO has developed a series of technical guidelines and documents in relation to the safety and the quality assurance of medicinal plants and herbal drugs preparations, such as "Quality Control Methods for Medicinal Plant Materials" (a collection of recommended test procedures for assessing the identity, purity and content of medicinal plant materials), "Guidelines on good agricultural and collection practices for medicinal plants", as well as "WHO guidelines for assessing quality of herbal medicines with reference to contaminants and residues". In turn, pharmaceutical laboratories have been investing in the enhancement of the quality for herbal products, aiming at the approval by governmental regulatory agencies, as a strategy to offer more reliable products, therefore conquering the confidence of health care professionals and consumers (Sahoo et al., 2010).

The interest in herbal drugs is continuously growing and they account for a significant share in the pharmaceutical market. The global herbal pharmaceutical industry (including drugs from herbal precursors and registered herbal medicines) invoices approximately US$ 50 billion/year (2008). In 2006, the best selling herbal products were: Ginseng (>U$ 1 billion global sales), Ginkgo (U$ 1 billion), Noni (U$ 1 billion), Saw Palmetto (U$ 600 millions) Echinacea (U$ 500 millions), Valerian (U$ 450 millions), and Green Tea (U $ 450 millions) (Gruenwald, 2008- Entrepreneur). The United States, China, Japan, Germany, South Korea and India, are the largest market. Medicinal plants have also been utilized as source of phytochemicals for the pharmaceutical, cosmetic and agrochemical industries. The most successful examples are paclitaxel (an anticancer drug from *Taxus baccata*), artemisinin (an antimalarial agent from *Artemisia annua*), vincristine/vinblastine (anticancer substances from *Catharanthus roseus*). The Pharmaceutical industry is interested in phytochemicals, however, the availability of quantities of pure chemical substances is normally a limiting factor, since the market demand for phytochemicals, usually reaches a scale from hundreds to thousands of kilograms per annum. (McChesney, 2007)

3. Medicinal plants threatened by extinction

The increasing demand for medicinal plants has endangered several species, since the main source of herbal drugs is the wild plant and the amount required from plant materials invariably exceeds the supply available from its natural source. Although the Convention on Biological Diversity (CBD), held in 1992, has established as goals, the conservation of biological diversity, the sustainable use of its components as well as the fair and equitable sharing of the benefits from the usage of genetic resources, it is still estimated that slightly more than 4000 medicinal plant species are under threat of extinction. The Convention on International Trade of Endangered Species of Wild Fauna and Flora (CITES), being the principal tool for monitoring or restricting the international trade of species threatened by over-exploitation, has published a biannual list of medicinal species like: *Taxus wallichiana, Panax quinquefolius, Dioscorea deltoidea, Hydrastis canadensis, Prunus africana , Rauvolfia serpentina* and *Pterocarpus santalinus* (Schippmann et al., 2002).

The overexploitation of a certain wild medicinal plant and consequent depletion of its raw material affect inevitably the economic feasibility of any phytopharmaceutical business in medium or long-term, since the production cost tends to be higher and the product supply become discontinuous. Furthermore, the extractivism provokes loss of genetic diversity, becoming the remaining plant population more vulnerable to diseases/pests and diminishing the variability of genotypes with features of interest such as yielding, bioactive substance content and resistance to biotic and abiotic factors (Rao et al., 2004). Hence, agencies concerned with conservation policies are recommending that wild species be brought into cultivation systems in order to assure the economic and environmental sustainability of herbal medicines trade (Schippmann et al., 2002). *Ginkgo biloba* and *Hypericum perforatum* are some of the top-selling medicinal plants, however they are not endangered, because their plant materials have been obtained by cultivation for a long time (Canter et al., 2005).

4. Cultivation of medicinal plants

The cultivation of medicinal plants is advocated as a means for meeting current and future demands for large quantities of herbal drugs, but also as a way to relieve the pressure of harvesting on wild populations (Schippmann et al., 2002). In China, one of the largest markets of herbal medicine, 380,000 ha of lands are utilized for farming of medicinal plants.

Medicinal plants are also cultivated for supplying phytochemicals. Bristol-Myers Squibb developed a system of production based upon isolation of a precursor of Taxol from the leaves or needles of cultivated *Taxus baccata* or *T. wallichiana* that provide the hundreds of kilograms of Taxol required per year for the treatment of cancer patients. (McChesney, 2007)

From the perspective of the market, domestication and cultivation provide a number of advantages over wild harvest for production of herbal drugs: (1) reliable botanical identification; (2) uniform and high quality raw material. As wild plants are dependent on many factors that cannot be controlled and the irregularity of supply is a common feature, the cultivation assures a steady source of raw material; (3) price and volume between farmer and pharmaceutical companies can be more easily negotiable, since the production forecast is more precise; (4) genetic breeding and biotechnology tools can lead to the development of plant materials with agronomically and commercially desirable features, permitting to optimize yield and to meet regulations as well as consumer preferences, respectively; (5) cultivated material can be easily certified as "organic product" (Schippmann et al., 2002; Canter et al, 2005).

Cultivated plants account for 60-90 % in terms of amount of plant material employed by Herbal medicines companies, but the number of wild species still is larger. Although the cultivation is apparently more advantageous than wild harvesting, only 130-140 species are cultivated in Europe, while just 20 out of 400 medicinal plants marketed in India are grown in field. Likewise, amongst 1000 plants more commonly used with medicinal purposes in China, only 100-250 species are sourced from cultivation. There are some reasons that can explain this low utilization of cultivated plants:

(1) Belief of that wild specimens are more potent than cultivated plants. Chinese believe that the physical appearance of wild roots to the human body symbolizes vitality and this feature is crucial for the potency of the ginseng roots, nevertheless cultivated roots do not exhibit this characteristic shape. Furthermore, some scientific studies support partly this hypothesis saying that secondary metabolites, the main responsible for therapeutic properties of herbal medicines, are biosynthesized by plants under particular conditions of stress and competition in their natural environments. Hence, perhaps the secondary metabolites would not be so expressed in monoculture conditions, therefore the active ingredient levels can be much lower in cultivated plant.

(2) Domestication of wild plant is not always technically possible. Many species are difficult to cultivate because of certain biological features or ecological requirements (slow growth rate, special soil requirements, low germination rates, susceptibility to pests, etc.).

(3) Economical feasibility. Domestication requires a long time of agronomical studies and high financial investment for the plantation. Generally, production costs through cultivation are higher than wild harvesting, thus few species can be marketed at a high sufficient price to make cultivation profitable, for instance *Garcinia afzelii*, *Panax quinquefolius*, *Saussurea costus* and *Warburgia salutaris*. Hence, many endangered medicinal plants only will bring into cultivation, if exists governmental incentive (Schippmann et al., 2002).

However, the cultivation of medicinal plant in agroforestry system can be a good alternative for more viable and environmentally sustainable farming. In China, ginseng (*Panax ginseng*) and other medicinal plants are grown in pine (*Pinus* spp.), *Paulownia tomentosa* and spruce (*Picea* spp.) forests; besides some medicinal herbs are often planted with bamboo (*Bambusa* spp.). In New Zealand, American ginseng showed better growth under *Pinus radiate*. The shade offered by forest species seems to favor the growth of medicinal plants. Likewise, quinine yields of *Cinchona ledgeriana* increase when it is protected by shade of other species, such as *Crotalaria anagyroides* and *Tephrosia candida*. In India, some medicinal plants that have also been successfully intercropped with fuel wood trees (e.g., *Acacia auriculiformis* and *Eucalyptus tereticornis*) and coconut. Intercropping gives some income to farmers during the period when the main trees have not started production. (Rao et al., 2004).

Application of traditional and biotechnological plant-breeding techniques can become the cultivation of medicinal plants a trade more attractive (eg. increasing the yielding) as well as it can improve features of the plant that affect the efficacy and safety of a herbal drug (eg. levels of bioactive compounds or presence of potentially toxic substances). *Mentha* spp (mints) have been engineered to modify essential oil production and to enhance the resistance of the plant to fungal infection and abiotic stresses. Genetic engineering allowed the enhancement of scopolamine and artemisinin in *Atropa belladonna* and *Artemisia annua*, respectively. (Canter et al., 2005)

5. Amburana cearensis

A. cearensis (Fabaceae) is a native tree from "Caatinga" (a kind of vegetation found in the Brazilian semi-arid region), where it is popularly known as "cumaru" or "imburana-de-cheiro" (Fig. 2). Because of these said popular names, *A. cearensis* is usually misidentified as *Dipteryx odorata* (Fabaceae) and *Commiphora leptophloeos* (Burseraceae). *A. cearensis* occurs widely in South America (from Peru to Argentina), along with another species of this taxon, *Amburana acreana*, which is found chiefly in the southwestern region of the Amazon Forest. *A. cearensis* can reach 15 m of height and 50 cm of diameter, but it is characterized by white flowers and dark pods containing only one seed each, besides its stem bark possessing reddish stains and a vanilla-like aroma of coumarin (**1**). At the early stage of development (seedlings), *A. cearensis* displays a hypertrophied and subterraneous tube-like structure, called xylopodium, which acts as a storage of water and nutrients, therefore it is considered an adaptive strategy for arid habitats (Lima, 1989; Cunha & Ferreira, 2003).

Given the various applications, *A. cearensis* has a great commercial importance in Northeastern region of Brazil. Its wood is used in the carpentry for the manufacturing of furniture, doors and crates, owing to its recognized durability, whereas the seeds are used as flavoring and insect repellents. The wood powder from it can be added to alcoholic beverage barrels for accelerating the aging process of sugar cane distilled spirits (cachaça) (Aquino et al, 2005). The seeds and stem bark are traditionally utilized for treating respiratory diseases, such as influenza, asthma and bronchitis due to anti-inflammatory, analgesic and bronchodilator properties. As far as folk medicine is concerned, *A. cearensis* is consumed as a homemade medication called "lambedô (a sugary drink), however in an industrial scale, the syrup is a pharmaceutical form, which is produced by the government and private laboratories (Fig. 3).

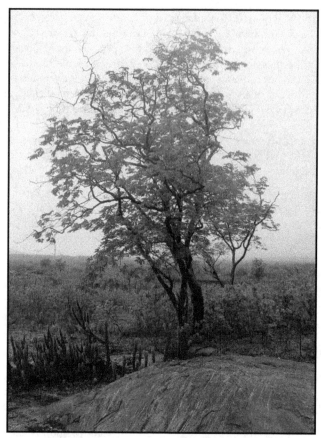

Fig. 2. A wild specimen of *Amburana cearensis* in its natural habitat.

The medicinal use of *A. cearensis* is based on scientific studies, which demonstrated that this plant possesses therapeutic properties that justify its recommendation for the treatment of respiratory illnesses. Preclinical tests demonstrated bronchodilator, analgesic and anti-inflammatory activities for the hydro-alcohol extract from the stem bark of the *A. cearensis*, which also showed to be free of toxicity in therapeutic doses. The chemical composition of the stem bark and seeds from it, consists basically of coumarin, flavonoids, phenol acids and phenol glucosides. Some of them were tested individually and showed pharmacological activities similar to the extract, hence they were considered the active principles of the *A. cearensis*.

However, the intense commercial use of *A. cearensis* has led to the threat of extinction for this specie. In order to ensure the conservation and the economic utilization of *A. cearensis*, we proposed the replacement of its stem bark of a wild adult plant for a young specimen, cultivated under controlled agronomic parameters. In an interdisciplinary study, ethanol extracts of cultivated plants were compared to the extracts of this wild plant through preclinical trials and phytochemical analysis.

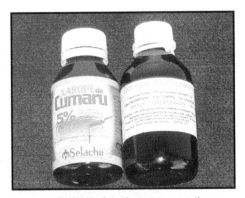

Fig. 3. Syrups made from the trunk bark of *Amburana cearensis*.

5.1 Agronomical study of *A. cearensis*

The agronomical study of *A. cearensis* was carried out with seedlings obtained by seed germination. Each plot consisted of six regularly spaced rows of 20 cm, whose sowing density was 50 seeds/row. The seedlings were transplanted to four garden beds (1.2m×10 m), fertilized prior to an organic fertilizer (2.8 kg m^{-2}), containing each of them 20 young plants.

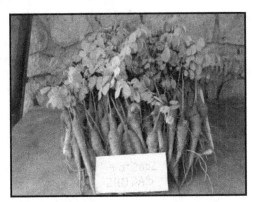

Fig. 4. Seedlings of *A. cearensis* harvested in 8th month of growth

Eight harvestings were performed monthly, starting on the 2nd month until the 9th month after the sowing. The plants harvested were evaluated with the following parameters: fresh plant weight, plant height, xylopodium diameter, root size, ethanol extract yield from the aerial part and xylopodium (Fig. 4). The fresh biomass production of *A. cearensis* seedlings increased almost eight-fold, during the 2nd through 9th month after the sowing. With reference to ethanol extract yield, there was a tendency of decrease for the extract weigh/xylopodium weight ratio over a period of time, while an oscillatory behavior was observed for yield of the ethanol extract from its aerial part, achieving a plateau on the 3rd and 7th month (Leal et al. 2011)

5.2 Phytochemistry of *A. cearensis*

5.2.1 Wild plant

While the pharmacological research about *A. cearensis* advanced, it was necessary to have a better understanding of the chemistry in this specie, previously limited to coumarin and a few phenol compounds, in order to discover its active principles. Bastos (1983), in her master thesis, found coumarin (1) as the most abundant component and described the isolation of isokaempferide (2), methyl 3,4-dimethoxy-cinnamate (3), afrormosin (4), 7-hidroxy-8,4'-dimethoxy-isoflavone (5), 24-methylenecycloartanol (6), β-sitosterol (7) and 6-hidroxy-coumarin (8). Additionally, the seeds presented a high oil content (23 %), which is composed of triglycerides of the following fatty acids: oleic acid (53 %), palmitic acid (19 %), stearic acid (8 %) and linoleic acid (7 %). Bravo et al. (1999) isolated amburosides A [(4-*O*-β-D-glucopyranosylbenzyl) protocatechuate] (9) and B [(4-*O*-β-D-glucopyranosylbenzyl) vanillate] (10) from the ethyl acetate extract of the trunk bark, utilizing just silica gel preparative Thin-Layer Chromatography (TLC) (Fig. 5)

Canuto & Silveira (2006) carried out a phytochemical investigation of the ethanol extract from the stem bark. The ethanol extract was partitioned with water and ethyl acetate. The aqueous phase showed to be very rich in sucrose (11), whereas the organic phase was dried and submitted to successive chromatographic columns on silica gel and dextran gels. These chromatographic separations led to the isolation of coumarin (1), two phenol acids [vanillic acid (12) and protocatechuic acid (13)], five flavonoids [isokaempferide (2), afrormosin (4), kaempferol (14), quercetin (15) and 4'-methoxy-fisetin (16)], amburoside A (9) and a mixture of β-sitosterol and stigmasterol glycosides (17-18). Later on, this same methodology was applied to isolate an isoflavone formononetin (19) and a novel coumarin 6-coumaryl protocatechuate (20) (Canuto et al., 2010) (Fig. 5). Continuing with the phytochemical study of *A. cearensis*, the seeds revealed high presence of phenol glucosides. Liquid-liquid partitioning from the ethanol extracts followed by chromatography on Sephadex LH-20 and a reversed-phase HPLC chromatography of the ethyl acetate fraction, resulted in the isolation of six new amburosides (C-H). 4-*O*-β-D-(6''-*O*-galloylglucopyranosyl)-benzyl protocatechuate (21), 4-*O*-β-D-(6''-*O*-acetylglucopyranosyl)-benzyl protocatechuate (22), 4-*O*-β-D-(6''-*O*-protocatechuoylglucopyranosyl)-benzyl protocatechuate (23), 4-*O*-β-D-(6''-*O*-feruloylglucopyranosyl)-benzyl protocatechuate (24), 4-*O*-β-D-(6''-*O*-vanilloylglucopyranosyl)-benzyl protocatechuate (25) and 4-*O*-β-D-(6''-*O*-sinapoylglucopyranosyl)-benzyl protocatechuate (26). Additionally, amburoside A (9), isokaempferide (2), vanillic acid (12), 6-hydroxycoumarin (8) and (*E*)-*o*-coumaric acid (27) were isolated from this same extract. (Canuto et al., 2010) (Fig. 5).

The isolation of 6-coumaryl protocatechuate (20) (trunk bark) and 6-hydroxycoumarin (8) (seeds) from *A. cearensis* presents an intriguing finding for biosynthesis of coumarins, since monoxygenated-coumarins are preferentially substituted at C-7 position (umbelliferone and its derivatives), according to biogenetic rules. This substitution pattern is due to the usual precursor of coumarins, *p*-coumaric acid, which is biosynthentized by the shikimate pathway from either tyrosine-deamination or *p*-hydroxylation of cinnamic acid (Dewick, 2002). Nevertheless, despite a large occurrence of simple coumarins oxygenated at the C-7 position, 6-hydroxycoumarin (8) was also found in some species like *Bidens parviflora* (Asteraceae), *Paeonia suffruticosa* (Paeoniaceae) and *Hydrangea chinensis* (Hydrangeaceae) (Tommasi et al., 1992; Wu et al., 2002; Khalil et al., 2003)

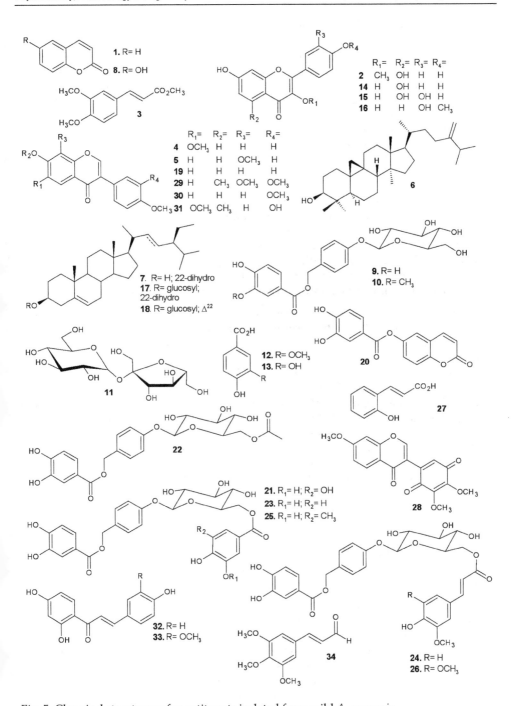

Fig. 5. Chemical structures of constituents isolated from wild *A. cearensis*.

Recently, Bandeira et al (2011) studied a resin exuded from the trunk of *A. cearensis* and found a flavonoid-rich material. The resin ethanol extract was partitioned with water and organic solvents, yielding an ethyl acetate fraction, which was chromatographed on silica gel. From this chromatography, a chloroform fraction was separated by a Sephadex LH-20, resulting in the isolation of a novel compound 3′,4′-dimethoxy-1′-(7-methoxy-4-oxo-4H-cromen-3-yl)-benzo-2′,5′-quinone (**28**), along with six known compounds:, 7,8,3′,4′-tetramethoxyisoflavone (**29**), 3′,4′-dimethoxy-7-hydroxyisoflavone (**30**) and 6,7,4′-trimethoxy-3′-hydroxyisoflavone (**31**), 4,2′,4′-trihydroxychalcone (**32**), 4,2′,4′-trihydroxy-3-methoxychalcone (**33**), 3,4,5-trimethoxycinnamaldehyde (**34**).

5.2.2 Cultivated plant

In order to seek a sustainable alternative for an economic utilization of *A. cearensis*, our research became focused on this *A. cearensis* cultivated plant. The chemical study of the cultivated *A. cearensis* was divided into two parts: (1) a Nuclear Magnetic Resonance (NMR) and the HPLC profiling of ethanol extracts obtained from the aerial part (EEAP) and xylopodium (EEX) of specimens cultivated according to the growing conditions described above; (2) A refined phytochemical analysis of EEAP and EEX extracts produced from specimens in 7 months of growth, where was chosen with basis on pharmacological results.

NMR profiling was performed with extracts of specimens from the 2nd through the 9th month of growth. ^{1}H NMR spectra, recorded in deuterated dimethylsulfoxide, revealed that the extracts from specimens with 2, 4, 7 and 9 months of growth, presented significantly different profiles, requiring further analysis. Hence, these extracts were duly analyzed comparatively with the wild plant extract by Photodiode Array detector (PDA)-HPLC profiling, utilizing constituents previously isolated from the wild *A. cearensis* as an analytical standard. The separations were performed on a C18 analytical column and the mobile phase was a gradient composed of H_2O (pH 3, H_3PO_4-Et$_3$N)/MeOH. The run time was 40 min and the chromatograms were observed at 254 nm. The qualitative analysis consisted of identification from analytical standards in the chromatograms of ethanol extracts, which were derived from the trunk bark (wild plant), xylopodium and the aerial part (cultivated plant) by retention time and UV spectra. Only 8 out of the 13 standards injected were detected in the samples. Coumarin (**1**) and vanillic acid (**12**) were the only substances present in all extracts of the *A. cearensis*. Amburoside B (**10**) and protocatechuic acid (**13**) were found in all extracts, except in the xylopodium extracts from specimens harvested in the 2nd and 4th month of growth, respectively. (*E*)-*o*-coumaric acid (**27**) and its glucoside (**35**), along with isokaempferide (**2**), afrormosin (**4**) and kaempferol (**14**) were not detected in any extracts. Ayapin (**36**) and (*Z*)-*o*-coumaric acid glucoside (**37**) were found only in cultivated plants (Table 2).

A quantitative analysis was carried out for four major constituents of the *A. cearensis* [coumarin (**1**), amburoside A (**9**), vanillic acid (**12**), protocatechuic acid (**13**)] in ethanol extracts from trunk bark (EETB) and seeds (EES) of the said wild plant, as well as the whole plant (EEWP), xylopodium (EEX), as well as the aerial part (EEAP) of cultivated specimens in the four following selected months (2, 4, 7 and 9), accounting for 10 samples. The HPLC method was developed in chromatographic condition similar to the once described above and validated according to analytical parameters, defined by the Brazilian Health Surveillance Agency and the Brazilian Institute of Metrology, Standardization and

Substances	Retention time (min.)	Trunk Bark	Xylopodium (month)				Aerial Part (month)			
			2	4	7	9	2	4	7	9
(Z)-Coumaric acid glucoside	3,85	-	+	+	+	+	-	-	-	-
p-Hidroxi-benzoic acid	4,99	+	+	+	+	+	-	-	-	-
Protocatechuic acid	7,36	+	+	-	+	+	+	+	+	+
Vanillic acid	10,87	+	+	+	+	+	+	+	+	+
Coumarin	13,98	+	+	+	+	+	+	+	+	+
Amburoside A	14,65	+	+	-	+	+	-	+	+	+
Ayapin	14,85	-	+	+	+	-	+	+	+	+
Amburoside B	17,17	+	-	+	+	+	+	+	+	+

Table 2. Distribution of some constituents in A. *cearensis* (+, presence; - ,not detected)

Industrial Quality: linearity, selectivity, accuracy, precision as well as the limit of detection and the limit of quantification. As can be noticed on Table 3, amburoside A (9) was the most abundant component in EETB, followed by coumarin (1), protocatechuic acid (13) and vanillic acid (12). However, coumarin (1) was the only component detected in EES. Among cultivated plants extracts, vanillic acid (12) was the principal component in 3 out of 4 periods analyzed through EEW, while coumarin (1) appeared as the major compound in the 7th month. Protocatechuic acid (13) and amburoside A (9) were below the limit of quantification in all extracts, except in the 9th month, whereby amburoside A (9) had a considerable content (Leal et al., 2011). In EEAP, vanillic acid (12) was the main constituent evaluated in all seasons, reaching the highest concentration in the 7th month (8520 mg/100g ext). On the other hand, coumarin (1) was the major component in xylopodium (4th month: 3760 mg/100g ext), except in the last month, when amburoside A (9) was the most abundant (680 mg/100g ext). Protocatechuic acid (13) presented measurable levels only in the EEAP of 4 months (360 mg/100g ext). Coumarin (1) and vanillic acid (12) were found preferentially in the aerial part, while amburoside A (9) was present mainly in the xylopodium. In comparison with wild plants, EEX of 9 months was the only cultivated plant extract which had amburoside A as the major component like EETB, even so at a concentration being three-fold lower than in the latter.

EEAP and EEX extracts harvested in the 7th month of growth were submitted to partition H_2O/EtOAc, yielding aqueous and ethyl acetate fractions from each extract. Isokaempferide (2), amburoside B (10), vanillic acid (12), p-hidroxy-benzoic acid (38) and the coumarin ayapin (36) were isolated from the ethyl acetate fraction derived from EEAP after being chromatographed on silica and dextran gels, while the aqueous fraction of EEAP yielded (E)-melilotoside (35) and amburoside B (10), again, through C18 solid-phase extraction (SPE) and C18 HPLC. On the flip side, adsorption and exclusion chromatography of the ethyl acetate fraction derived of EEX, afforded the isolation of amburoside A (9) and protocatechuic acid (13), whereas (Z)-melilotoside (37) was isolated by Sephadex LH-20 followed with the purification through C18 HPLC (Fig. 6). (E/Z)- melilotoside (35 and 37) are trivial names for o-coumaric acid glucoside in allusion to the genus *Melilotus*, where these compounds were firstly identified. Interestingly, the E and Z-melilotosides were found in different parts of the A. *cearensis*: (E)-stereoisomer exclusively in the aerial part, while (Z)-

Extracts	Concentration (mg/100g extract)– CV (%)			
	Protocatechuic acid	Vanillic acid	Coumarin	Amburoside
Wild Plant				
Trunk bark	320 (6,3)	200 (5,6)	1340 (6,8)	2180 (5,5)
Seeds	ND	ND	23520 (3,9)	ND
Cultivated Plant				
Whole				
2 months	ND	1520 (1,3)	1020 (5,7)	ND
4 months	ND	2680 (13,4)	2000 (7,0)	ND
7 months	ND	3440 (4,3)	4060 (6,5)	ND
9 months	ND	1520 (6,1)	660 (1,8)	400 (5,7)
Aerial Part				
2 months	ND	4780 (10,6)	1540 (3,0)	ND
4 months	360 (3,3)	6120 (4,8)	1660 (2,0)	260 (8,7)
7 months	ND	8520 (1,0)	6060 (7,9)	ND
9 months	ND	3460 (6,3)	1500 (3,3)	ND
Xylopodium				
2 months	ND	780 (5,3)	1320 (1,0)	380 (5,3)
4 months	ND	760 (7,5)	3760 (0,9)	ND
7 months	ND	1380 (2,9)	2500 (4,2)	300 (10,4)
9 months	ND	540 (9,8)	420 (10,8)	680 (9,4)

Table 3. Concentrations of four major compounds of *A.cearensis* in different extracts.

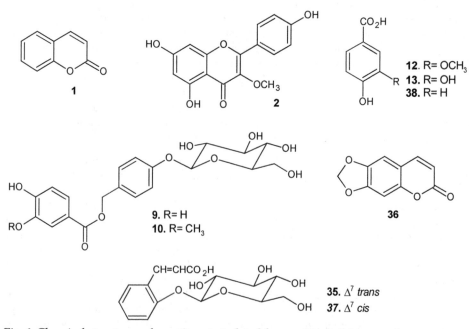

Fig. 6. Chemical structures of constituents isolated from cultivated *A. cearensis*.

stereoisomer was present only in xylopodium. In *Melilotus alba* (a legume), the melilotosides are considered the precursors of coumarin, being one of the major constituents of *A. cearensis*. (*E*)-melilotoside (**35**) exposed to UV radiation (sunlight) may be converted to the less stable stereoisomer (Z), which do undergo enzyme-catalyzed lactonization to yield coumarin (**1**) (Dewick et al., 2002).

As part of our effort for finding out which substances are responsible by medicinal properties of *A. cearensis*, isokaempferide (**2**), afrormosin (**4**), amburoside A (**9**), vanillic acid (**12**) and protocatechuic acid (**13**) obtained from this work were assayed in diverse pharmacological tests, which will be discussed briefly. The chemical structures of the new compounds were elucidated by means of spectroscopic techniques such as IR, HRMS, 1D and 2D NMR (COSY, HSQC, HMBC and NOESY).

5.3 Pharmacology of *A. cearensis*

The literature reports several toxicological and pharmacological studies carried out with the extracts and substances isolated from wild and cultivated *A. cearensis*. The focus of them is on the anti-inflammatory, antioxidant, smooth muscle relaxant, antinociceptive, neuroprotector and platelet antiaggregant effects (Leal, 1995; 2006; Leal et al., 1997; 2000; 2001; 2003ab; 2005; 2006ab; 2008).

A toxicological study carried out with the hydroalcoholic extract (HAE) from the trunk bark of the *A. cearensis* administered to rats by the oral route did not show any toxic effects (Leal et al., 2003). Further studies demonstrated that the HAE administered to rats daily for 50 days did not interfere with the pregnancy rate and development during the 1st as well as the 2nd generation of animals (Leal et al., 2003a, Leal et al., 2006a). The cytotoxicity of isokaempferide (**2**), kaempferol (**14**), amburoside A (**9**) and protocatechuic acid (**13**) from the *A. cearensis*, were evaluated on tumor cell lines and on the sea urchin egg development, as well as their lytic properties on mouse erythrocytes. The results showed that isokaempferide (**2**) and kaempferol (**14**), but not amburoside A (**9**) and protocatechuic acid (**13**), inhibited the sea urchin egg development, as well as tumor cell lines. However, only protocatechuic acid (**13**) induced lysis on mouse erythrocytes (Costa-Lotufo et al., 2003).

Previous studies (Leal et al., 1997; 2000) reported the antinociceptive, antiedematogenic and smooth muscle relaxant properties of HAE, coumarin (**1**), and the flavonoid fraction, from wild *A. cearensis*. The antiedematogenic activity was manifested in inflammatory process dependents on polimorphonuclear cells, while the antinociceptive effect of coumarin (**1**) and HAE seems to occur by a mechanism at least in part dependent on the opioid system. Nevertheless, the nitridergic system has also an important role in the coumarin nociception. Additional studies about the pharmacological potential of the HAE, coumarin (**1**) and the flavonoid fraction emphasized the anti-inflammatory potential of these species, which seems to be related to the presence of coumarin (**1**) in the plant (Leal et al., 2003).

Like other medicinal plants containing coumarin (**1**) such as *Justicia pectoralis*, *Pterodon polygaliflorus*, *Hybanthus ipecacuanha* and *Eclipta alba*, *A. cearensis*, also has a relaxing activity on isolated guinea pig tracheal muscles (Leal et al., 2000). Confirming this as particular effect, it was recently (Leal et al., 2006) demonstrated the relaxant action of the isokaempferide (**2**). The relaxation of the guinea-pig isolated trachea, induced by isokaempferide (**2**), was a direct and an epithelium-independent phenomenon, resulting from several intracellular actions through a common pathway e.g., the opening of Ca^{2+} and ATP-sensitive K^+ channels.

Previous studies (Leal et al., 2003; Leal, 2006) showed that the anti-inflammatory activity of HAE, coumarin (1), isokaempferide (2) and amburoside A (9) from *A. cearensis*, seems to occur by an inhibitory action on the release of inflammatory mediators, and/or alternatively by interfering with a certain phase of the neutrophil migration into the inflammatory focus. Other data (Leal et al., 2008) corroborated this hypothesis showing that both the isokaempferide (2) and amburoside A (9) exert their anti-inflammatory activities mainly by inhibiting the lipopolysaccharide-induced release of TNF-α, although the involvement of other inflammatory mediators cannot be excluded. Furthermore, inhibitions of some biological functions of neutrophils, namely, accumulation of cells and activity of hydrolytic enzymes, as myeloperoxidase, may also play a role.

Amburoside A (9) showed a hepatoprotective property in the CCl_4-induced liver toxicity model in rats. This effect may be due to its capacity to modulate the oxidative stress, especially by reducing of the lipid peroxidation, as well as by a significant restoration to normal levels of the catalase activity and GSH contents as observed in CCl_4-intoxicated rats after the amburoside A (9) treatment (Leal et al., 2008).

The large-scale usage and demand for the wild *A. cearensis*, as a medicinal plant by communities in the Northeastern of Brazil, governmental programs of phytotherapy as well as the pharmaceutical industry, are contributing to decrease availability on these species, presently considered as endangered ones. In this sense, our laboratory has conducted comparative studies on the pharmacological profile of the ethanolic extract (EtOHE) or vanillic acid (12) from the wild and cultivated *A. cearensis*, by evaluating their antinociceptive and antiedematogenic activities in several experimental models, such as the formalin test, carrageenan or dextran-induced edema and carragenan-induced neutrophil migration into the rat peritoneal cavity (Leal et al., 2010).

The acute treatment with both the EtOHE prepared from all parts of the cultivated *A. cearensis* (4, 7 or 9 months) or the wild *A. cearensis*, present antinociceptive and anti-inflammatory activities (Fig. 7). In addition, vanillic acid (12), which together with coumarin (1) are the major compounds present in cultivated *A. cearensis*, also showed an antinociceptive activity by inhibiting both phases of the formalin test in mice, and this effect was partially blocked by naloxone. Thus, the data suggest that antinociceptive effect of vanillic acid (12) occur by a mechanism at least in part dependent on the opioid system (Leal et al., 2010).

Coumarin (1) has been found in several Brazilian medicinal plants including *J. pectoralis*, *M. glomerata* and *A. cearensis*. It has been reported that the antinociceptive and the anti-inflammatory activities of these species seems to be related at least in part to the presence of coumarin (1) (Leal et al., 1997; 2003; Leal et al., 1997; Lino et al., 1997; Leal et al., 2000; Freitas et al., 2008). The biological effects of coumarin (1) include antibacterial, antiviral, antiedematogenic, antioxidant, lipoxygenase inhibition, lipid peroxidation inhibition, and scavenging of superoxide hydroxyl radicals (Hoult & Paya, 1996; Chang et al., 1996; Casley-Smith et al., 1993; Rajarajeswari & Pari, 2011).

Recently (Leal et al., 2010), it was also determined that the anti-inflammatory effect of vanillic acid (12) is isolated from the cultivated *A. cearensis*. This compound orally administered to rats, was shown to significantly inhibit the carrageenan, but not the dextran-induced edema. It also reduced the accumulation of PMN into the peritoneal cavity of rats and this effect was comparable to that observed with dexamethasone, used as a standard drug (Fig. 7).

Vanillic acid (12) is a benzoic acid derivative that is used as a flavoring agent. It is an intermediate in the production of vanillin from ferulic acid (Prince et al., 2011; Kim et al., 2011). Previous studies have shown antifilarial, antibacterial, antioxidant, hepatoprotective and anti-inflammatory (Kim et al., 2011; Prince et al., 2011; Itoh et al., 2009) effects of the vanillic acid. This compound exerts its anti-inflammatory effect by suppressing the production of prostaglandin E2, nitric oxide and cytokines. Furthermore, it also suppressed the activation of nuclear-factor-kappa B and caspase (Kim et al., 2011; Itoh et al., 2009). These findings confirm the anti-inflammatory activity of vanillic acid (12) as demonstrated by our laboratory.

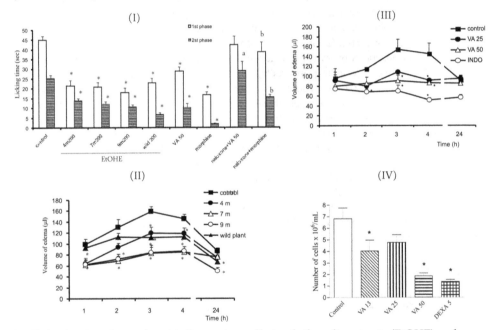

Fig. 7. Antinociceptive and anti-inflammatory effects of ethanolic extracts (EtOHE) and vanillic acid (VA) from *Amburana cearensis* in rodents.[1]

A growing body of evidence suggests that the extract and chemical constituents from the wild *A. cearensis* have pharmacological properties which justify at least in part its traditional use in the treatment of asthma. Among others, the anti-inflammatory activity is possible due

[1] I : effects of EtOHE (cultivated, (4, 7 and 9 months(m) or wild plants: 200 mg/kg, p.o.), VA (50 mg/kg, p.o.) or morphine (MP, 5 mg/kg, s.c.) on the formalin-induced nociception in mice (6-18 animals/group). II, III and IV: anti-inflammatory effects of EtOHE and VA on the carrageenan (Cg)-induced mice paw edema and Cg-inuced rat peritonitis.

to their capacity to modular several responses, especially those related to oxidative stress, the production of inflammatory mediators, and the accumulation and/or activation of inflammatory cells as neutrophils.

The preliminary pharmacological study of the cultivated *A. cearensis* (Leal et al., 2010) showed that both cultivated and wild plants have antinociceptive and anti-inflammatory activities in rodents. Coumarin (1) and vanillic acid (12) are possibly responsible for the pharmacological activities of the cultivated *A. cearensis* extracts, however the pharmacological importance of other chemical constituents present in the cultivated species cannot be ruled out.

6. Conclusions

The interdisciplinary study of the *A. cearensis* revealed that its ethanol extracts from cultivated and wild sources have similar phytochemical profiles, as consequence, both extracts possess similar pharmacological activities. Hence, these findings support the idea of the utilization of cultivated plants for the manufacturing of herbal drugs preparations by pharmaceutical laboratories, favoring the uniform and constant supply of high quality raw material, as well as the conservation of the wild specimens in the original biome. Indeed, this research indicates promising prospects for the rational use of the *A. cearensis*, however, it is still needed to be advanced in some issues concerning with agronomical, phytochemical and pharmacological knowledge of these species. The influence of some agronomic parameters (plant spacing, shading or sunlight exposure, water supply, etc) on the chemical composition will be performed. Chemical markers or a metabolomic approach will be developed in order to evaluate the influence of the aforementioned agronomic parameters on chemical composition. Pharmacological testing with other types of inflammation experimental models and clinical trials will be carried out aiming to elucidate the mechanisms of action of the *A. cearensis* active principles as well as to evaluate the efficacy in human beings. Additionally, an economic analysis should be performed in order to evaluate the economic feasibility in the production of *A. cearensis* herbal drug preparations from cultivated source.

7. Acknowledgements

This work was supported by Conselho Nacional de Desenvolvimento Científico e Tecnológico (CNPq) and by Banco do Nordeste do Brasil (BNB).

8. References

Aquino, F.W.B., Rodrigues, S., Nascimento, R.F. & Casimiro, A.R.S. (2005). Phenolic compounds in imburana (*Amburana cearensis*) powder extracts, *European Food Research and Technology* Vol. 221: 739-745.

Bandeira, P.N., Farias, S.S., Lemos, T.L.G., Braz-Filho, R., Santos, H.S., Albuquerque, M.R.J.R. & Costa, S.M.O. (2011). New isoflavone derivative and other flavonoids from the resin of *Amburana cearensis*, *Journal of the Brazilian Chemical Society* Vol. 22: 372-375.

Bastos, C.R.V. (1983). *Contribuição ao conhecimento químico de Torresea cearensis* (Fr. All.) (Master Thesis), Universidade Federal do Ceará, Fortaleza, pp.

Bravo, J.A., Sauvain, M., Gimenez, A., Muñoz, V., Callapa, J., Le Men-Olivier, L., Massiot, G., & Lavaud, C. (1999). Bioactive phenolic glycosides from *Amburana cearensis*, *Phytochemistry* Vol. 50: 71-74.

Calixto, J.B. (2000). Efficacy, safety, quality control, marketing and regulatory guidelines for herbal medicines (phytotherapeutic agents), *Brazilian Journal of Medical and Biological Research*. Vol. 33: 179-189.

Canter, P.H., Thomas, H. & Ernst, E. (2005). Bringing medicinal plants into cultivation: opportunities and challenges for biotechnology, *TRENDS in Biotechnology* Vol. 23: 180-185.

Canuto, K.M., Lima, M.A.S. & Silveira, E.R., (2010). Amburosides C-H and 6-O-protocatechuoyl coumarin from *Amburana cearensis*, *Journal of the Brazilian Chemical Society* Vol. 21: 1746-1753.

Canuto, K.M., Silveira, E.R. & Bezerra, A.M.E., (2010). Estudo Fitoquímico de espécimens cultivados de cumaru (*Amburana cearensis* A. C. Smith), *Química Nova* Vol. 33: 662-666.

Canuto, K.M. & Silveira, E.R., (2006). Chemical constituents of trunk bark of *Amburana cearensis* A.C. Smith., *Química Nova* Vol. 29: 1241-1243.

Carvalho, P.E.R. (1994). *Espécies florestais brasileiras: recomendações silviculturais, potencialidades e uso da madeira*, EMBRAPA, Brasília, pp.

Casley-Smith, J.R., Morgan, R.G. & Piller, N.B. (1993). Treatment of lymphedema of the arms and legs with 5,6-benzo-[α]pyrone. The *New England Journal of Medicine* Vol. 329: 1158–1163

Chang, W.S., Lin, C.C., Chuang, S.C. & Chiang, H.C. (1996). Superoxide anion scavenging effect of coumarins. *The American Journal of Chinese Medicine* Vol. 24: 11-17

Costa-Lotufo, L.V., Jimenez, P. C., Wilke, D.V., Leal, L.K.A.M., Cunha, G.M.A., Silveira, E.R., Canuto, K.M., Viana, G.S.B., Moraes, M.E.A., Moraes, M.O. & Pessoa, C., (2003). Antiproliferative effects of several compounds isolated from *Amburana cearensis* A.C. Smith. *Zeitschrift fur Naturforschung C* Vol. 58c: p. 675-680.

Cunha, M.C.L. Ferreira, R.A. (2003). Aspectos morfológicos da semente e do desenvolvimento da planta jovem de *Amburana cearensis* A.C. Smith- Leguminosae Papilionoideae. Revista Brasileira de Sementes Vol. 25: 89-96.

Dewick, P.M. (2002). *Medicinal Natural Products: a biosynthetic approach*, 2nd ed., John Wiley & Sons, New York, 515 p.

Freitas, T.P., Silveira, P.C., Rocha, L.G., Rezin, G.T., Rocha, J., Citadini-Zanette, V., Romao, P. T., Dal-Pizzol, F., Pinho, R.A., Andrade, V.M. & Streck, E.L. (2008). Effects of *Mikania glomerata* Spreng. and *Mikania laevigata* Schultz Bip. ex Baker (Asteraceae) extracts on pulmonary inflammation and oxidative stress caused by acute coal dust exposure. *Journal of Medicinal Food* Vol. 11: 761-766.

Gobbo-Neto, L., Lopes, N.P. (2007). Medicinal plants: factors of influence on the content of secondary metabolites. *Química Nova*, Vol. 30: 374-381, 2007

Gruenwald, J. (2008). The global herbs & botanicals market; Herbs and botanicals are currently showing the most potential in functional foods and cosmetics. *Entrepreneur* URL: http://www.entrepreneur.com/tradejournals/article/181916708_1.html

Guedes, R.S., Alves, E.U., Gonçalves, E.P., Viana, J.S., Moura, M.F. & Costa, E.G. (2010). Emergence and vigor of *Amburana cearensis* (Allemão) A.C. Smith seedling in function of the sowing position and depth, *Semina: Ciências Agrárias* Vol. 31: 843-850.

Guedes, R.S., Alves, E.U., Gonçalves, E.P., Viana, J.S., França, P.R.C. & Santos, S.S. (2010b) .Physiological quality of *Amburana cearensis* (Allemão) A.C. Smith seeds stored, *Semina: Ciências Agrárias* Vol. 31: 331-342.

Hoult, J.R.S. and Paya, M. (1996). Pharmacological and biochemical actions of simple coumarins: natural products with therapeutic potential. *General Pharmacology* Vol. 27: 713-722.

Itoh, A., Isoda, K., Kondoh, M., Kawase, M., Kobayashi, M., Tamesada, M. & Yagi, K., (2009). Hepatoprotective effect of syringic acid and vanillic acid on concanavalin a-induced liver injury. *Biological & Pharmaceutical Bulletin* Vol. 32: 1215-1219.

Khalil, A.T., Chang, F.R., Lee, Y. H., Chen, C.Y., Liaw, C.C., Ramesh, P., Yuan, S.S.F., & Wu, Y.C. (2003). Chemical constituents from the *Hydrangea chinensis*. *Archives Pharmacal Research* Vol. 31: 15-20.

Kim, M.C., Kim, S.J., Kim, D.S., Jeon, Y.D., Park, S.J., Lee, H.S., Um, J.Y., & Hong, S.H. (2011). Vanillic acid inhibits inflammatory mediators by suppressing NF-κB in lipopolysaccharide-stimulated mouse peritoneal macrophages *Immunopharmacology and Immunotoxicology* Vol. 33:1-8

Koeppe, D.E., Rohrbaugh, L.M., Rice, E.L. & Wender, S.H. (1970). Effect of age and chilling temperature on the concentration of scopolin and caffeoylquinic acids in tobacco, *Physiologia Plantarum* Vol. 23: 258-266.

Leal, L.K.A.M., Pierdoná, T.M., Góes, J.G.S., Fonsêca, K.S., Canuto, K.M., Silveira, E.R., Bezerra, A.M.E., Viana, G. S. B. (2011). A comparative chemical and pharmacological study of standardized extracts and vanillic acid from wild and cultivated *Amburana cearensis* A.C. Smith. *Phytomedicine* Vol. 18: 230-233.

Leal, L.K.A.M., Canuto, K.M., Costa, K.C.S., Nobre-Júnior, H.V., Vasconcelos, S.M., Silveira, E.R., Ferreira, M.V.P., Fontenele, J.B., Andrade, G. M., Viana, G. S. B. (2009). Effects of amburoside A and isokaempferide, polyphenols from *Amburana cearensis*, on rodent inflammatory processes and myeloperoxidase activity in human neutrophils. *Basic & Clinical Pharmacology & Toxicology* Vol. 104: 198.

Leal, L.K.A.M., Fonseca, F.N., Pereira, F.A., Canuto, K.M., Felipe, C.F.B., Fontenele, J. B., Pitombeira, M.V., Silveira, E.R., Viana, G.S.B., (2008). Protective effects of amburoside A, a phenol glucoside from *Amburana cearensis*, against CCl₄-induced hepatotoxicity in rats. *Planta Medica* Vol. 74: 497.

Leal, L.K.A.M., Costa, M.F., Pitombeira, M., Barroso, V.M., Silveira, E.R., Canuto, K.M., Viana, G.S.B., (2006). Mechanisms underlying the relaxation induced by isokaempferide from *Amburana cearensis* in the guinea-pig isolated trachea. *Life Sciences* Vol. 79: 98-104.

Leal, L.K.A.M., Nobre, H.V., Cunha, G.M.A., Moraes, M.O., Pessoa, C., Oliveira, R.A., Silveira, E.R., Canuto, K.M., Viana, G.S.B., (2005). Amburoside A, a glucoside from *Amburana cearensis*, protects mesencephalic cells against 6-hydroxydopamine-induced neurotoxicity. *Neuroscience Letters* Vol. 388, 86-90.

Leal, L.K.A.M., Nechio, M., Silveira, E.R., Canuto, K.M., Fontenele, J.B., Ribeiro, R.A., Viana, G.S.B., (2003a). Anti-inflammatory and smooth muscle relaxant activities of the hydroalcoholic extract and chemical constituents from *Amburana cearensis* A. C. Smith. *Phytotherapy Research* Vol. 17: 335-340.

Leal, L.K.A.M; Oliveira, F.G.; Fontenele, J.B.; Ferreira, M.A.D. & Viana, G.S.B. (2003b). Toxicological study of hydroalcoholic extract from *Amburana cearensis* in rats. *Pharmaceutical Biology* Vol. 41: p. 308-314.

Leal, L.K.A.M., Ferreira, A.A.G. & Viana G.S.B. (2000). Antinociceptive, anti-inflammatory and bronchodilador activities of Brazilian medicinal plants containing coumarin: a comparative study. *Journal of Ethnopharmacology* Vol. 70: 151-9.

Leal, L.K.A.M, Matos, M.E.; Matos, F.J.A., Ribeiro, R.A., Ferreira, F.V. & Viana, G.S.B. (1997). Antinociceptive and antiedematogenic effects of the hydroalcoholic extract and coumarin from *Torresea cearensis* Fr. All. *Phytomedicine* Vol. 4: p. 221-227.

Lima, D.A. (1989) *Plantas das caatingas*, Academia Brasileira de Ciências Rio de Janeiro, 243 p.

Lino, C.S., Taveira, M.L., Viana, G.S.B. & Matos, F.J.A. (1997). Analgesic and antiinflammatory activities of *Justicia pectoralis* Jacq and its main constituents: coumarin and umbelliferone. *Phytotherapy Research* Vol. 11: 211-215.

McChesney, J.D., Venkataraman, S.K., & Henri, J.T. (2007). Plant natural products: Back to the future or into extinction? *Phytochemistry* Vol. 68: 2015–2022

Menković, N., Šavikin-Fodulović, K. & Savin, K. (2000). Chemical composition and seasonal variations in the amount of secondary compounds in *Gentiana lutea* leaves and flowers, *Planta Medica* Vol. 66: 178-180

Prince, P.S.M., Dhanasekar, K. & Rajakumar, S. (2011). Preventive effects of vanillic acid on lipids, Bax, Bcl-2 and myocardial infarct size on isoproterenol-induced myocardial infarcted rats: a biochemical and in vitro study, *Cardiovascular Toxicology* Vol. 11: 58–66.

Rajarajeswari, N & Pari, L. (2011). Antioxidant Role of Coumarin on Streptozotocin-Nicotinamide-Induced Type 2 Diabetic Rats, *Journal of Biochemical and Molecular Toxicology* Vol. 25: 1-7.

Rao, M.R., Palada, M.C. & Becker, B.N. (2004). Medicinal and aromatic plants in agroforestry systems, *Agroforestry Systems* Vol. 61: 107–122.

Sahoo, N., Manchikanti, P. & Dey, S. (2010). Herbal drugs: Standards and regulation *Fitoterapia* Vol. 82: 462–471.

Schippmann, U., Leaman, D.J. & Cunnningham, A.B. (2002). *Impact of cultivation and gathering of medicinal plants on biodiversity: global trends and issues.* FAO, Rome, pp. 1-21.

Silva, M.G.V., Craveiro, A.A.; Matos, F.J.A., Machado, M.I.L. & Alencar, J.W. (1999). Chemical variation during daytime of constituents of the essential oil of *Ocimum gratissimum* leaves, *Fitoterapia* Vol. 70: 32-34.

Southwell, I.A. & Bourke, C.A. (2001). Seasonal variation in hypericin content of *Hypericum perforatum* L. (St. John's Wort), *Phytochemistry* Vol. 56: 437-.441

Tommasi, N., Feo, V., Pizza, C. & Zhou, Z.I. (1992). Constituents of *Bidens parviflora*. *Fitoterapia* Vol. 63: 470.

Wagner, H. (2011). Synergy research: Approaching a new generation of phytopharmaceuticals. *Fitoterapia* Vol. 82: 34–37.

Williams, R.D. & Ellis, B.E. (1989). Age and tissue distribution of alkaloids in *Papaver somniferum*, *Phytochemistry* Vol. 28: 2085-2088.

Wu, S.; Ma, Y., Luo, X., Hao, X. & Wu, D. (2002). Studies on chemical constituents in root back of *Paeonia suffruticosa*. *Zhongcaoyao*, Vol. 33: 679-680.

Zobayed, S.M.A., Afreen, F., Kozai, T. (2007). Phytochemical and physiological changes in the leaves of St. John's wort plants under a water stress condition. *Environmental and Experimental Botany* Vol. 59: 109–116

5

Alkaloids and Anthraquinones from Malaysian Flora

Nor Hadiani Ismail, Asmah Alias and Che Puteh Osman
Universiti Teknologi MARA,
Malaysia

1. Introduction

The flora of Malaysia is one of the richest flora in the world due to the constantly warm and uniformly humid climate. Malaysia is listed as 12th most diverse nation (Abd Aziz, 2003) in the world and mainly covered by tropical rainsforests. Tropical rainforests cover only 12% of earth's land area; however they constitute about 50% to 90% of world species. At least 25% of all modern drugs originate from rainforests even though only less than 1% of world's tropical rainforest plant species have been evaluated for pharmacological properties (Kong, et al., 2003). The huge diversity of Malaysian flora with about 12 000 species of flowering plants offers huge chemical diversities for numerous biological targets. Malaysian flora is a rich source of numerous class of natural compounds such as alkaloids, anthraquinones and phenolic compounds. Plants are usually investigated based on their ethnobotanical use. The phytochemical study of several well-known plants in folklore medicine such as *Eurycoma longifolia*, *Labisia pumila*, *Andrographis paniculata*, *Morinda citrifolia* and *Phyllanthus niruri* yielded many bioactive phytochemicals. This review describes our work on the alkaloids of *Fissistigma latifolium* and *Meiogyne virgata* from family Annonaceae and anthraquinones of *Renellia* and *Morinda* from Rubiaceae family.

2. The family *Annonaceae* as source of alkaloids

Annonaceae, known as *Mempisang* in Malaysia (Kamarudin, 1988) is a family of flowering plants consisiting of trees, shrubs or woody lianas. This family is the largest family in the Magnoliales consisting of more than 130 genera with about 2300 to 2500 species. Plants of the family Annonaceae are well known as source of a variety of alkaloids (Cordell, 1981). Many alkaloids have important physiological effects on human and exhibit marked pharmacological activity which is useful as medicine. For examples, atropine is used widely as an antidote to cholinesterase inhibitors such as physostigmine. Morphine and codeine are narcotic analgesics and antitusive agent while caffeine, which occurs in coffee, tea and cocoa is a central nervous system stimulant. Caffeine is also used as cardiac and respiratory stimulant andbesides as an antidote to barbiturate and morphine poisoning (Parker, 1997). The first report on phytochemical studies of alkaloids from Malaysian Annonaceae plants was on the leaves of *Desmos dasymachalus* which has led to the isolation of new 7-hydroxyaporphine, dasymachaline (Chan & Toh, 1985).

The phytochemical investigation of Malaysian Annoaceous plants for their alkoloidal content continue to flourish. Phytochemical survey of the flora of the Peninsula Malaysia and Sabah, with systematic screening for alkaloids resulted in reports on chemical constituents of several plants from Annonaceae illustrating great interest in this field (Teo, *et al.*, 1990). Lavault *et al.*, (1981) analysed the alkaloid content of three Annonaceae plants; *Disepalum pulchrum*, *Polyalthia macropoda* and *Polyalthia stenopetala* which led to the isolation of several isoquinoline compounds. Isolation of two new 7,7'-bisdehydroaporphine alkaloids; 7,7'-bisdehydro-*O*-methylisopiline and 7-dehydronornuciferine-7'-dehydro-*O*-methylisopiline from bark of *Polyalthia bullata* was reported by Connolly *et al.*, (1996). Kam (1999) reviewed the alkaloids derived from Malaysian flora in a book entitled chemical and biological approach of alkaloids.

In Malaysia, eight species of *Fissistigma* are known. They are *F. mobiforme*, *F. cylindrium*, *F. fulgens*, *F. kingii*, *F. lanuginosum*, *F. latifolium*, *F. munubriatum* and *F. kinabaluensis* (Nik Idris *et al.*, 1994). Not much has been reported on the phytochemical studies of *Fissistigma* species. The studies on the alkaloids from *Fissistigma fulgens* have led to the isolation of aporphine, oxoaporphine and protoberberine alkaloids. Liriodenine, anonaine, argentinine, discretamine and kikemanine were found from this species (Awang, *et al.*, 2000). The phytochemical work on alkaloidal composition of the Malaysian *Fissistigma manubriatum* by Saaid and Awang (2005) yielded two oxoaporphines, lanuginosine and liriodenine together with two tetrahydroprotoberberines, tetrahydropalmatine and discretine. We studied the alkaloids of *Fissistigma latifolium* and reported the isolation of nine alkaloids including a new aporphine compound (Alias *et al.*, 2010).

Meiogyne cylindrocarpa, *Meiogyne monosperma* and *Meiogyne virgata* are the only three *Meiogyne* species found in Malaysia. Only *Meiogyne virgata* was studied by Tadic *et al.* (1987). The sample collected from Mount Kinabalu, Sabah was reported to contain azafluorene alkaloid, kinabaline, together with liriodenine, cleistopholine and other aporphine alkaloids. Our work on *Meiogyne virgata* from Hulu Terengganu yielded nine alkaloids from aporphine, oxoaporphines and azaanthracene groups.

2.1 Alkaloids of *Fissistigma latifolium* and *Meiogyne virgata*

Since the last three decades, a large number of alkaloidal compounds have been isolated from some Annonaceae species. Tertiary and quaternary isoquinoline and quinoline alkaloids are pharmacologically important compounds commonly found in Annonaceae plants. Continuing our interest on this family of plants, we pursued phytochemical investigation on *Fissistigma latifolium* and *Meiogyne virgata*.

2.1.1 Alkaloids of *Fissistigma latifolium*

Fissistigma latifolium (Dunal) Merr. from the genus *Fissistigma* is a climbing shrub found in lowland forest of Malaysia, Sumatra, Borneo and Philippines (Verdout, 1976). The genus *Fissistigma* (Annonaceae) consists of about 80 species and is widely distributed in Asia and Australia (Sinclair, 1955). Several species of the genus *Fissistigma* have been used in Southeast Asia as traditional medicines (Perry, 1980). They have been used for muscular atrophy, hepatomegaly and hepatosplenomegaly (Kan, 1979). In Malaysia, the medicinal uses of *Fissistigma* species was briefly mentioned by Burkill as the treatment for childbirth, malaria, wounds, ulcer and rheumatism (Kamarudin, 1988).

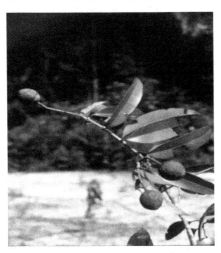

Fig. 1. *Fissistigma latifolium*

Previous studies on *F. fulgens* and *F. manubriatum* have resulted in the isolation of aporphine, oxoaporphine and protoberberine alkaloids. Similarly, the studies on alkaloids from *Fissistigma latifolium* led to the isolation of a new aporphine alkaloid, (-)-*N*-methylguattescidine **1** (Alias, *et al.*, 2010). This alkaloid, together with eight known alkaloids, namely liriodenine **2**, lanuginosine **3**, (-)-asimilobine **4**, dimethyltryptamine **5**, (-)-remerine **6**, (-)-anonaine **7**, columbamine **8** and lysicamine **9**, were obtained from the methanol extract of the bark of the plant. The new compound was characterized by analysis of spectroscopic methods such as NMR (Nuclear Magnetic Resonance), IR (Infrared) and GC-MS (Gas-Chromatography-Mass Spectrometry).

(-)-*N*-Methylguattescidine **1** exhibited a molecular formula of $C_{19}H_{17}O_4N$ based on the HRESIMS spectrum (positive mode), which showed a pseudomolecular ion at m/z 324.3581 [M+H]+ (calcd. 324.3595). The UV spectrum showed an absorption band at 310 nm, suggesting the compound was an aporphine alkaloid with substitutions at position 1 and 2. The IR spectrum indicated the presence of C-H aromatic at 3056, C-O at 1266 and OH at 3409 cm-1, respectively. The absorption of methyl group appeared at 2945 and 2833. The 13C-NMR spectrum showed presence of 19 carbons. The signal at δ 198.0 ppm confirmed the presence of the carbonyl group, while the signal at δ 153.1 ppm is evidence for the oxygenated aromatic carbon. The DEPT spectrum revealed three methylene carbons at δ 26.9 ppm, 41.4 ppm and 96.9 ppm. Signal at δ 96.9 ppm is indicative of a methylenedioxy carbon. This is consistent with two doublets at δ 5.99 ppm (J = 1.2 Hz) and δ 6.07 ppm (J = 1.2 Hz) in the 1H-NMR spectrum for the protons of methylenedioxy group which is typically located at positions 1 and 2. The characteristic ABD aromatic signals of H-11, H-10 and H-8 of aporphine alkaloid were observed at δ 8.24 ppm (*d, J* = 8.7 Hz), δ 7.13 ppm (*dd, J* = 8.7, 2.7 Hz) and δ 7.39 ppm (*d, J* = 2.7 Hz), respectively. The 1H-NMR spectrum also exhibited an *N*-methyl signal at δ 2.34 ppm and another methyl group attached to C-6a gave a singlet at δ 1.52 ppm. The assignment of this methyl group at the 6a position is confirmed through its HMBC correlation with C-6a at δ 62.7 ppm, C-1b at δ 118.3 ppm and C-7 at δ 198.0 ppm. HMQC spectrum shows two cross peaks at δ 26.9 ppm (C-4) axis, represented the correlations of C-4 to H-4 (δ 2.55 ppm) and H-4′ (δ 3.00 ppm). At δ 41.4 ppm (C-5) axis, two cross peaks showed the correlations between C-5 and H-5 (δ 2.99 ppm) and H-5' (δ 3.01 ppm). The quaternary carbon signals were assigned based on HMBC experiment. C-1a at δ 108.9 ppm, C-7a at δ 126.0 ppm and C-9 at δ 153.1 ppm were assigned based on their correlations with H-11 at δ 8.24 ppm, while C-1b at δ 118.3 ppm and C-2 at δ 143.2 ppm showed correlations with H-3 at δ 6.54 ppm. (-)-N-methylguattescidine, is a rare 6a-methylated-7-oxo-aporphine alkaloid, having only been previously reported by Reynald *et al.* in 1982. Presented below are structures and spectroscopic data of the isolated compounds.

(1)

(-)-N-Methylguattescidine (**1**). yellow amorphous solid; [α] $^{30}_D$: -20° (c = 0.1 mg mL^{-1}, CHCl$_3$); MS m/z: 324.1242, C$_{19}$H$_{17}$O$_4$N; UV λ_{max} nm EtOH: 235, 310; IR υ_{max} cm^{-1}: 3409, 1710, 1266; ^{1}H NMR (CDCl$_3$, 300 MHz) δ ppm : 8.24 (1H, d, J = 8.7 Hz, H-11), 7.39 (1H, d, J = 2.7 Hz, H-8), 7.13 (1H, dd, J_o = 8.7 Hz; J_m = 2.7 Hz, H-10), 6.54 (1H, s, H-3), 6.07 (1H, d, J = 1.2 Hz, H-2), 5.99 (1H, d, J = 1.2 Hz, H-1), 3.52 (1H, m, H-11a), 3.01 (1H, m, H-5), 3.00 (1H, m, H-4), 2.99 (1H, m, H-5'), 2.55 (1H, m, H-4'); ^{13}C NMR (CDCl$_3$, 75 MHz) δppm : 153.1 (C-9), 143.2 (C-2), 138.8 (C-1), 126.0 (C-7a), 125.3 (C-3a), 123.1 (C-11a), 122.7 (C-11), 122.2 (C-10), 118.3 (C-1b), 110.3 (C-8), 108.9 (C-1a), 103.9 (C-3), 96.9 (O-CH$_2$-O), 62.7 (C-6a), 41.4 (C-5), 34.1 (N-CH$_3$), 26.9 (C-4), 25.0 (CH$_3$).

(2)

Liriodenine (**2**), yellow needles; MS m/z : 275, C$_{17}$H$_9$O$_3$N; UV λ_{max} nm EtOH : 215, 246, 268, 395, 412; IR υ_{max} cm^{-1} : 3054, 1726, 1421, 1265; ^{1}H NMR (CDCl$_3$, 300 MHz) δ ppm : 8.9 (1H, d, J = 5.1 Hz, H-5), 8.66 (1H, dd, J_o = 7.2 Hz; J_m = 1.2 Hz, H-11), 8.59 (1H, dd, J_o = 7.8 Hz; J_m = 1.2Hz, H-8), 7.79 (1H, d, J = 5.1 Hz, H-4), 7.76 (1H, td, J_o = 7.8 Hz; 7.2 Hz; J_m = 1.5 Hz, H-10), 7.59 (1H, td, J_o = 7.8 Hz;7.2; J_m = 1.2 Hz, H-9), 7.16 (1H, s, H-3), 6.40 (2H, s, O-CH$_2$-O); ^{13}C NMR (CDCl$_3$, 75 MHz) δppm : 151.7 (C-2), 147.9 (C-1), 146 (C-6a), 145.4 (C-3a), 144.9 (C-5), 135.7 (C-1a), 133.9 (C-10), 132.9 (C-7a), 131.3 (C-11a), 128.8(C-8), 128.6 (C-9), 127.4 (C-11), 124.2 (C-4), 108.2 (C-1b), 103.3 (C-3), 102.4 (O-CH$_2$-O), 182.4 (C-7).

(3)

Lanuginosine (**3**), yellow needles; MS m/z : 305, C$_{18}$H$_{11}$O$_4$N; UV λ_{max} nm EtOH : 246, 271, 315, 258, 283, 334; IR υ_{max} cm^{-1} : 3055, 2987, 2306, 1712, 1635, 1363, 1265, 1046, 896; ^{1}H NMR (CDCl$_3$, 300MHz) δ ppm : 8.85 (1H, d, J = 5.4 Hz, H-5), 8.58 (1H, d, J_o = 9.0 Hz, H-11), 8.04 (1H, d, J = 3 Hz, H-8), 7.79 (1H, d, J = 5.4 Hz, H-4), 7.32 (1H, dd, J_o = 9.0 Hz; J_m = 3 Hz, H-10), 7.17 (1H, s, H-3), 6.47 (2H, s, O – CH$_2$ – O); ^{13}C NMR (CDCl$_3$, 75MHz) δ ppm : 158.0 (C-9), 151.0 (C-2), 146.0 (C-1), 144.9 (C-5), 144.0 (C-6a), 136.0 (C-3a), 133.0 (C-7a), 131.9 (C-1b), 129.1 (C-11), 126.2 (C-11a), 124.3 (C-4), 122.6 (C-10), 110.2 (C-8), 109.0 (C-1a), 102.3 (C-3), 55.8 (OCH$_3$), 102.5 (O – CH$_2$ – O), 182.0 (C-7).

(4)

Asimilobine (**4**), brownish amorphous; MS m/z : 267, $C_{17}H_{17}O_2N$; UV λ_{max} nm EtOH : 274, 308; IR υ_{max} cm^{-1} : 3390, 1675, 1600, 1225; ^{1}H NMR (CDCl$_3$, 300MHz) δ ppm : 8.30 (1H, d, J = 7.8 Hz, H-11), 7.36 – 7.25 (3H, m, H-8, H-9, H-10), 6.73 (1H, s, H-3), 3.92 (1H, m, H-6a), 3.50 (1H, m, H-5′), 3.08 (1H, d, H-4′), 3.04 (1H, d, H-5), 2.99 (1H, m, H7), 2.85 (1H, m, H7), 2.74 (1H, d, H-4), 3.61 (3H, s, OCH$_3$), 2.00 (1H, s, N-H); ^{13}C NMR (CDCl$_3$, 75MHz) δ ppm : 148.6 (C-2), 143.0 (C-1), 135.6 (C-7a), 131.7 (C-11a), 129.4 (C-16), 128.1 (C-3a), 127.7 (C-8), 127.4 (C-10), 127.3 (C-9), 127.2 (C-11), 125.5 (C-1a), 114.6 (C-3), 53.4 (C-6a), 42.8 (C-5), 36.7 (C-7), 28.2 (C-4), 60.4 (OCH$_3$).

(5)

Dimethyltryptamine (**5**), reddish amorphous; MS m/z : 188, $C_{12}H_{16}N_2$; UV λ_{max} nm EtOH : 240, 252; IR υ_{max} cm^{-1} : 3945, 3055, 2305, 1634, 1422, 1265, 1046, 896; ^{1}H NMR (CDCl$_3$, 300MHz) δ ppm : 7.60 (1H, d, J_o = 5.7 Hz, H-7), 7.38 (1H, d, J_o = 7.1 Hz, H-4), 7.20 (1H, td, J_o = 6.9Hz; J_m0.9 Hz, H-5), 7.12 (1H, td, J_o = 6.9 Hz; J_m = 0.9 Hz, H-6), 3.03 (2H, m, H-8), 2.80 (2H, m, H-9), 8.28 (1H, brs, N-H), 2.49 (6H, s, 2(CH$_3$); ^{13}CNMR (CDCl$_3$, 75MHz) δ ppm : 136.0 (C-7), 127.0 (C-3a), 122.0 (C-6), 121.7 (C-2), 119.2 (C-5), 118.7 (C-4), 59.4 (C-9), 44 (C-3), 22.9 (C-8), 44.9 (2CH$_3$).

(6)

Remerine (**6**), yellow amorphous; MS m/z : 279, $C_{18}H_{17}O_2N$; UV λ_{max} nm EtOH : 234, 264; IR υ_{max} cm^{-1} : 1401, 1361, 1053, 942; ^{1}H NMR (CDCl$_3$, 300MHz) δ ppm : 8.09 (1H, d, J_o = 7.5 Hz, H-11), 7.34 – 7.24 (3H, m, H-8, H-9, H-10), 6.59 (1H, s, H-3), 4.000 (1H, m, H-6a), 3.4 (1H, m, H-5′), 3.10 (1H, m, H-4′), 3.00 (1H, m, H-5), 2.90 (1H, m, H-7′), 2.80 (2H, m, H-7, H-4), 6.11 (1H, d, J_m = 1.2 Hz, CH-O), 5.96 (1H, d, J_o = 1.2 Hz, CH-O), 2.62 (3H, s, CH$_3$); ^{13}C NMR (CDCl$_3$, 75MHz) δppm : 146.7 (C-2), 142.8 (C-1), 136.3 (C-7a), 128.1 (C-8), 128.0 (C-1b), 127.6 (C-9), 127.0 (C-10), 127.0 (C-11), 125.4 (C-3a), 126.5 (C-1a), 126.0 (C-11a), 125.4 (C-3a), 62.4 (C-6a), 53.3 (C-6a), 43 (C-5), 36.9 (C-7), 28 (C-4), 100.7 (O – CH$_2$ – O), 39.0 (CH$_3$).

(7)

Anonaine (**7**), yellow amorphous; MS m/z : 265, $C_{17}H_{13}O_2N$; UV λ_{max} nm EtOH : 234, 272, 315; IR υ_{max} cm^{-1} : 1040, 945; ^{1}H NMR (CDCl$_3$, 300MHz) δ ppm : 8.09 (1H, d, J_o = 7.5 Hz, H=11), 7.36 – 7.19 (3H, m, H-8, H-9, H-10), 6.6 (1H, s, H-3), 4.04 (1H, dd, H-6a), 3.48 (1H, m, H-5′), 3.1 (1H, m, H-4′), 3.07 (1H, m, H-5), 3.02 (1H, m, H-7′), 6.12 (1H, d, J_m = 1.5, CH – O), 5.97 (1H, d, J_m = 1.5, CH – O); ^{13}C NMR (CDCl$_3$, 75MHz) δ ppm : 147.0 (C-2), 143.0 (C-1), 135.4 (C-7a), 131.4 (C-11a), 129.0 (C-1b), 128.0 (C-3a), 127.8 (C-8), 127.7 (C-9), 127.0 (C-10), 126.1 (C-11), 116.3 (C-1a), 53.6 (C-6a), 43.6 (C-5), 37.4 (C-7), 29.6 (C-4), 100.6 (O –CH$_2$– O).

(8)

Columbamine (8), red amorphous solid; MS m/z : 338, $C_{20}H_{20}O_4N$; UV λ_{max} nm EtOH : 206, 225, 265, 345; IR υ_{max} cm^{-1} : 3390, 1600; ^{1}H NMR (CDCl$_3$, 300MHz) δ ppm : 9.00 (1H, s, H-8), 8.08 (1H, s, H-13), 7.65 (1H, d, J_o = 9.0 Hz, H-11), 7.61 (1H, d, J_o = 8.7 Hz, H-12), 7.27 (1H, s, H-1), 6.79 (1H, s, H-4), 4.68 (2H, t, J_o = 6.6 Hz; 6.3 Hz, H-6), 3.18 (2H, t, J_o = 6.0 Hz, H-5), 4.02 (3H, OCH$_3$), 3.99 (3H, OCH$_3$), 3.92 (3H, OCH$_3$). ; ^{13}C NMR (CDCl$_3$, 75MHz) δ ppm : 163.0 (C-10), 151.0 (C-3), 150.0 (C-4a), 149.0 (C-2), 142.0 (C-9), 140.0 (C-8), 139.0 (C-11), 132.0 (C-14), 129.0 (C-12a), 126.0 (C-1a), 123.3 (C-12), 120.0 (C-13), 119.0 (C-8a), 111.0 (C-4), 108.0 (C-1), 56.0 (C-6), 27.0 (C-5), 60.0 (OCH$_3$), 58.0 (OCH$_3$), 57.0 (OCH$_3$).

(9)

Lysicamine (9), yellow amorphous; MS m/z : 291, $C_{18}H_{13}O_3N$; UV λ_{max} nm EtOH : 214, 250, 255, 261, 319; IR υ_{max} cm^{-1} : 1675, 1600, 1225; ^{1}H NMR (CDCl$_3$, 300MHz) δ ppm : 9.10 (1H, d, J_o = 5.1 Hz, H-11), 8.70 (1H, d, J_o = 6.9 Hz, H-5) 8.48 (1H, dd, J_o = 7.5 Hz; J_m = 1.5 Hz, H-8), 7.76 (1H, td, J_o = 7.2 Hz; J_m = 1.5 Hz, H-10), 7.7 (1H, d, J_o = 6.9 Hz, H-4), 7.55 (1H, td, J_o = 7.2 Hz; J_m = 1.2 Hz, H-9), 7.24 (1H, s, H-3), 4.05 (3H, s, OCH$_3$), 3.97 (3H, s, OCH$_3$); ^{13}C NMR (CDCl$_3$, 75MHz) δppm : 156.7 (C-6a), 152.0 (C-2), 145.2 (C-1), 139.0 (C-5), 135.3 (C-3a), 134.7 (C-11a), 132.0 (C-7a), 130.9 (C-10), 125.7 (C-9), 122.0 (C-1b), 119.6 (C-1a), 108.7 (C-3), 65.1 (OCH$_3$), 56.8 (OCH$_3$), 182.5 (C=O).

Table 1.

2.1.1 Alkaloids of *Meiogyne virgata*

Meiogyne virgata is a rainforest tree grows in Peninsular Malaysia, Borneo, Java and Sumatera. The genus *Meiogyne* (Annonaceae) consists of about 24 species and widely distributed in Indo-china, Thailand, Peninsular Malaysia, Sumatra, Java, Borneo and the Philippines. There is no formal report on the traditional uses of *Meiogyne virgata* in Malaysia. However, being an alkaloid rich species, it could be useful medicinally.

We have conducted phytochemical work on *Meiogyne virgata*. Six of the aporphine alkaloids in *Fissistigma latifolium* were also found in *Meiogyne virgata* collected from the Peninsular Malaysia. Isolation and purification of alkaloids from the bark of *Meiogyne virgata* afforded nine alkaloids; four oxoaporphines, liriodenine 2, lanuginosine 3, asimilobine 4 and lysicamine 9; four aporphines, anonaine 7, remerine 6, nornuciferine 10 and norushinsunine 11; and one azaanthracene alkaloid, cleistopholine 12.

Most of the compounds are yellowish or colorless hygroscopic liquid at room temperature while impure samples will appear brownish. They have low solubility in water but dissolve well in methanol, chloroform, acetone, dichloromethane and other common organic solvent. They are also soluble in dilute acid as the protonated derivative. The melting point of these thype of compounds in range 100-300 °C.

Most of oxoaporphine and aporphine alkaloids showed IR spectra typified by the 7-oxo group with absorption band in the 1635-1660 cm^{-1} region. The UV spectra data for these type of compounds are quite characteristic for the skeletal type. There is indication that they may also be diagnostic for a particular oxygenation pattern. For example, 1, 2-methylenedioxy

(10)

Nornuciferine (**10**), Colourless crystalline solid; MS m/z : 281 (M$^+$); UV λ_{max} nm EtOH : 234, 272, 315; IR υ_{max} cm^{-1} : 1040, 945

^{1}H NMR (CDCl$_3$, 300 MHz) δ ppm : 8.39 (1H, d,J= 7.8 Hz, H-11), 7.33-7.20 (3H, m, H-8, H-9, H-10), 6.65 (1H, s, H-3), 3.98 (1H, dd, J= 13.4; 5.2 Hz, H-6a), 3.41 (1H, dd, J= 12.3; 6.3 Hz, H-5'), 3.90 (3H, s, OMe-2), 3.68 (3H, s, OMe-1), 3.08 (1H, dd, J=13.2 Hz, H-4), 3.04 (1H, td, J= 12.3; 5.1 Hz, H-5), 2.85 (1H, dd, J= 13.4 ; 5.2 Hz, H-7'), 2.68 (1H, dd, J= 13.2; 6.0 Hz, H-4'), 2.64 (1H, t, J= 13.4 Hz, H-7).; ^{13}C NMR (CDCl$_3$, 125 MHz) δ ppm : 152.3 (C-2), 145.2 (C-1), 135.0 (C-7a), 132.1 (C-1b), 132.1 (C-11a), 131.2 (C-3a), 128.4 (C-8), 127.8 (C-10), 127.4 (C-9), 127.1 (C-11), 126.6 (C-1a), 111.8 (C-3), 60.3 (OMe-1), 55.9 (OMe-2), 53.6 (C-6a), 43.0 (C-5), 37.2 (C-7), 29.7 (C-4).

(11)

Norushinsunine (**11**), Colourless crystalline solid; MS m/z : 281; UV λ_{max} nm EtOH : 217, 247, 252, 259, 273, 319; IR υ_{max} cm^{-1} : 3488, 3355, 1574, 1215; ^{1}H NMR (CDCl$_3$, 300MHz) δ ppm : 8.16 (1H, dd, J = 7.2;1.2 Hz, H=11), 7.45 (1H, td, J = 8.7;1.2 Hz, H-10), 7.40 (1H, dd, J = 8.1;0.9 Hz, H-8), 7.34 (1H, td, J = 7.2;1.2 Hz, H-9), 6.59 (1H, s, H-3), 6.11 (1H, d, J =1.5 Hz, O – CH$_2$ – O), 5.95 (1H, d, J = 1.2 Hz, O – CH$_2$ – O), 4.61 (1H, d, J = 3.0 Hz, H-7), 4.06 (1H, d, J = 3.3 Hz, CH – O). 3.37 (1H, ddd, J = 5.0;3.9;1.2 Hz, H-4', 2.68 (1H,dd, J=16.2;3.9 Hz, H-4); ^{13}C NMR (CDCl$_3$, 75MHz) δ ppm : 147.1 (C-1), 142.6 (C-2), 135.6 (C-1a), 130.3 (C-7a), 129.4 (C-9), 129.1 (C-3a), 123.6 (C-1b), 115.6 (C-11a), 108.4 (O – CH$_2$ – O), 71.0 (C-7), 57.2 (C-6a), 43.1 (C-5), 29.2 (C-4).

(12)

Cleistopholine (**12**), yellow glassy solid; MS m/z : 281 (M$^+$); UV λ_{max} nm EtOH : 234, 272, 315; IR υ_{max} cm^{-1} : 1040, 945; ^{1}H NMR (CDCl$_3$, 400 MHz) δ ppm : 8.95 (1H, d,J= 4.8 Hz, H-2), 8.31 (1H, dd,J= 8.5;2.2 Hz, H-5), 8.21 (1H, dd,J= 8.5;2.2 Hz, H-8), 7.79 (1H, m, H-6), 7.79 (1H, m, H-7), 2.89 (1H, s, CH3); ^{13}C NMR (CDCl$_3$, 100.6 MHz) δ ppm : 184.7 (C-9), 181.9 (C-10), 153.4 (C-2), 151.6 (C-4), 150.1 (C-9a), 134.6 (C-7), 134.2 (C-6), 132.6 (C-10a), 131.2 (C-3), 129.1 (C-4a), 127.4 (C-5), 127.2 (C-8), 22.8 (CH3).

Table 2.

derivative in compound **2** gives increase to a bathochromic shift in the 235-250 nm bands on comparison with the corresponding compound **9**. The addition of acid will gives a substantial bathochromic shift of the longest-wavelength band. In oxoaporphine and aporphine, position 1 and 2 are constantly oxygenated. It is frequent to find further oxygen substituent at C-9, C-10 and C-11 and occasionally at C-8. Other than that, H-4 and H-5 will give a characteristic AB system with doublet of doublet at about 7.6 ppm and 8.7 ppm with a coupling constant about 5.4 Hz. The small J value is due to the adjacent of electronegative nitrogen atom. The methylenedioxyl group gives singlet peak at about 6.0 ppm due to the inductive effect cause by existence of the neighboring C-7 carbonyl. The C-11 proton usually the most deshielded and the C-3 protons always appeared at a higher field then the aromatic hydrogen (Cordell, 1981). Presented below are structures and spectroscopic data of the isolated compounds.

3. The family of Rubiaceae as source of anthraquinones

Rubiaceae is among the largest flowering plants family comprising of 450 genera and 13,000 species. In Malaysia, 70 genera and 555 species of Rubiaceous plants were reported (Wong, 1989). Most Rubiaceous plants are shrubs or small trees and infrequently herbs (Hutchinson, 1973). Rubiaceous plants are distributed worldwide but they are mainly tropical. They are easily recognized at family level by decussate, entire leaves, presence of stipules, actinomorph flowers and inferior ovary.

Rubiaceous plants are known to accumulate substantial amount of anthraquinones particularly in the roots (Han, *et al.*, 2001). Anthraquinones containing plants are used traditionally for various ailments and health complaints such as diarrhea, loss of appetite, fever, wounds and cancer. The plant extracts are used in form of poultice, lotion and decoction from various plant parts. *Morinda, Hedyotis, Primatomeris* and *Rennellia* are among anthraquinone containing-genera that are widely used in Malaysian traditional medicine (Ismail, *et al.*, 1997; Jasril, *et al.*, 2003; Ahmad, *et al.*, 2005; Lajis, *et al.*, 2006; Osman, *et al.*, 2010).

Morinda comprises of approximately 80 species, distributed worldwide in tropical areas. It is considered to be highly nutritious plant and is used as traditional medicine. In Malaysia *M. citrifolia* and *M. elliptica* are widely used. The roots of *M. elliptica* are used to treat jaundice and gastric complaints and the leaves are used to treat flatulence and fever. *Prismatomeris* and *Hedyotis* species on the other hand are recorded in various traditional medicine systems such as Traditional Chinese Medicine. Several well-known *Prismatomeris species* used in folk medicine in Malaysia are *P. glabra* and *P. malayana*. *P. glabra* is claimed to be aphrodisiac and widely used in the east coast of Malaysia. *P. Malayana* contained the anthraquinones, rubiadin and rubiadin-1-methyl ether (Lee, 1969). *Hedyotis* plants are generally consumed as tonic or febrifuge for treatment of diarrhea and dysentery (Lajis, et al., 2006). Several species of *Hedyotis* native to Malaysia are *H.capitellata, H. Herbaceae, H.dichtoma, H. diffusa* and *H. verticillata*. Besides anthraquinones, *Hedyotis* also contain β-cabolline alkaloids, flavonoids and triterpenes. *Rennellia* is another small genus of Rubiaceae family. Consists of shrubs and small trees, the plants may be found in lowland tropical rainforest of Peninsular Malaysia and Sumatra. *R. elliptica*, is used for general health improvements and dubbed as Malaysian Ginseng most likely due to the appearance of its yellow roots.

Anthraquinones of the Malaysian Rubiaceae are generally of the *Rubia* type. Rings A and B of the anthraquinone skeleton are biosynthetically derived from chorismic acid and *a*-ketoglutarate *via* o-succinylbenzoic acid, whereas ring C is formed from isopentenyl diphosphate *via* the terpenoid pathway (Han, *et al.*, 2001). Chorismate is first converted to isochorismate, and then to *o*-succinoylbenzoic acid (OSB) in the presence of α-ketoglutarate and thiamine diphosphate. OSB is activated at the aliphatic carboxyl group to produce an OSB-CoA ester. It is the ring closure of OSB-CoA which results in the formation of 1,4-dihydroxy-2-naphthoic acid (DHNA) leading to ring A and B. The prenylation of DHNA at C-3, leads to naphthoquinol or naphthoquinone. The ring C formation is a consequence of the cyclization *via* C-C bond between the aromatic ring of the naphthoquinone and an isoprene unit, isopentenyl diphosphate (IPP) or 3,3-dimethylallyl diphosphate (DMAPP).

Of the anthraquinone from Malaysian Rubiaceeae are substituted only on ring C while the remaining are substituted on both ring A and ring C. Anthraquinones from genus *Morinda* are typically substituted at C-1, C-2, and C-5, C-6 or C-7, C-8 and C-1, C-2 and C-3

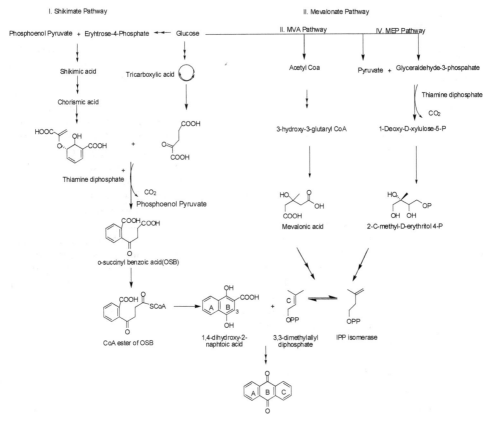

Fig. 2. Biosynthetic Pathway of Anthraquinones

meanwhile anthraquinones from *Hedyotis* are differed by rare substitution at C-1, C-2 and C-4. Anthraquinones from *Hedyotis* displayed wide structural variation. *H. capitellata* contains furanoanthraquinones (Ahmad, *et al.*, 2005) and *H. dichotoma* was reported to contain both 9,10- and 1,4-anthraquinone (Hamzah & Lajis, 1998). Genus *Rennellia* is closely related to *Morinda* and anthraquinones reported from *R. elliptica* are similar to those from genus *Morinda* (Osman *et al.*, 2010). One particular difference is the occurrence of anthraquinone with methyl substitution at C-6 which is characteristic to this plant.

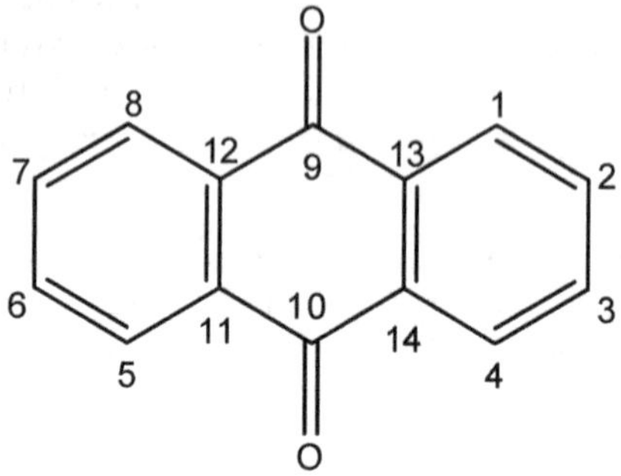

Fig. 3. Basic Skeleton of Anthraquinones

There are several characteristic spectroscopic data that distinguished anthraquinones from other types of compounds. In mass spectra, the major fragmentations are due to two consecutive loss of carbonyls, $[M-CO]^+$ and $[M-2CO]^+$. In the IR spectra, the unchelated carbonyl only viewed as one sharp stretching band at 1670 cm^{-1} due to symmetrical character of 9,10-anthraquinone (Derksen, *et al.*, 2002). Anthraquinones substituted with hydroxyl at *peri* position displayed two carbonyl absorption bands at about 1670 cm^{-1} and 1630 cm^{-1}. Anthraquinones give several chracteristic UV absorptions at 265-280 nm and 285-290 nm due to electron transfers bonds of benzoid chromophore and at 430-437 nm due local excitation of quinoid carbonyls. The location hydroxyl substituent can be distinguished by observing the absorption maxima in UV spectra. Addition of dilute sodium hydroxide solution caused bathchromic shift of absorption maxima. The shift is useful in distinguishing substitution pattern of polyhydroxyanthraquinones. Proton NMR spectra of 9,10-anthraquinones shows typical A_2B_2 substitution pattern of *ortho*-substituted aromatic ring. An unsubstituted anthraquinone ring can be easily distinguished by the presence of at least two sets of multiplets at ca. δ_H 8.10 and ca. δ_H 7.20 in the aromatic region. Anthraquinones substituted at both rings A and C will give several doublets in the aromatic region. The two carbonyl groups in the molecule can be easily distinguished if hydroxyl substituents present in *para* position. Hydroxyl groups adjacent to carbonyl can be seen as sharp singlets much downfield at δ_H 12-14 due to strong intramolecular hydrogen bonding to the adjacent carbonyl. The presence of hydroxyl adjacent to carbonyl cause significant shift of carbonyl carbon resonance to downfield region at 186-189 ppm.

3.1 Anthraquinones of *Rennellia elliptica* Korth.

R. elliptica Korth. was also previously known as *R. elongata* (King & Gamble) Ridl. It is a shrub of about 2 m tall. This shrub can be found in lowland to hill forest to c. 500m above sea level. *R. elliptica* Korth. is widely distributed from Southern Myanmar to West Malaysia.

R. elliptica is used for general health improvements and dubbed as Malaysian Ginseng may be due to the appearance of its yellow roots. Its medicinal uses were documented as treatment of body aches, after-birth tonic and aphrodisiac (Mat Salleh & Latiff, 2002). The root extract of *R. elliptica* was reported to be antimalarial (Osman, *et al.*, 2010) and antioxidant (Ahmad, *et al.*, 2010). Further study is warranted to investigate the antimalarial potential of roots of *R. elliptca*.

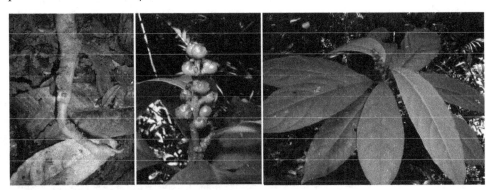

Fig. 4. Rennellia elliptica Korth

Phytochemical studies of the roots of *R. elliptica* Korth. resulted a new anthraquinone 1,2-dimethoxy-6-methyl-9,10-anthraquinone **18**, along with ten known ones. The known anthraquinones were nordamnacanthal **13**, 2-formyl-3-hydroxy-9,10-anthraquinone **14**, damnacanthal **15**, 1-hydroxy-2-methoxy-6-methyl-9,10-anthraquinone **16**, lucidin-ω-methyl ether **17**, 3-hydroxy-2-methoxy-6-methyl-9,10-anthraquinone **19**, rubiadin **20**, 3-hydroxy-2-methyl-9,10-anthraquinone **21**, rubiadin-1-methyl ether **22** and 3-hydroxy-2-hydroxymethyl-9,10-anthraquinone **23**.

Anthraquinone **18**, 1,2-dimethoxy-6-methyl-9,10-anthraquinone, isolated for the first time as bright yellow amorphous solid. The HREIMS of **18** displayed a [M + H]⁺ peak at 283.0968 [calc 283.3067] suggesting a molecular formula of $C_{17}H_{14}O_4$. The absorption maxima in the UV spectrum were observed at 373, 341 and 257 nm, indicative of an anthraquinone moiety. The IR spectrum did not show presence of chelated carbonyl and hydroxyl groups. The sp^2 C-H stretch for the aromatic ring was observed at 3,081 cm⁻¹. With the exception of the sharp singlet in the downfield region for the hydrogen-bonded hydroxyl group, the ¹H NMR spectrum resembles that of compound **16**, suggesting a similar substitution pattern. Splitting pattern of the five aromatic proton signals suggested substitutions on both rings. Two overlapping doublets centered at δ_H 8.17 are due to H-8 (*d, J* = 7.8 Hz) and H-4 (*d, J* = 8.7 Hz), the *peri*-hydrogens. A doublet at δ_H 7.28 (*J* = 8.7 Hz) is due to H-3, meanwhile H-7 gave another doublet of doublet at δ_H 7.58 (J_o = 7.8 Hz, J_m = 1.7 Hz). These assignments were confirmed by their respective correlations in the COSY spectrum. H-5 resonated as a singlet at 8.06 ppm. In addition, two sharp singlets at δ_H 2.53 (3H, *s*) and 4.02 (6H, *s*) due to a methyl and two methoxy groups, respectively, were also observed. The location of the methoxy groups were established at C-1 and C-2 of ring C based on its NOE correlation with H-3. Thus, the only possible location for the methyl substituent is at C-6. This assignment was confirmed through NOE correlations of the methyl group with H-5 and H-7. The placement of methyl group at C-6 was further confirmed by HMBC experiment

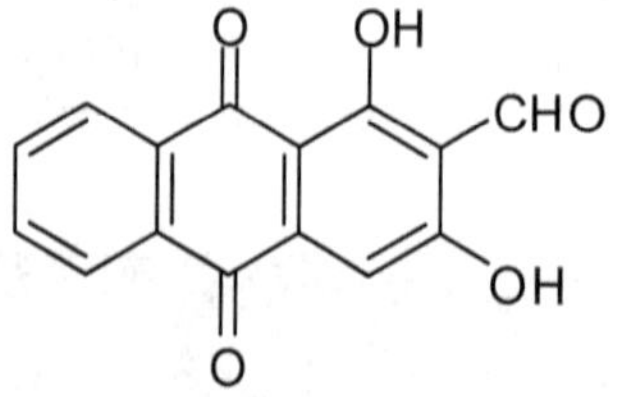

(13)

Nordamnacanthal. (13) Orange crystals. Mps 216-219 ° [lit. 220 ° C (Me₂CO) Chang (1984)]. UVλ$_{max}$ EtOH nm: 421, 295, 259. UVλ$_{max}$ EtOH/ -OH nm: 512, 357, 283. IR v$_{max}$ (KBr) cm⁻¹ :3460, 1646, 1627, 1382. MS m/z 268 [M⁺], 240, 212, 184, 138. ¹H NMR (CDCl₃, 300MHz): 14.05 (1H, s, 1-OH), 12.70 (1H, s, 3-OH), 10.52 (1H, s, 2-CHO), 8.30 (2H, m, H-5, H-8), 7.88 (2H, m, H-6, H-7), 7.36 (1H, s, H-4). ¹³C NMR (CDCl₃, 75.5 MHz): 193.9 (2- CHO), 186.8 (C=O, C-9), 181.4 (C=O, C-10), 169.2 (C-OH,C-1), 168. 1 (C-OH, C-3), 139.1 (C-2), 134.8 (C-7), 134.7 (C-6), 133.3 (C-14), 133.2 (C-13), 127. 8 (C-8), 127.0 (H-5), 112.1 (C-14), 109.4 (C-4), 109.1 (C-13)

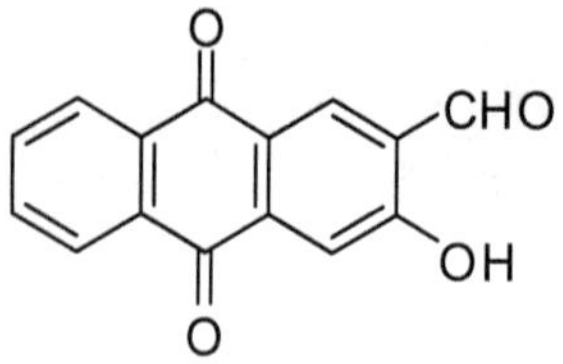

3-Formyl-2-hydroxy-9,10-anthraquinone (14). Bright orange needle crystals. Mps 212-214 °C [259-260°C, Rath et al.(1995)]. UVλ$_{max}$ EtOH nm: 380, 277, 246. UVλ$_{max}$ EtOH/ -OH nm: 466, 392, 310, 254. IR v$_{max}$ (KBr) cm⁻¹: 3467, 1655, 1657, 1564. MS m/z 252 [M⁺], 229, 206, 167, 139. ¹H NMR (CDCl₃, 300MHz): 11.45 (1H, s, 3-OH), 10.17 (1H, s, 2-CHO), 8.68 (1H, s, H-4), 8.35 (2H, m, H-5, H-8), 7.88 (2H, m, H-6, H-7), 7.86(1H, s, H-1) .¹³C NMR (CDCl₃, 75.5 MHz): 196.8 (2-CHO), 181.0 (C=O, C-9, C-10), 165.3 (C-OH, C-3), 139.1, 134.8 (C-4), 134.8, 133.3, 127.6, 127.5, 127.3, 126.1, 124.5, 123.4, 116.5 (C-1)

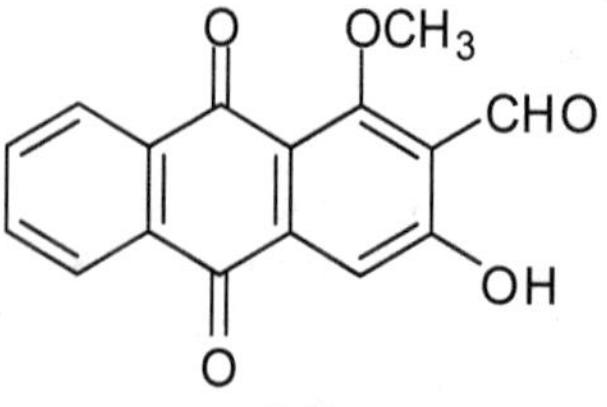

(14)

Damnacanthal (15). Yellow crystals. Mps 208-211°C [lit. 218-218.5 ° C (Me₂CO) Chang (1984)]. UVλ$_{max}$ EtOH nm: 381, 284, 250, 213. UVλ$_{max}$ EtOH/ -OH nm: 460, 379, 315, 262, 250. IR v$_{max}$ (KBr) cm⁻¹: 3437, 1644, 1561. MS m/z: 282 [M⁺], 254, 225, 196. ¹H NMR (CDCl₃, 300MHz): 12.29 (1H, s, 3-OH), 10.49 (1H, s, 2-CHO), 8.25 (2H, m, H-5, H-8), 7.84 (2H, m, H-6, H-7), 7.68 (1H, s, H-4), 4.14 (3H, s, 1-OCH₃)

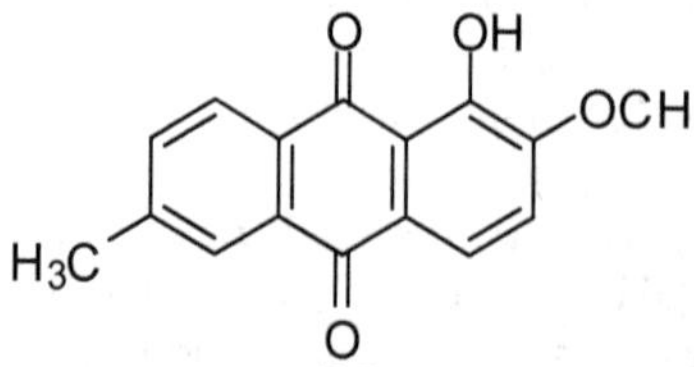

(15)

1-Hydroxy-2-methoxy-6-methyl-9,10-anthraquinone (16). Red needle crystals. Mps 220-221 °C. UVλ$_{max}$ EtOH nm: 421, 278, 262, 231. UVλ$_{max}$ EtOH/ -OH nm: 505, 314, 258. IR v$_{max}$ (KBr) cm⁻¹: 3467, 1653, 1637. MS m/z: 268 [M⁺], 239, 197, 169,139, 115. ¹H NMR (CDCl3, 300MHz): 13.20 (1H, s, 1-OH), 8.23 (1H, d, J=8.1, H-8), 8.12 (1H, s, H-5), 7.89 (1H, d, J=8.4, H-4), 7.61 (1H, d, J=8.1, H-7), 7.19 (1H, d, J=8.4, H-3), 4.04 (3H, s, 2-OCH₃), 2.56 (3H, s, 6-CH₃). ¹³C NMR (CDCl3, 75.5 MHz): 189.1(C=O, C-9), 181.8 (C=O, C-10), 154.0 (C-OH, C-1), 152.7 (C-OCH₃, C2), 146.2 (C-6), 134.6 (C-7), 134.0 (C-11), 131.10 (C-12), 127.8 (C-5), 127.1 (C-8), 125.5 (C-14), 121.0 (C-4), 116.1 (C-13), 115.6 (C-3), 56.4 (2-OCH₃), 22.0 (6-CH₃)

(16)

Lucidin-ω-methyl ether (17). Yellow crystals. Mps 175-179°C [lit 170°C, Dictionary of Natural Products (1995); 163-166°C, Leistner (1975)]. UVλ_{max} EtOH nm: 412, 280, 24. UVλ_{max} EtOH/ -OH nm: 491, 314, 242 IR ν_{max} (KBr) cm^{-1}: 3428, 2927, 1668, 162. MS m/z: 284 [M$^+$], 263, 241, 213, 185. ^{1}H NMR (CDCl$_3$, 300MHz): 13.29 (1H, s, 1-OH), 9.39 (1H, s br, 3-OH), 8.27 (2H, m, H-5, H-8), 7.80 (2H, m, H-6, H-7), 7.32 (1H, s, H-4), 4.90 (2H, s, 2-CH$_2$OCH$_3$), 3.59 (3H, s, 2-CH$_2$OCH$_3$). ^{13}C NMR (CDCl$_3$, 75.5 MHz): 186.9 (C=O, C-9), 182.2 (C=O, C-10), 164.1 (C-1), 161.7 (C-3), 134.1 (C-11), 134.1 (C-12), 133.6 (C-6), 133.5 (C-7), 126.8 (C-2), 114.4 (C-4), 109.7 (C-8), 109.7 (C-13), 109.6 (C-5), 109.6 (C-14), 68.9 (2-CH$_2$OCH$_3$), 59.3 (2-CH$_2$OCH$_3$)

1,2-Dimethoxy-6-methyl-9,10-anthraquinone (18). Bright yellow crystals. Mps 193-196 °C. UVλ_{max} EtOH nm: 373, 341, 257, 222. UVλ_{max} EtOH/ -OH nm: 373, 342, 257, 222. IR ν_{max} (KBr) cm^{-1}:1666, 1601, 1327, 1267MS m/z: 282 [M$^+$], 253, 221, 194, 165, 139. ^{1}H NMR (CDCl$_3$, 300MHz): 8.17 (2H, dd, J=8.7, 7.8, H-4, H-8), 8.06 (1H, s, H-5), 7.58 (1H, d, J=7.8, H-7), 7.28 (1H, d, J=8.7, H-3), 4.02 (6H, s, 1-OCH$_3$, 2-OCH$_3$), 2.53 (3H, s, 6-CH$_3$).^{13}C NMR (CDCl$_3$, 75.5 MHz): 182.7 (C=O, C-9), 182.7 (C=O, C-10), 159.1 (C-1), 149.6 (C-2), 144.6 (C-6), 134.8 (C-7), 132. 9 (C-11), 132.9 (C-12), 127.5 (C-14), 127.4 (C-13), 127.1 (C-8), 126.9 (C-5), 125.2 (C-4), 115.9 (C-3), 61.3 (1-OCH$_3$), 56.3 (2-OCH$_3$), 21.8 (6-CH$_3$)

2-Hydroxy-3-methoxy-6-methyl-9,10-anthraquinone (19) Light yellow amorphous solid. Mp 210-215 °C. UVλ_{max} EtOH nm: 393, 286, 244. UVλ_{max} EtOH/ -OH nm: 509, 316, 250. IR ν_{max} (KBr) cm^{-1}: 3203, 2927, 2869, 1666, 1265. MS m/z: 268 (M$^+$], 239, 207, 169. ^{1}H NMR (CDCl$_3$, 300MHz): 8.18 (1H, d, J=8.1, H-8), 8.08 (1H, s, H-5), 7.79 (1H, s, H-1), 7.76 (1H, s, H-4),7.57 (1H, d, J=8.1, H-7), 6.23 (1H, s br, 2-OH), 4.11 (3H, s, 3-OCH$_3$), 2.54 (3H, s, 6-CH$_3$). ^{13}C NMR (CDCl$_3$, 75.5 MHz): 182.4 (C=O), 162.8(C-OH, C-2), 151.4 (C-OCH$_3$, C-3), 144.9, 134.5, 133.6, 127.4, 127.2, 112.6, 108.3, 56.6 (3-OCH$_3$), 21.9 (6-CH$_3$)

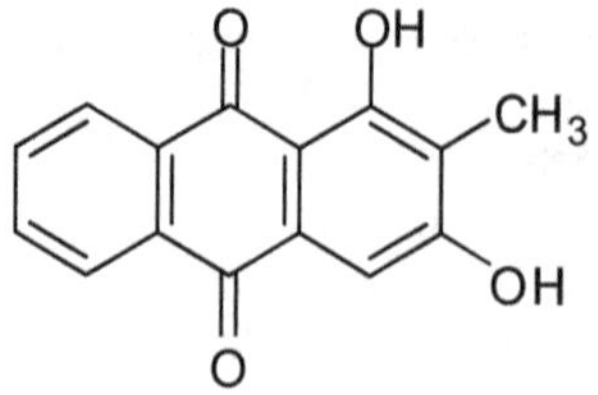

(20)

(21)

(22)

(23)

Rubiadin (**20**). Yellow crystals. Mps 250-258 °C [lit. 280-283 ° C, Leistner (1975)]. UVλ$_{max}$ EtOH nm: 413, 279. UVλ$_{max}$ EtOH/ -OH nm: 496, 314, 241 IR v$_{max}$ (KBr) cm^{-1}: 3436, 1653, 1626. MS m/z: 254 [M+], 226, 197, 152, 115. ^{1}H NMR (Acetone-d6, 300MHz): 13.20 (1H, s, 1-OH), 8.31 (1H, m, H-8), 8.23 (1H, m, H-5), 7.92 (2H, m, H-6, H-7), 7.38 (1H, s, H), 2.20 (3H, s, 2-CH$_3$). ^{13}C NMR (Acetone-d6, 75.5 MHz): 186.9 (C=O,C9), 181.8 (C=O, C-10), 163.2 (C-OH, C-1), 162.4 (C-OH, C-3), 134.3, 134.2, 133.5, 133.5, 132.4, 126.8, 126.5, 117.9, 107.17, 7.3

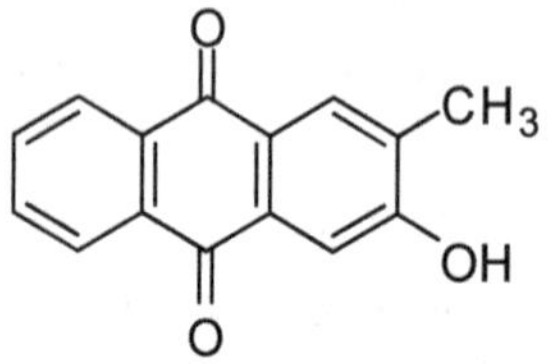

3-Hydroxy-2-methyl-9,10-anthraquinone (**21**). Yellow crystals. Mps 138- 142 ° C. UVλ$_{max}$ EtOH nm: 379, 329, 274, 245, 239. UVλ$_{max}$ EtOH/ -OH nm: 496, 314, 246 . IR v$_{max}$ (KBr) cm^{-1}: 3436, 1663, 651. MS m/z 238 [M+], 238, 210, 181, 152, 105. ^{1}H NMR (Acetone-d6, 300MHz): 8.23 (2H, m, H-5, H-8), 8.05 (1H, s, H-1), 7.89 (2H, m, H-6, H-7), 7.67 (1H, s, H-4), 2.39 (3H, s, 2-CH$_3$). ^{13}C NMR (Acetone-d6, 75.5 MHz): 182.6 (C=O, C-10), 181.5 (C=O, C-9), 161.0 (C-OH, C-3), 134.1 (C-2), 133.8 (C-14), 133.7 (C-7), 133.6 (C-6), 132.2 (C-13), 130.1 (C-1),126.6 (C-5), 126.5 (C-8), 111.4 (C-4), 15.6 (2-CH$_3$)

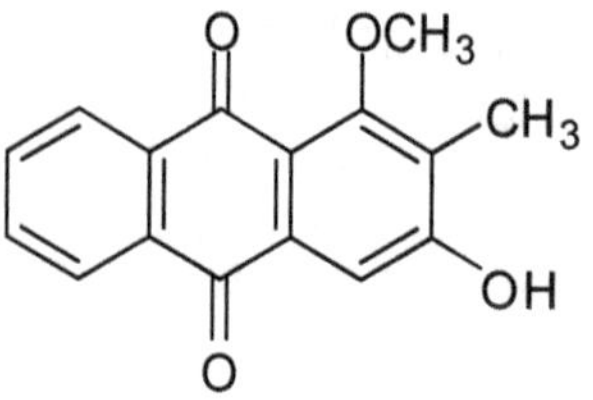

Rubiadin-1-methyl ether (**22**). Light yellow crystal. Mps 302-304 ° C [282-284, Briggs (1976); 300 ° C, Roberts (1977)]. UVλ$_{max}$ EtOH nm: 354, 332, 279. UVλ$_{max}$ EtOH/ -OH nm: 440, 314, 246. IR v$_{max}$ (KBr) cm^{-1}: 3437, 2913, 2847, 1668, 1651. MS m/z : 268, 239, 207, 181. ^{1}H NMR (Acetone-d6, 300MHz): 9.50 (1H, s, br, 3-OH), 8.20 (2H, m, H-5, H-8), 7.87 (2H, m, H-6, H-7), 7.63 (1H, s, H-4), 3.90 (3H, s, 1-OCH$_3$), 2.27 (3H, s, 2-CH$_3$). ^{13}C NMR (Acetone-d6, 75.5 MHz): 182.7 (C=O), 180.4 (C=O), 161.2 (C-OH), 140.6, 134.4, 134.2, 133.0, 132.6, 126.8, 126.0, 60.4 (OCH$_3$), 8.4 (CH$_3$)

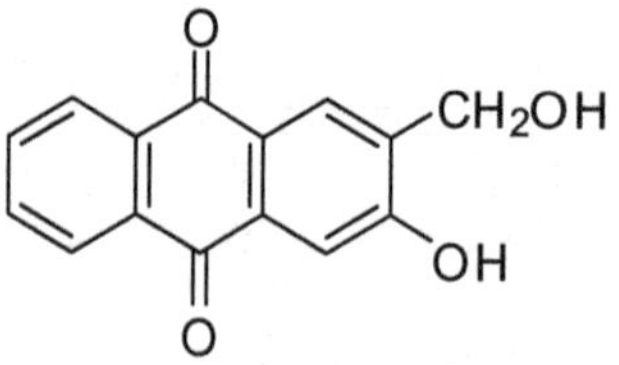

3-Hydroxy-2-hydroxymethyl-9,10-anthraquinone (**23**). Light yellow solid . UVλ$_{max}$ EtOH nm: 374, 274, 238. UVλ$_{max}$ EtOH/ -OH nm: 481, 311, 246 IR v$_{max}$ (KBr) cm^{-1}: 3468, 1628. ^{1}H NMR (Acetone-d6, 300MHz): 8.38 (1H, s, H-4), 8.24 (2H, m, H-5, H-8), 7.89 (2H, m, H-6, H-7), 7.63 (1H, s, H-1), 4.803 (2H,s, 2-CH$_2$OH). ^{13}C NMR (Acetone-d6, 75.5 MHz): 182.9 (C=O, C-9), 181.7 (C=O, C-10), 160.1 (C-OH, C-3), 136. 1 (C-2), 134.2 (C-14), 134.1 (C-11), 133.8 (C-6), 133.7 (C-7), 133.6 (C-12), 126.7 (C-4), 126.6 (C-5), 125.9 (C-13), 125.6 (C-8), 111.5 (C-1), 59.0 (2-**CH$_2$OH**)

Table 3.

which showed a ^3J correlation with H-7. The methine carbons (C-3, C-4, C-5, C-7 and C-8) were assigned through HMQC correlations while the quaternary carbons (C-1, C-2, C-6, C-11, C-12, C-13 and C-14) were assigned based on careful analysis of HMBC spectrum. Both carbonyl carbons in this compound resonated very closely to each other with only 0.01 ppm difference at δ_C 182.70 and 182.71, which further confirmed the unchelated nature of the carbonyls. Presented below are structures and spectroscopic data of the isolated compounds.

3.2 Anthraquinones of *Morinda elliptica*

Morinda elliptica or locally known as 'mengkudu kecil' is a shrub or small tree and it is very common in wild state of Malay Peninsula and northwards Burma (Burkill, 1966). It can be seen growing wild in newly developed areas, bushes and lowland secondary forest throughout the peninsula. *M. elliptica* is very common and always available and mostly used by the Malays for medicinal purposes. Traditionally, different parts of the plant are used in various ways for a number of health problems and ailments. The leaves may be added to rice for loss of appetite and taken for headache, cholera, diarrhea and wounds. Sometimes a lotion is made and used for hemorrhoid and applied upon body after childbirth (Burkill, 1966). The extracts and anthraquinones isolated from *M. elliptica* were reported to possess wide spectrum of biological activities such as antioxidant (Ismail, *et al.*, 2002; Jasril, *et al.*, 2003), antimicrobial, anti-HIV and anticancer (Ali, *et al.*, 2000).

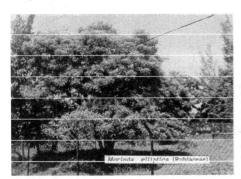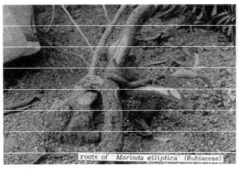

Fig. 5. *Morinda elliptica*

Five anthraquinones in roots of *M. elliptica* which are nordamnacanthal **13**, damnacanthal **15**, lucidin-ω-methyl ether **17**, rubiadin **20** and rubiadin-l-methyl ether **22** are the same constituents found in *R. elliptica*. The others are 1-hydroxy-2-methylanthraquinone **23**, soranjidiol **25**, morindone **26**, morindone-5- methyl ether **27** and alizarin-1-methyl ether **28**. In addition, 2-formyl-1-hydroxyanthraquinone **24** was reported as a new naturally occuring anthraquinone from roots of *M. elliptica*. HR-MS of **24** showed molecular ion peak at 252.0414 consistent with molecular formula of $C_{15}H_{14}O_4$. A bathchromic shift (407 to 531 nm) upon adding NaOH suggested the presence of OH at C-1 of the anthraquinone skeleton. The presence of hydroxyl group was evident from the broad stretching band observed at 3448 cm^{-1}. Two sharp stretching vibrations due to chelated and unchelated carbonyls were observed at 1638 and 1676 cm^{-1}, respectively. In the proton NMR, the signal for chelated hydroxyl group is at δ_H 13.26. The splitting pattern of ^1H NMR suggest substitution pattern

(24)

(25)

(26)

(27)

2-Formyl-1-hydroxy-9,10-anthraquinone (**24**). Mps 183-185° C [lit. 259-260 ° C, Rath et al. (1995)]. UVλmax EtOH nm: 229, 278, 331, 407. UVλmax EtOH/ -OH nm: 229, 280, 308, 531. IR vmax (KBr) cm-1: 3448 (OH), 1696 (aldehyde), 1676 (C=O unchelated), 1638 (C=O chelated), 1592 (C=C aromatic). MS m/z 252 (M+), 2224, 196, 168. ^{1}H NMR (CDCl$_3$, 500MHz): 13.26 (1H,s, 1-OH), 10.63 (1H, s, CHO), 8.35 (1H, m, H-8), 8.32 (1H, m, H-5), 8.23 (1H, d, J= 8.0 Hz, H-3), 7.89 (1H, d, J= 8.0 Hz, H-4), 7.88 (2H, m, H-6, H-7). 13C NMR(CDCl3, 125 MHz): 164.5 (C-1), 128.4 (C-2), 135.4 (C-3), 118.7 (C-4), 127.7 (C-5), 134.7 (C-6), 135.3 (C-7), 127.2 (C-8), 188.9 (C-9), 181.8 (C-10), 117.4 (C-11), 137.2 (C-12), 134.8 (C-13), 133.3 (C-14) and 188.0 (C-15).

Soranjidiol. Yellow-orange neddles (**25**) Mps 276-273°C [lit. 271-272 ° C, Adesogan (1973)]. UVλ$_{max}$ EtOH nm: 265, 409. UVλ$_{max}$ EtOH/ -OH nm: 308, 489. IR v$_{max}$ (KBr) cm^{-1}: 3401 (OH), 1667 (C=O unchelated), 1635 (C=O chelated), 1593 (C=C aromatic). MS m/z 254 (M$^+$), 226, 197, 115. ^{1}H NMR (DMSO$_{-d6}$, 500 MHz): 13.10 (1H,s, 1-OH), 11.21 (1H, s, 6-OH), 7.63 (1H, d, J= 7.57 Hz, H-3), 7.57 (1H, d, J=7.57 Hz, H-4), 7.25 (1H, dd, J$_{7,8}$ = 8.55 Hz, J$_{7,5}$ = 2.69 Hz, H-7), 7.45 (1H, d, J= 2.69 Hz, H-5), 2.27 (3H, s, CH3). ^{13}C NMR (DMSO$_{-d6}$, 125 MHz): 187.6 (C=O), 181.8 (C=O), 163.8 (C-OH), 160.0 (C-OH), 136.9, 135.6, 134.2, 131.1, 129.8, 124.5, 121.4, 118.6, 114.7, 112.5, 15.8 (CH$_3$)

Morindone (**26**). Orange needles. Mps 240-241 ° C (CHCl3) [lit. 248-249.5 ° C, Leistner (1975)]. UVλ$_{max}$ EtOH nm: 260, 299, 448. UVλ$_{max}$ EtOH/ -OH nm: 260, 302, 338, 558. IR v$_{max}$ (KBr) cm^{-1}: 3462 (OH), 1628 (C=O chelated). MS m/z 270 (M$^+$), 242, 135.^{1}H NMR (CDCl$_3$, 500MHz): 13.21 (1H, s, 1-OH), 12.95 (1H, s, 5-OH), 7.85 (1H, d- J=8.2 Hz, H-8), 7.75 (1H, d, J= 7.7 Hz, H-4), 7.52 (1H, d, J=7.6Hz, H-3), 7.26 (1H, d, J=8.2 Hz, H-7), 6.32 (1H, s, 6-OH), 2.39 (3H, s, CH$_3$). ^{13}C NMR (CDCl$_3$, 125 MHz): 186.6 (C=O),179.9 (C=O), 170.4 (C-OH), 169.8 (C-OH), 161.4 (C-OH), 151.3, 149.4, 136.6, 130.9, 121.3, 119.8, 118.9, 115.3, 16.3 (CH$_3$)

Morindone-5-methyl ether (**27**). Orange cystals. Mp 232°C [lit. 223 ° C, Chang & Lee (1984)]. UVλ$_{max}$ EtOH nm: 410, 497. UVλ$_{max}$ EtOH/ -OH nm: 314, 388, 498. IR v$_{max}$ (KBr) cm^{-1}: 3389 (OH), 2926, 1672 (C=O unchelated), 1630 (C=O chelated), 1581 (C=C aromatic). MS m/z 284 (M$^+$), 266, 238, 197. ^{1}H NMR (CDCl$_3$, 500MHz): 13.02 (1H, s, 1-OH),8.14 (1H, d, J=8.55 Hz, H-8), 7.70 (1H, d, J= 8.06 Hz, H-4), 7.51 (1H, d, J=7.81 Hz, H-3), 7.35 (1H, d, J=8.54 Hz, H-7), 6.73

(1H, s, 6-OH), 4.03 (3H, s, OCH_3), 2.37 (3H, s, CH_3). ^{13}C NMR ($CDCl_3$, 125 MHz): 187.8 (C=O), 182.0 (C=O), 160.6 (C-OH), 155.9, 146.8, 136.9, 134.5, 132.3, 127.1, 125.9, 125.5, 112.0, 118.9, 114.7, 62.3 (OCH_3), 16.1 (CH_3)

Alizarin-1-methyl ether. Yellow-orange crystals (28). Mp 164 [lit 178-179 °C, Chang & Lee (1984)]. UVλ_{max} EtOH nm: 313, 378, 485. UVλ_{max} EtOH/ -OH nm: 315, 333, 493. IR v_{max} (KBr) cm^{-1}: 3443 (OH), 2926, 1671 (C=O unchelated), 1589 (C=C) aromatic. MS m/z 254 (M$^+$), 236, 208, 183. ^{1}H NMR (DMSO$_{-d6}$, 500MHz): 8.28 (2H, m, H-5, H-8), 8.15 (1H, d, J= 8.55 Hz, H-4), 7.78 (2H, m, H-7, H-6), 7.37 (1H, d, J = 8.54 Hz, H-3), 6.70 (1H, s, 2-OH), 4.04 (3H, s, OCH_3). ^{13}C NMR (DMSO$_{-d6}$ 125 MHz): 182.7 (C=O), 182.1 (C=O), 155.5, 146.6, 131.4, 133.9, 132.9, 127.5, 127.1, 126.8, 125.8, 125.6, 120.2, 62.3 (OCH_3)

(28)

on ring C only. H-3 and H-4 appeared as doublets at δ_H 8.23 and 7.89 respectively. A formyl group (δ_H 10.63) is attached to C-2. HMBC correlations of C-10 with H-3 and H-5 confirmed the assignment of the protons at their respective positions and supported by their respective COSY correlations. ^{13}C NMR showed fifteen carbons peaks as expected. One of the chelated carbonyl carbon was further downfield at δ_C 188.9 (C-9), confirming the chelated nature of this carbonyl. The assignment of carbons were accomplished using FGHMQC and FGHMBC experiment. Presented below are structures and spectroscopic data of the isolated compounds.

4. Conclusion

The phytochemical study on *Fissistigma latifolium* and *Meiogyne virgata* (Annonaceae) yielded twelve alkaloids; (-)-*N*-methylguattescidine 1, liriodenine 2, lanuginosine 3, (-)-asimilobine 4, dimethyltryptamine 5, (-)-remerine 6, (-)-anonaine 7, columbamine 8, lysicamine 9, nornuciferine 10, norushinsunine 11 and cleistopholine 12. Tryptamine alkaloids have never been reported from *Fissistigma* species, whereas (-)-*N*-methylguattescidine 1 represents a rare finding of a naturally occurring 6a-methylated-7-oxo-aporphine alkaloid. Alkaloids 3, 6, 9 and 10 have never been reported from *Meiogyne* species.

Rennellia and *Morinda* are often confused with each other due to their similar traditional usage. Both plants are traditionally used for fever, postpartum and body ache treatment. Our phytochemical study on roots extract of *R. elliptica* showed significant similarities of major anthraquinones with those found in Morinda species. The major constituents of *R. elliptica*, nordamnacanthal, damnacanthal, rubiadian, rubiadin methyl ether and lucidin-ω-methyl ether are also present in *M. elliptica* and *M. citrifolia*.

5. Acknowledgment

Universiti Teknologi MARA, Universiti of Malaya, Ministry of Higher Education for Research grants and Ministry of Science, Technology and Innovation Malaysia for scholarship awarded to Alias,A.

6. References

Abd Aziz, R. (2003). *Siri Syarahan Perdana Professor*. Skudai: Universiti Teknologi Malaysia.

Adesogan, E.K. (1973). Anthraquinones and anthraquinols from *Morinda lucida*. The biological significance of oruwal and oruwalol, *Tetrahedron* 29 (1973), p. 4099.

Ahmad, R., Mahbob, E. N. M., Noor, Z. M., Ismail, N. H., Lajis, N. H., & Shaari, K. (2010). Evaluation of antioxidant potential of medicinal plants from Malaysian Rubiaceae (subfamily Rubioideae). *African Journal of Biotechnology, 9*(46), 7948-7954.

Ahmad, R., Shaari, K., Lajis, N. H., Hamzah, A. S., Ismail, N. H., & Kitajima, M. (2005). Anthraquinones from *Hedyotis capitellata*. *Phytochemistry, 66*(10), 1141-1147.

Ali, A. M., Ismail, N. H., Mackeen, M. M., Yazan, L. S., Mohamed, S. M., Ho, A. S. H., et al. (2000). Antiviral, Cytotoxic and Antimicrobial Activities of Anthraquinones Isolated from the Root of *Morinda elliptica*. *Pharmaceutical Biology, 38*, 298-301.

Alias, A., Hazni, H., Mohd Jaafar, F., Awang, K. and Ismail, N. H. (2010). Alkaloids from *Fissistigma latifolium* Dunal Merr. *Molecules*, 15, 4583-4588.

Awang, K.; Hamid, A.; Hadi, A. (2000). Protoberberine Alkaloids From *Fissistigma fulgens* Merr. (Annonaceae). *Malaysian J. Sci., 19*, 41–44.

Briggs, L.H., Beachen, J.F., Cambie, R.C., Dudman, N.P.B., Steggles, A.W. & Rutledge, P.S. (1976) Chemistry of *Coprosma* genus. Part XIV. Constituents of five New Zealand species. *J. Chem. Soc. Perkin Trans. I*, 1789-1792

Burkill, I. H. (1966). *A Dictionary of the Economic Product of the Malay Peninsular*. Volumes I & II. Ministry of Agriculture and Cooperatives, Kuala Lumpur.

Chan, K. C. & Toh, H. T. (1985). A new aporphinoid from *Desmos dasymachallus*. In: *Proceedings of the 2nd Meeting of the Natural Products Group*, edited by Said, I.M. & Zakaria, Z. 17-20. Jabatan Kimia, Fakulti Fizis dan Gunaan, Universiti Kebangsaan Malaysia, Bangi.

Chang, P. and Lee, K., Cytotoxic antileukemic anthraquinones from *Morinda parvifolia*. *Phytochemistry*, 23, 1733-1736. (1984).

Connolly, J. D., Haque, M. D. E., Kadir, A. A. (1996): Two 7,7-bisdehydroaporphine alkaloids from *Polyalthia bullata*. *Phytochemistry* 43: 295-297.

Cordell, G.A. (1981). *Introduction to Alkaloid: A Biogenetic Approach;* John Wiley & Sons: New York, NY, USA, 6–19.

Derksen, G. C. H., Van Beek, T. A., & Atta ur, R. (2002). Rubia tinctorum L *Studies in Natural Products Chemistry* (Vol. Volume 26, Part 7, pp. 629-684): Elsevier.

Hamzah, A. S., & Lajis, N. H. (1998). Chemical Constituents of Hedyotis herbaceae. *ARBEC, Article II*, 1-6.

Han, Y.-S., der Heiden, R. V., & Verpoorte, R. (2001). Biosynthesis of Anthraquinones in Cell Cultures of the Rubiaceae. *Plant Cell, Tissue and Organ Culture, 67*, 201-220.

Hutchinson, J. (1973). *The Families of Flowering Plants* (3rd ed.): Oxford University Press.

Ismail, N. H., Ali, A. M., Aimi, N., Kitajima, M., Takayama, H., & Lajis, N. H. (1997). Anthraquinones from *Morinda elliptica*. *Phytochemistry, 45*(8), 1723-1725.

Ismail, N. H., Mohamad, H., Mohidin, A., & Lajis, N. H. (2002). Antioxidant Activity of Anthraquinones from *Morinda elliptica*. *Natural Product Science, 8*(2), 48-51.

Jasril, Lajis, N. H., Lim, Y. M., Abdullah, M. A., Sukari, M. A., & Ali, A. M. (2003). Antitumor Promoting and Antioxidant Activities of Anthraquinones Isolated from the Cell

Suspension Culture of *Morinda elliptica*. *Asia Pacific Journal of Molecular Biology and Biotechnology, 11*(1), 3-7.

Kan, W. S. (1979). In *Pharmaceutical Botany*; National Research Institute of Chinese Medicine: Taiwan, 268.

Kam, T. S. (1999). Alkaloids from Malaysian Flora, in Alkaloids: Chemical and Biological Perspectives, S. W. Pelletier (Ed.), Pergamon, Amsterdam, Volume 14, Chapter 2, 285-435.

Kamaruddin, M. S. (1998). Proceedings Malaysian Traditional Medicine, 10-11 June 1998, Universiti Malaya, Kuala Lumpur, 80.

Kong, J.-M., Goh, N.-K., & Chia, T.-F. (2003). Recent Advances in Traditional Plant Drugs and Orchids. *Acta Pharmacologica Sinica, 24*(1), 17-21.

Lajis, N. H., Ahmad, R., & Atta-ur, R. (2006). Phytochemical studies and pharmacological activities of plants in genus Hedyotis/oldenlandia *Studies in Natural Products Chemistry* (Vol. Volume 33, Part 13, pp. 1057-1090): Elsevier.

Lavault, M., Cabalion, P. and Bruneton, J. (1981). Alkaloids of Uncaria guianensis. *Planta Med.* 42, 50.

Lee, H. H. (1969). Colouring matters from Prismatomeris malayana. *Phytochemistry, 8*(2), 501-503.

Leistner,E.,1975. Isolation,identifica tion and biosynthesis of anthraquinones in cell suspension cultures of Morinda citrifolia. Planta Med. (Suppl.) 214–224.

Mat Salleh, K., & Latiff, A. (2002). *Tumbuhan Ubatan Malaysia*: Universiti Kebangsaan Malaysia & Kem, Sains, Teknologi dan Alam Sekitar.

Nik Idris, Y., Lim, S. Y., Zaemah, J. and Ikram, M. S. (1994). *Alkaloid daripada Batang Fissistigma latifolium (Annonaceae) dan Potensinya Sebagai Dadah Anti-Leukaemia*, Laporan Teknik FSFG 4 : 199-204

Osman, C. P., Ismail, N. H., Ahmad, R., Ahmat, N., Awang, K., & Jaafar, F. M. (2010). Anthraquinones with Antiplasmodial Activity from the Roots of Rennellia elliptica Korth. (Rubiaceae). *Molecules, 15*(10), 7218-7226.

Parker, Sybil P. (1997). *Chemistry; Dictionaries*. McGraw-Hill (New York).

Perry, L. M. (1980). *Medicinal Plants of Southeast Asia*. MIT: Cambridge, 19.

Rath, G., Ndonzao, M., & Hostettmann, K. (1995). Antifungal Anthraquinones from *Morinda lucida*. *Int J. Pharmacogn., 33*, 107-114.

Roberts, J. L., Rutledge, P. S., and Trebilcock, M. J. (1977). Experiments Directed Towards the Synthesis of Anthracyclinones. I Synthesis of 2-Formylmethoxyanthraquinones *Aust. J. Chem.*, , 30, 1553.

Saaid M., and Awang, K. (2005) Alkaloids of *Fissistigma manubriatum*. Malaysian *Journal of Science.* 24 (1), 41-45.

Sinclair, J., (1955) A revision of the Malayan Annonaceae. *The Gardens' Bulletin Singapore, 14*, 149-69.

Tadic, D., Cassels, B. K., Leboeuf, M. and Cavé, A. (1987). Kinabaline and the aporphinoid biogenesis azaanthracene and azafluorene alkaloids. *Phytochemistry, 26*, 537–541.

Teo, L.E., Pachiaper, G., Chan, K.C., Hadi, H.A., Weber, J.F., Deverre, J.R., David, B. & Sevenet, T. (1990). A new phytochemical survey of Malaysia V. Preliminary screening and plant chemical studies. *J. Ethnopharmacol.* 28(1) : 63-101.

Verdout, B. (1976). *Annonaceae, Flora of Tropical East Africa*; Crown Agents for Oversea Government and Administrations: London, UK, pp. 101–102.

Wong, K. M. (1989). Rubiaceae (from the genus Rubia). In F. S. P. Ng (Ed.), *Tree Flora of Malaya; A Manual for Foresters* (Vol. 4, pp. 324-337, 404-405): Longman Malaysia.

6

General Introduction on Family Asteracea

Maha Aboul Ela, Abdalla El-Lakany and Mohamad Ali Hijazi
Dept. of Pharmacognosy, Faculty of Pharmacy,
Beirut Arab University,
Beirut,
Lebanon

1. Introduction

Asteraceae is the largest family of the plant kingdom, very abundant and also a diverse one. The Asteraceae plants are the most widely distributed of all the families (Porter, C.L. (1969); Evans W. (1989); Hutchinson, J.(1973); Core, E. L. (1955) of the angiosperms. It includes about 1400 genera and over 25000 species (Harborne , J. B., Turner, B.L. (1984); Aboul Ela, M. A.,(1991), forming approximately 10% of the flowering plants.

Asteaceae has characteristic taxonomical characters (Muschler, R. (1912). Members of the family are generally herbs of annul or perennial habits and some tropical forms occur as shrubs. Flowers are grouped in heads known as capitula, surrounded by involucres. It is of two kinds of florets; tubular or disc florets with tubular corolla and mostly hermaphrodite, and ligulate or ray floret, with starp like corolla and mostly female.

2. Chemistry of genus Matricaria

Genus Matricaria comprises plants with various secondary metabolites of different chemical nature recorded mainly in *Matricaria chamomilla.*German chamomile flowers contain 0.24- to 2% volatile oil which is blue in color. Chamomile also contains up to 8% flavone glycosides and flavonol; up to 10 percent mucilage polysaccharides; up to 0.3 percent choline; and approximately 0.1 percent coumarines. The tannin level in chamomile is less than one percent. (Alternative Medicine Review (2008))

Following is a review of the chemical compounds that have been isolated previously from genus Matricaria (Tables 1, 2, 3, and 4).

2.1 Volatile oil

Name	Source	Structure	References
a) Azulene derivatives			

Chamazulene	M. chamomilla		Alternative Medicine Review 2008, Ness, A.,Metzger, J. W., Shmidt, P. C. (1996)
Chamazulene Carboxylic acid	M. chamomilla	HOOC	Stahl, E. (1954)
Chamavioline	M. chamomilla	O═ H	Motl, O. ,Repcak, M. (1979), Motl, O. ,Repcak, M. ,Ubik, K. (1983)
Matricin (proazulene)	Ligulate and tubular floret only of M. chamomilla	H₃C HO OCOCH₃ O O	Alternative Medicine Review (2008), S˘orm, F.,Nowak, J., Herout, V.(1953), Cekan, Z., Herout, V., Sorm, F.,(1957)
Matricarin	M. chamomilla	H₃C OCOCH₃ O O	Alternative Medicine Review (2008)
b) Sesquiterpenes i) Oxygenated sesquiterpenes			

(1R*,2R*,3R*,6R*,7R*)1,2 ,3,6,7-pentahydroxy-bisabolol-10(11)-ene	M. aurea	R1	R2	R3	Ahmed A. Ahmed, Maha A. Abou Elela (1999)
		H	H	H	
(1R*,2R*,3R*,6R*,7R*)1,2 ,3,6,7-tetrahydroxy-1-acetoxy-bisabolol-10(11)-ene	M. aurea	Ac	H	H	Ahmed A. Ahmed, et al.(1993)
(1R*,2R*,3R*,6R*,7R*)1,2 ,3,6,7-tetrahydroxy-2-acetoxy-bisabolol-10(11)-ene	M. aurea	H	Ac	H	Ahmed A. Ahmed, Maha A. Abou Elela (1999)

(1R*,6R*,7R*)1,6,7-trihydroxy-bisabolol-2,10- diene	M. aurea	R	Ahmed A. Ahmed, et al.(1993)
		H	
(1R*,6R*,7R*)1,6,7-trihydroxy-1-acetoxybisabolol-2,10-diene	M. aurea	Ac	Ahmed A. Ahmed, et al.(1993)

(-)-α-bisabolol	*M. chamomilla*		Alternative Medicine Review (2008), S˘orm, F.,Zaoral M.,Herout, V.(1951)
(-)-α-bisabolol oxide A	*M. chamomilla*		Alternative Medicine Review 2008, Sampath , V., et al (1969)
(-)-α-bisabolol oxide B	*M. chamomilla*		Alternative Medicine Review (2008), Sampath ,V.,Sabata, et al ,(1969)
(-)-α-bisabolol oxide C	*M. chamomilla*		Schilcher, H., et al (1976)
α-bisabolone oxide	*M. chamomilla* growing in turkey		Hölzl, J., Demuth, G.(1973)

Spathulenol	*M. chamomilla*	HO	Alternative Medicine Review (2008), Motl, O., et al(1977)
Caryophyllene epoxide	*M. chamomilla*		Reichling, J., et al (1983)
ii) Unsaturated sesquiterpenes			
β-bisabolene	*M. chamomilla*		Anne ORAV, Tiiu KAILAS, and Kaire IVASK (2001)
Trans-β- farnesene	*M. chamomilla*		Alternative Medicine Review (2008), Lemberovics, E. (1979)
Trans -α-farnesene	*M. chamomilla*		Lemberovics, E. (1979)

β-selinene	*M. chamomilla*		A.Pizard, et al.(2006)
Germacrene D	*M. chamomilla*		Anne ORAV, Tiiu KAILAS, and Kaire IVASK (2001) A.Pizard, et al.(2006)
Germacrene A	*M. chamomilla*		A.Pizard, et al.(2006)
Bicyclo germacrene	*M. chamomilla*		A.Pizard, et al.(2006)
Cadinene	*M. chamomilla*		Alternative Medicine Review (2008), Anne ORAV, Tiiu KAILAS, and Kaire IVASK (2001)
α-muurolene,	*M. chamomilla*		Motl, O., Repcak, M.(1979)

Calamemene	*M. chamomilla*		Motl, O., Repcak, M.(1979)
β-caryophyllene	In the root oil of *M. chamomilla*		Reichling, J., et al (1983)
c) Monoterpenes			
α-pinene	*M. chamomilla*		Anne ORAV, Tiiu KAILAS, and Kaire IVASK (2001), A.Pizard, et al.(2006)
α-Terpinene	*M. chamomilla*		A.Pizard, et al.(2006)

Myrcene	*M. chamomilla*		Stransky, K., et al., (1981)
Sabinene	*M. chamomilla*		Anne ORAV, Tiiu KAILAS, and Kaire IVASK (2001) , A. Pizard, et al.(2006)
Gerianol	*M. chamomilla*	CH_2OH	Stransky, K., et al., (1981)
Spiroethers			
Cis (Z)-enyne dicycloether *cis*-2-[hexadiyne)- (2,4)-ylidene]-1,6-dioxaspiro-[4,4]-nonene)	*M. chamomilla*		Alternative Medicine Review (2008), Bohlmann, F., Zdero, C. (1982), Bohlmann, F., et al ,(1961)

| Trans (E)-enyne dicycloether *trans*-2-[hexadiyne)-(2,4)-ylidene]-1,6-dioxaspiro-[4,4]-nonene | *M. chamomilla* | 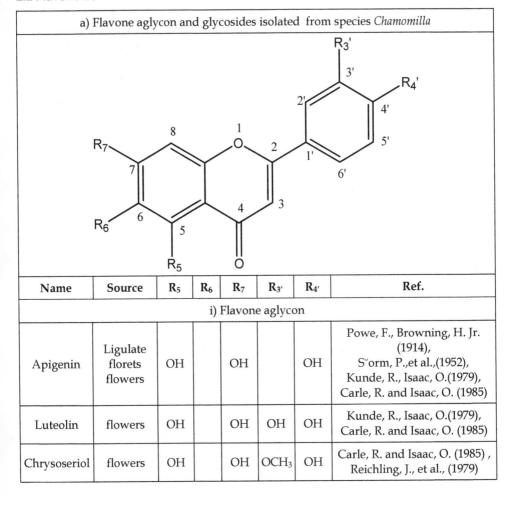 | Alternative Medicine Review (2008), Bohlmann, F., et al ,(1961), Bohlmann, F., Zdero, C. (1982) |
| (3S*,4S*,5R*)-(E)-3,4-dihydroxy-2-(hexa-2,4-diynyliden)-1,6-dioxaspiro-(4,5) decane | *M. aurea* | | Ahmed A. Ahmed, Maha A. Abou Elela (1999) |

Table 1. Volatile components isolated from Matricaria species

2.2 Flavonoids

a) Flavone aglycon and glycosides isolated from species *Chamomilla*

Name	Source	R₅	R₆	R₇	R₃′	R₄′	Ref.
				i) Flavone aglycon			
Apigenin	Ligulate florets flowers	OH		OH		OH	Powe, F., Browning, H. Jr. (1914), Sˇorm, P.,et al.,(1952), Kunde, R., Isaac, O.(1979), Carle, R. and Isaac, O. (1985)
Luteolin	flowers	OH		OH	OH	OH	Kunde, R., Isaac, O.(1979), Carle, R. and Isaac, O. (1985)
Chrysoseriol	flowers	OH		OH	OCH₃	OH	Carle, R. and Isaac, O. (1985) , Reichling, J., et al., (1979)

ii) Flavone glycosides								
Luteolin-7-glucoside	Egyptian chamomile floret (leaves) Ligulate florets	OH		OGlu	OH		OH	Kunde, R., Isaac, O.(1979), Elkiey, M. A.,et al., (1963), Greger, H. (1975)
Luteolin-4'-glucoside		OH			OH	OH	OGlu	
Chrysoseriol-7-glucoside	Leaves	OH		OGlu	OCH_3		OH	Greger, H. (1975)
Apigenin-7-glucoside (Apigetrin)	Ligulate floret	OH		OGlu			OH	Kunde, R., Isaac, O.(1979), Lang, W., Schwandt, K. (1957), Hörhammer, L., Wagner, H., Salfner, B. (1963)
Apigenin-7-(6''-O-acetyl)-glucoside	Ligulate florets	OH		OGlu-ac.			OH	Kunde, R., Isaac, O.(1979), Redaelli, C., Formentini, L., Santaniello, E. (1979)
Apigenin-7-(6''-O-apiosyl)-glucoside (apiin)	Ligulate florets	OH		OGlu-Apio.			OH	Kunde, R., Isaac, O.(1979), Wagner, H., Kirmayer, W. (1957)

b) Flavonol aglycones and glycosides isolated from *Chamomilla* species

Name	Source	R_3	R_5	R_6	R_7	$R_{3'}$	$R_{4'}$	Ref.
— i) Flavonol aglycones								
Lutuletin	Tubular floret flowes	OH	OH	OCH_3	OH	OH	OH	Kunde, R., Isaac, O.(1979), Carle, R. and Isaac, O. (1985), Ahmed A. Ahmed, Maha A. Abou Elela (1999)
Quercetin	Leaves Tubular floret flowers	OH	OH		OH	OH	OH	Kunde, R., Isaac, O.(1979), Carle, R. and Isaac, O. (1985), Greger, H. (1975)
Chrysosplenol	Chamomile flower	OCH_3	OH	OCH_3	OCH_3	OH	OH	Carle, R. and Isaac, O. (1985), Exner, J., et al., (1981), Hänsel, R., Rimpler, H., Walther, K. (1966)
Chrysosplenit in	Flowers	OCH_3	OH	OCH_3	OCH_3	OCH_3	OH	Carle, R. and Isaac, O. (1985), Hänsel, R., Rimpler, H., Walther, K. (1966)
Eupatoletin	Chamomile flower Ligulate florets	OH	OH	OCH_3	OCH_3	OH	OH	Kunde, R., Isaac, O.(1979), Carle, R. and Isaac, O. (1985), Exner, J., et al., (1981), Hänsel, R., Rimpler, H., Walther, K. (1966)
Eupalitin	Chamomile flower	OH	OH	OCH_3	OCH_3		OH	Carle, R. and Isaac, O. (1985), Exner, J., et al., (1981), Hänsel, R., Rimpler, H., Walther, K. (1966)
— ii) Flavonol glycosides								
Quercetin-7-glucoside (Quercimeritri n)	Tubular floret	OH	OH		OGlu	OH	OH	Kunde, R., Isaac, O.(1979), Lang, W., Schwandt, K. (1957) , Horhammer, L.,

								Wagner, H., Salfner, B. (1963)
Quercetin-3-rutinoside	Chamomile flower	OGlu-Rham	OH		OH	OH	OH	Elkiey, M. A.,et al., (1963)
Quercetin-3-galactoside	Chamomile flower	OGal	OH		OH	OH	OH	Elkiey, M. A.,et al., (1963)

Table 2. Flavone and flavonol aglycon and glycosides isolated from species *Chamomilla*

2.3 Coumarines and other polyphenolic compounds

a) Coumarines

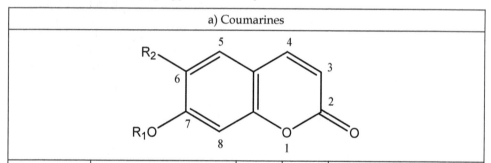

Name	Source	R₁	R₂	Ref.
Herniarin	Ligulate and Tubular floret of *M. chamomilla*	CH₃	H	Schilcher, H. (1985)
Umbelliferone	Ligulate and Tubular floret of *M. chamomilla*	H	H	Schilcher, H. (1985)
Isoscopoletin	*M. chamomilla*	CH₃	H	Kotov, A. G., et al., (1991)
Esculetin	*M. chamomilla*	H	OH	Kotov, A. G., et al., (1991)
Scopoletin	*M. chamomilla*	H	OCH₃	Kotov, A. G., et al., (1991)

b) Phenyl carboxylic acid

Name	Source	R_1	R_2	R_3	R_4	Ref.
Synergic acid	Ligulate and tubular floret of M. chamomilla	COOH	OCH_3	OH	OCH_3	Reichling, J., et al., (1979)
Vanillic acid	Ligulate and tubular floret of M. chamomilla	COOH	H	OH	OCH_3	Reichling, J., et al., (1979)
Anisic acid	M. chamomilla	COOH	H	OCH_3	H	Reichling, J., et al., (1979)
Caffeic acid	M. chamomilla	$CH_2=CH_2COOH$	OH	OH	H	Reichling, J., et al., (1979)

Table 3. Coumarines and other polyphenolic compounds isolated from genus Matricaria

2.4 Miscellaneous substances

Chamomile contains up to 10% mucilage polysaccharides (Alternative Medicine Review (2008)).The main chain of the polysaccharide consists of α-1-> 4 connected D-galacturone acids (Carle, R. and Isaac, O.,(1985)). In addition to xylose, arabinose, galactose, glucose, rhamnnose (Janecke, H., Weiser, W. (1964))(Janecke, H., Weiser, W.(1965)).

Recently, three polysaccharides were isolated and showed remarkable antiphlogistic activity against mouse ear edema induced by crotone oil (Füller, E., (1992)) as fructane (74.3% fructose and 3.4% glucose, similar to inulin), rhamnogalacturonane (28% uronic acid, 3.2% protein, similar to pectin), and arabino-3, 6-galactane glycoproteins.

- Chamomile contains up to 0.3% choline ((Alternative Medicine Review (2008)), (Bayer, J. et al. (1958)) which is supposed to be participating in the antiphlogistic activity of the extract.
- More than 13 amino acids were detected (Schilcher, H.,(1980)) from the fresh chamomilla herb as L-leucine, DL-methionine, DL-α-alanine, glycine, L-histidine, L-(+)-lysine, DL- threonine, DL-serine, and L-glutaminic acid.
- Tannin level is less than 1% (Alternative Medicine Review (2008).

3. Some reported pharmacological activity of the chemical constituents of Matricaria

Several pharmacological actions have been assigned for German chamomile, based primarily on *in vitro* and animal studies. Such actions include antibacterial, antifungal, anti-inflammatory, antispasmodic, anti-ulcer, antiviral, carminative, and sedative effects (Alternative Medicine Review 2008). It is important to mention that therapeutic effectiveness is mainly due to the combined pharmacological and biochemical effects of several chamomile constituents (Schilcher, H.,(1987)).

3.1 Apoptotic effect against cancerous cell

- Darra et al. in 2008 showed that α-bisabolol is able to rapidly, efficiently and selectively induce apoptosis in malignant tumor cells by targeting lipid rafts on cell membranes. Thereafter, α-bisabolol could interact with Bid protein (one of pro-apoptotic Bcl-2 family proteins, analyzed either by Surface Plasmon Resonance method or by intrinsic fluorescence measurement) recruited in lipid rafts region after α-bisabolol treatment, which may be involved in the transduction pathway from plasma membranes to intracellular compartments including mitochondria. However, toxicity towards normal cells or in animals was absent. (Elena Darra, et al., (2008))
- In 2007, Farnesol had been demonstrated by Joo et al. to inhibit proliferation and induce apoptosis in a number of neoplastic cell lines from different origins (J.H. Joo,et al., (2007)) with preferential action in transformed cells versus untransformed cells (Adany, Cancer Lett. (2000)) and (Srivastava JK, Gupta S. (2007))
- Other preliminary study by Srivastava et al. in 2007 recorded that *in vitro* exposure to chamomile results in differential apoptosis in cancerous cells but not in normal cells at similar doses; apigenin and apigenin glycosides appear to be the key components responsible for these effects, (Deendayal patel et al. (2007))
- Moreover, Patel *et al in 2007* identified many mechanisms of action for apigenin-mediated cancer prevention and therapy, including estrogenic/anti-estrogenic activity, anti-proliferative activity, induction of cell-cycle arrest and apoptosis, prevention of oxidation, induction of detoxification enzymes, regulation of the host immune system, and changes in cellular signaling. This suggests that apigenin possesses enormous potential for development as a promising cancer chemopreventive agent in the near future for breast, cervical, colon, lung, prostate, ovarian, skin, endometrial, thyroid, and gastric, hepatocellular, and adrenocortical cancers as well as leukemia. Pre-clinical studies of various animal models of cancer that closely simulate human cancers are still needed (Barton, H. 1959).

3.2 Sedative and anxiolytic effect

- Shinomiya et al. (Kazuaki S. et al., (2005)) investigated the hypnotic activities of chamomile and passiflora extracts using sleep-disturbed model rats. A significant decrease in sleep latency was observed with chamomile extract at a dose of 300 mg/kg. His findings strongly suggested that chamomile is a herbal product possessed both hypnotic and anxiolytic activity in animals.
- (Avallone R.,et al., (2000) showed that apigenin, a flavonoid isolated from *Matricaria chamomilla*, significantly reduced the locomotor activity in the open field test of rats.
- (Viola H., et al.,(1995) , in a study about intraperitoneal administration of chamomile extract in mice, concluded that apigenin functions as a ligand for benzodiazepine receptors, resulting in anxiolytic and mild sedative effects, but no muscle relaxant or anticonvulsant effects. He also reported that apigenin extracted from chamomile flowers inhibited [3H]-flunitrazepam binding in the bovine cerebral cortex.
- Gould L., et al.,(1973) reported that hospitalized patients were given a strong chamomile tea, and ten of the twelve patients immediately fell into a deep sleep lasting 90 minutes.
- Della Loggia, R., et al.,(1981)) also demonstrated that chamomile extract caused a significant prolongation of sleeping time induced by barbiturates in mice.

3.3 Antispasmodic effect

Both flavonoids and essential oil contribute to the musculotropic antispasmodic effect of chamomile. Apigenin, alpha-bisabolol, and the cis-spiroethers appear to provide the most significant antispasmodic effects. (Alternative Medicine Review (2008).

- Maschi *et al.* in 2008 reported the spasmolytic activity of chamomile was through inhibition of cAMP-PDE for the first time. Human platelet cAMP-PDE and recombinant PDE5A1 were assayed in the presence of chamomile infusions. Chamomile inhibited cAMP-PDE activity (IC50) 17.9-40.5 μg/mL), while cGMP-PDE5 was less affected (-15% at 50 μg/mL). Among the individual compounds tested, flavonoids showed an inhibitory effect (IC50) 1.3-14.9 μM), contributing to around 39% of the infusion inhibition.
- Carle, R., Gomaa, K. in 1992 demonstrated that the chamomile oil itself, (-)-α- bisabolol, the bisabolol oxides A and B, and the enyne dicycloethers have a papaverine-like musculotropic spasmolytic activity. In addition, the coumarin derivates umbelliferone and herniarin are also antispasmodically active,(Acheterrath-Tuckermann,et al., 1980)
- In Tests that was performed using rat or rabbit duodenum, where the contractions were induced by barium chloride, acetyl choline, and histamine (Hava M., Janku J. (1957), (Janku, J. (1981), apigenin inhibits the contractions of smooth muscle and those of seminal vesicle of cavy and of rabbit uterus. 10 mg of apigenin were equieffective to about 1 mg of papaverine as for musculotropic effect. (Della Loggia, R. 1985)
- Other flavonoids contribute to the smooth muscle relaxation but to lesser degree. They can be classified in descending activity as follows: apigenin, quercetin, luteolin, kaempferol, luteolin-7-glucoside, and apigenin-7-glucoside. (Hörhammer, L.,et al., (1963)

3.4 Antimicrobial effect

Preliminary *in vitro* studies on the antimicrobial activity of chamomile have yielded promising results.

- Annuk H,et al., in 1999 proved that chamomile extract at concentration 2.5 mg/ml killed trichomonads effectively. It also blocked aggregation of various strains of *Escherichia coli.*
- Shikov, A., et al., in 1999 demonstrated that chamomile oil extract inhibited the production of urease at *H. pylori*. It was suggested that the mechanism of therapeutic action of chamomile oil is based on inhibition of colony activity of *H. pylori* and an inhibiting effect on adhesion of this microorganism of phospholipid – lecithin.
- Turi M. *et al.* in 1997 showed that chamomile extract inhibited the growth of poliovirus and herpes virus while chamomile esters and lactones demonstrated activity against *Mycobacterium tuberculosis* and *Mycobacterium avium.*
- Berry M. in 1995 showed that chamomile oil, at a concentration of 25 mg/mL, demonstrated antibacterial activity against such Gram-positive bacteria as *Bacillus subtilis, Staphylococcus aureus, Streptococcus mutans,* and *Streptococcus salivarius,* as well as some fungicidal activity against *Candida albicans*
- The strongest antibacterial activity was recorded for α- bisabolol. It is active in low concentrations against *Staphylococcus aureus, Bacillus subtilis, Escherichia coli,*

Streptococcus faecalis, and *Pseudomonas aeruginosa* and inhibits the growth of strains of *Bacterium phlei* that were resistant against standard anti-infectives (Szabo-Szalontai, M., et al., (1976) and (Szalontai, M.,et al., (1975). Bisabolol, together with enyne dicycloethers, also showed fungistatic activity against *Candida albicans, Trichophytone menthagrophytes,* and *Trichophytone rubrum* at a concentration of 100µg/ml. Chamazulene also had this fungistatic activity, but at higher concentrations (Szalontai.,M., Verzar-petri, G., Florian, E. (1977).

3.5 Anti inflammatory effect

- Recent study in 2009 by Srivastava *et al.* done on aqueous extract of chamomile flowers growing in Egypt, where LPS-activated RAW 264.7 macrophages were used as in vitro model, Chamomile treatment inhibited the release of LPS-induced PGE2 in RAW 264.7 macrophages. This effect was found to be due to inhibition of COX-2 enzyme activity by chamomile. In addition, chamomile extract caused reduction in LPS-induced COX-2 mRNA and protein expression, without affecting COX-1 expression. This suggested that mechanism of action of chamomile on the inhibition of PGE2 production was due to the suppression of the COX-2 gene expression and direct inhibition of COX-2 enzyme activity which is similar to non-steroidal anti inflammatory drugs.
- (-)-α- bisabolol was capable of inhibiting both 5-lipoxygenas and cyclooxygenase (Szelenyi J., Isaac, O., Thiemer, K., (1979)). It has antipyretic activity against yeast-induced pyrexia of the rat (Büchi, O. (1959)). Other experiments showed that (-)-α-bisabolol was capable of inhibiting the formation of ulcers induced by indomethacin, stress, or alcohol (Szelenyi J., Isaac, O., Thiemer, K., (1979))
- Regarding azulenes, their anti inflammatory effect was proven (Zierz, P., Kiessling, W (1953), (Zierz, P., et al. (1957) through inhibition of histamine liberation, inhibition of 5-hydroxytryptamine liberation, anti-hyaluronidase effect, and a decrease of the capillary activity (Uda, T.(1960). This is besides to the activation of the ACTH production (Kato, et al. (1959).
- Chamazulene was identified as the antiphlogistic principle of chamomile oil in a test system of chemosis caused by mustard oil in rabbit and cavy eye (Heubner, et al. (1933) and Pommer (1942)). It was proved by Ammon et al. in 1996 to inhibit 5-lipoxygenase.
- Antiphlogistic activity of flavonoids was proved much later (Baumann, J., et al., (1980)), (Carle, R., Gomaa, K. (1992), (Della loggia, R. (1985)), Della loggia, R., et al., (1984)), (Della loggia R., et al., (1986), Wurm, G., (1982). Apigenin even exceeded the activity of indomethacin and phenylbutazone. The experiments further showed that apigenin had both a positive influence on the vascular phase of the inflammation (e.g., edema) and on the cellular phase (e.g., the migration of leucocytes). Antiphlogistic activity of flavonoids decreased in the following order: Apigenin > luteolin > quercetin > myricetin > apigenin-7-glucoside > rutin.

3.6 Anti ulcerative effect

Torrado S, et al., in 1995 reported that significant protective effect against gastric toxicity of 200 mg/kg acetylsalicylic acid where achieved after oral administration of chamomile oil to rats at doses ranging from 0.8-80 mg/kg bisabolol. Moreover, *in vitro* studies revealed that alpha-bisabolol inhibited gastric ulcer formation induced by indomethacin, ethanol, or stress, Szelneyi I, Isaac O., thiemer K. (1979)

3.7 Other Pharmacological actions

3.7.1 Inhibition of Aflatoxin G1 production

Yoshinari et al. in 2008 showed that the spiroethers of German chamomile inhibited production of aflatoxin G1 AFG1 by *Aspergillus parasiticus* with inhibitory concentration 50% (IC50) values of 2.8 and 20.8 mM respectively. This is through inhibiton of cytochrome P450 monooxygenase CYPA and without inhibiting fungal growth. In addition, it also inhibited production of 3-acetyldeoxynivalenol 3-ADON by *Fusarium graminearum* by inhibiting TRI4. The inhibitory activity of the (E)-spiroether isomer was much stronger than that of the (Z)-spiroether in both cases. Inhibition of TRI4 by the spiroethers showed that TRI4 may be a good target for inhibiting biosynthesis of trichothecene mycotoxins.

3.7.2 Protective effect on diabetic complications

- Kato et al. in 2008 investigated the effects of chamomile hot water extract and its major components on the prevention of hyperglycemia and the protection or improvement of diabetic complications in diabetes mellitus. Results suggested that a suppressive effect of chamomile on blood glucose level was independent of the inhibition of intestinal α-glycosidases but depended on the inhibition of hepatic glycogen phosphorylase (GP). Furthermore, chamomile extract has good inhibitory potency against aldose reductase (ALR2), which plays key roles in the polyol pathway and its activation promotes the progress of diabetic complications. Chamomile components, umbelliferone, esculetin, luteolin, and quercetin, could inhibit sorbitol accumulation in human erythrocytes. Therefore, daily consumption of chamomile tea with meals could be potentially useful in the prevention and self-medication of hyperglycemia and diabetic complications. ATSUSHI KATO,et al ., (2008)

3.7.3 Antioxidant effect

- Lado *et al.* in 2004 studied the volatile oil of several plants and their main components to determine their antioxidant activity. This was done by using the modified method of ferric reducing ability of plasma (FRAP). The reducing ability of juniper, yarrow, and chamomile (145.107 ± 0.007mmol/kg) was very significant and it was twice as high as the average values of the other plants (Lavander, salvia, rosemary, etc). The reducing abilities of the components of volatile oils are lower than those of volatile oils; therefore, the reducing capacities of volatile oils not only attributed solely to terpenes, but also other biologically active compounds may also contribute to ferric reduction and in electron scavenging (Cristina Lado, et al.,(2004)).

3.7.4 Inhibition of morphine dependence

- Gomaa *et al.* in 2003 showed that co-administration of *M. chamomilla* extract containing 0.3% apigenin with morphine not only inhibited dependence to morphine but also prevented the increase in plasma cAMP induced by naloxone-precipitated abstinence. Furthermore, naloxone precipitated morphine withdrawal behavior syndrome was abolished by acute *M. chamomilla* treatment before naloxone challenge, indicating that *M. chamomilla* extract has an inhibitory effect on the expression of naloxone-precipitated morphine withdrawal syndrome.

3.7.5 Tachykinin receptor antagonist

- Yamamoto et al. in 2002 discovered a novel and potent nonpeptide tachykinin NK1 receptor antagonist in the extract of dried flowers of *Matricaria chamomilla.* . It has a unique structure of a polyacylated Spermine which was established as $N1$, $N5$, $N10$, $N14$-tetrakis [3-(4-hydroxyphenyl)-2-propenoyl]-1, 5, 10, 14-tetraazatetradecane (tetracoumaroyl spermine). The Ki values of 1a, estimated from the inhibitory action on the substance P (SP)-induced contraction of the guinea pig ileum and the inhibition of the binding of [3H][Sar9, Met(O2)11]SP to human NK1 receptors, were 21.9 nM and 3.3 nM, respectively.

4. Clinical indications of *Matricaria chamomilla*

German chamomile is a well-known and widely used herb in different parts of the world. Few well designed, randomized, double-blind; placebo-controlled studies are available to fully assess its therapeutic benefit. (Alternative Medicine Review 2008)

4.1 Gastrointestinal effect

- De la Motte S, (1997) conducted a prospective, randomized, multicenter, double-blind, parallel group trial, where 79 children (ages six months to five years) with acute, non complicated diarrhea received either a commercial preparation of apple pectin and chamomile extract or placebo for three days, in addition to a typical rehydration and re-alimentation diet. At the end of three days, significantly more children in the pectin/chamomile group (85%) experienced diarrhea alleviation compared to the placebo group (58%) (p<0.05). The pectin/chamomile combination experienced a significant 5.2-hour shorter duration of symptoms compared to the placebo group. Weizman Z. et al. in 1993 in double-blind studies observed the efficacy of a herbal decoction consisting of German chamomile, vervain, licorice, fennel, and balm mint on 68 healthy infants with colic. For seven days the infants (ages 2-8 weeks) received 150 mL of the herbal preparation or placebo with each colic episode, but no more than three times daily. After seven days, 57 percent of the infants receiving the herbal preparation experienced colic relief compared to 26 percent in the placebo group (p<0.01).
- Schmid et al. in 1975 showed that chamomile extract is successfully applied in pediatrics due to its carminative and spasmolytic effect with diseases of the gastrointestinal tract and the effect as such is said to set in immediately after taking the preparation. The internal administration of chamomile tea or preparations from chamomile extracts is appropriate in different gastric troubles that can be classed under term of "dyspepsia," as recorded by Weiss in 1987.

4.2 General anti-inflammatory effect

- In 1999 Schilcher demonstrated that chamomile extract therapy is advisable in pediatrics for sensitive skin care of babies, treatment of an inflamed skin or skin defects (as dermatitis ammoniacalis, scald and burn areas and exfoliative dermatitis), and for the treatment of inflammations of the nose and the paranasal sinus by application of a chamomile bath and inhalation.
- Nasemann et al. in 1991 reported about the antiphlogistic effect of Kamillosan® ointment in comparison with a nonsteroidal ointment in case of episiotomies, with

colpitis senilis, and about the improvement of the healing of wounds after surgical operations carried out by laser in gynecology after taking a chamomile (hip) bath.
- Carle et al. in 1987, and according to reports of various gynecological hospitals, showed that chamomile extract is a suitable remedy for the treatment of bartholinitis, vulvitis, and mastitis and in rare cases secondarily healing episiotomies.

4.3 Dermatologyical effect

- Stechele in 1991 and according to a pediatrician's open report showed that very good results could be achieved by using chamomile ointment for the treatment of napkin dermatitis.
- Aertgeerts P et al. in 1985, in an open, bilateral comparative trial, 161 patients with eczema on their hands, forearms, and lower legs initially treated with 0.1-percent diflucortolone valerate received one of four treatments: chamomile cream (Kamillosan), 0.25-percent hydrocortisone, 0.75-percent fluocortin butyl ester (a glucocorticoid), or 5.0-percent bufexamac (a nonsteroidal anti-inflammatory). After 3-4 weeks, the chamomile cream was found to be as effective as hydrocortisone and demonstrated superior activity to bufexamac and fluocortin butyl ester.
- As for Born in 1991, chamomile extract was applied for the irrigation of undermined margins of a wound, pouches, sinus tracts, and hip baths, correspondingly diluted or in concentrated form for swabbing inflammatory lesions of the mucosa.
- Contzen in 1975 proved that the chamomile bath can be used successfully with the local treatment of deep second-degree burns. Apart from an accelerated cleansing process of a wound a significant improvement of the granulation is also observed. Deep necroses are excised; superficial ones heal without proteolytic ferments.
- Glowania HJ et al. in 1987and through a double-blind trial examined the therapeutic efficacy of a topical chamomile extract on 14 patients with weeping dermabrasions from tattoo applications. Those using chamomile noted a statistically significant decrease in the weeping wound area and increased drying compared to the placebo group.

4.4 Sleep enhancement

In an open case study to examine the cardiac effects of two cups of chamomile tea on patients undergoing cardiac catheterization, Gould L. et al. observed that 10 of 12 patients in the study achieved deep sleep within 10 minutes of drinking the tea, Gould L, et al. (1973). The patients had a small but significant increase in mean brachial artery pressure. No other significant hemodynamic changes were observed.

4.5 Radiation therapy

- Fidler P. et al. in 1996 conducted a randomized, double-blind study with 164 cancer patients taking 5-fluorouracil (5-FU) chemotherapy. The patients rinsed three times daily with either a chamomile mouthwash or placebo. After 14 days, no difference was observed between the two groups in the incidence of stomatitis induced by 5-FU.
- Carl W. et al. 1991 examined the effect of 15 drops of Kamillosan Liquidum, a German chamomile mouthwash preparation, in 100 mL of water taken three times daily, for radiation and/or chemotherapy-induced mucositis (characterized by inflammation and ulceration of the gastrointestinal tract including the mouth). Cancer patients (n=98)

were divided into two groups. One group of 66 patients (20 undergoing radiation therapies, 46 undergoing chemotherapy) participated in prophylactic oral care with the mouthwash. The remaining 32 patients underwent chemotherapy and were treated therapeutically after mucositis had developed. Of the 20 patients undergoing radiation, only one developed high-grade (grade 3) mucositis in the final week of treatment, 65 percent developed intermediate grade mucositis, and 30 percent developed low-grade mucositis. Of the 46 patients concurrently receiving chemotherapy and the mouthwash, 36 remained free of any clinically significant mucositis. Of the 32 patients with existing mucositis, all noted immediate relief from mouth discomfort, and within seven days almost all patients had no clinical sign of mucositis.

-   Maiche AG et al. in 1991 carried out a double-blind, randomized, placebo-controlled study, where 48 women receiving radiation therapy for breast cancer were treated topically with either chamomile cream or placebo (almond oil) to protect the radiation-treated area. While there were no significant differences between the two groups in objective scores of skin irritation, the patients preferred the chamomile containing cream to the placebo for its rapid absorption and stainlessness.
-   According to Bulmenberg, E.-W., Hoefer-Janker, H. (1972), the reactions of mucosa of the rectum resulting from a highly dosed radiation therapy, frequently felt to be unendurable; can also be treated successfully with chamomile extract. For that purpose enema is given three times a week; besides antiphlogistic properties, this also has a mild cleaning effect

4.6 Other uses

-   According to Hinz in 1995, a standardized ethanolic-aqueous chamomile flower extract is suitable for the adjuvant therapy of *Angina lacunaris* and for the symptomatic treatment of herpangina often occurring in (early) childhood. In addition has a pain-alleviating effect in cases of inflammatory and painful esophageal diseases.

5. Photograph of the two matricaria specie

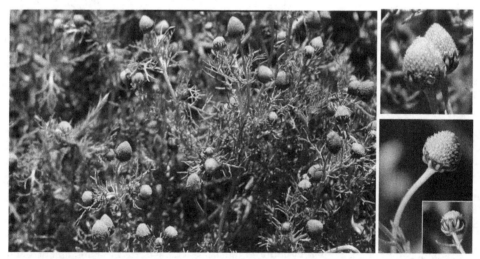

Fig. 1. Photograph of *Matricaria aurea*

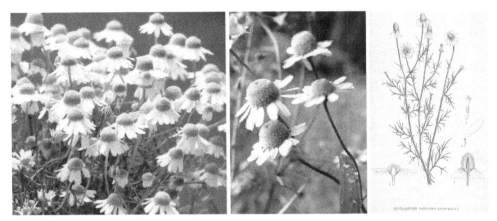

Fig. 2. Photograph of *Matricaria chamomilla*.

(10-40cm in height, with erect, branching stems .the capitulum (to 1.5cm in diameter) comprises 12-20 white ligulate florets surrounding a conical hollow receptacle on which numerous yellow tubular (disk) florets are inserted (Bruneton J. (1995))

6. Conclusions and recommendations

A lot of studies have been conducted on *Matricaria chamomilla* all over the world where many important biologically active compounds have been separated and identified. However, very few studies are available for *Matricaria aurea* world wide. Nowadays, researches are focusing on exploring the pharmacological profile of compounds from natural origin, where promising results aroused. Challenges remain in finding ways to benefit from these biologically important compounds in treating human health problems.

7. References

[1] Porter, C.L. "Taxonomy of flowering plants", Eurasia Publishing House (Pvt.) Ltd., Ram Nagar, New Delhi, India, 410 (1969)

[2] Evans, W. "Pharmacognosy"; 13th Edition, Bailleire Tinadall., London, Philladelphis, Toronto, Sydney and Tokyo, 226 (1989).

[3] Hutchinson, J. "The families of flowering plants", 2nd Edition, Oxford University Press, Ely House, London, 482 (1973).

[4] Core, E.L. "Plant taxonomy", Engle Cliffs, N.J. Prentice-Hall inc., 423 (1955).

[5] Harborne, J. B.; Turner, B.L. "Plant Chemosystematics", Academic Press, London, 113 (1984).

[6] Aboul Ela, M. A; "A Thesis of Doctor of Philosophy degree in Pharmaceutical sciences"; Faculty of Pharmacy, Alexandria University, Alexandria, Egypt 4 (1991).

[7] Muschler, R. "A manual Flora of Egypt", Berlin, Freid Laender and sohn Karlstrase, Volume II (1912).

[8] Alternative Medicine Review Volume 13, Number 1 2008

[9] Ness, A., Metzger, J. W., Schmidt, P. C. (1996) Pharm. Acta Helvet., 71, 265-271. 83. Piesse, S. (1863) Comptes Rend. hebdom. Séances Acad. Sciences, 57, 1016.

[10] Stahl, E. (1954) Chem. Ber., 87, 202, 205, 1626.

[11] Motl, O., Repcak, M. (1979) Planta Med., 36, 272.

[12] Motl, O., Repcak, M., Ubik, K. (1983) Arch. Pharm., 316, 908.

[13] S̆o rm, F., Nowak, J., Herout, V. (1953) Chem. Listy, 47, 1097.

[14] Cekan, Z., Herout, V., ˇSorm, F. (1954) Chem. Listy, 48, 1071.

[15] Cekan, Z., Herout, V., ˇSorm, F. (1954) Collect Czechoslov. Chem. Commun., 19, 798.

[16] Cekan, Z., Herout, V., ˇSorm, F. (1957) Collect Czechoslov. Chem. Commun., 22, 1921.

[17] Ahmed A. Ahmed, Maha A. Abou Elela, "Highly oxygenated bisabolenes and acetylene from Matricaria aurea". Phytochemistry 51 (1999) 551-554

[18] Ahmed A. Ahmed, J. Jakupovic, Maha A. Abou Elela, Ahmed A. seif El-Din and Nadia S. Hussein, (1993)" Two Bisabolanes from Matricaria aurea". Natural product letters 3(4): 277-281

[19] S̆orm, F., Zaoral, M., Herout, V. (1951) Collect Czechoslov. Chem. Commun., 16, 626-638.

[20] Sampath, V., Trivedi, G. K., Paknikar, S. K., Bhattacharyya, S. C. (1969) Indian J. Chem., 7, 100

[21] Sampath, V., Trivedi, G. K., Paknikar, S. K., Sabata, B. K., Bhattacharyya, S. C. (1969) Indian J. Chem., 7, 1060

[22] Schilcher, H., Novotny, L., Ubik, K., Motl, O., Herout, V. (1976) Arch. Pharm., 309, 189.

[23] Hölzl, J., Demuth, G. (1973) Dtsch. Apoth. Ztg., 113, 671.

[24] Motl, O., Felklova, M., Lukes, V., Jasikova, M. (1977) Arch. Pharm., 310, 210.

[25] Anne ORAV, Tiiu KAILAS, and Kaire IVASK, "Volatile Constituents of Matricaria recutita L. f". Proc. Estonianrom Estonia" Acad. Sci. Chem., 2001, 50, 1, 39-45

[26] Reichling, J., Bisson, W., Becker, H., Schilling, G. (1983) Z. Naturforsch., 38 c, 159.

[27] Lemberovics, E. (1979) Sci. Pharm., 47, 330.

[28] A.Pizard, H. Alyari, M.R. Shakiba , S. Zehtab-Salmasi and A. Mohammadi, "Essential Oil content and composition of German Chamomile (Matricaria chamomilla L.) at Different Irrigation Regimes. Journal of Agronomy 5 (3): 451-455, 2006

[29] Stransky, K., Streibel, M., Ubik, K., Kohoutova, J., Novotny, L. (1981) Fette, Seifen, Anstrichmittel, 83, 347.

[30] Kumar, S., Das, M., Singh, A., Ram, G., Mallavarapu, G. R., Ramesh, S. (2001) J. Med. Arom. PlantSciences, 23, 617–623.

[31] Bohlmann, F., Herbst, P., Arndt, Ch., Schönowski, U., Gleinig, H. (1961) Chem. Ber., 94, 3193.

[32] Bohlmann, F., Zdero, C. (1982) Phytochemistry, 21, 2543-9.

[33] F.Bohman and H. Kapteyn (1967): Die Polyine aus Chrysanthemum carintum. Chemical Berichte, 100, 1927

[34] F.Bohman and H. Kapteyn (1967): Die Polyine aus Chrysanthemum carintum. Chemical Berichte, 100, 1927

[35] Yamazaki, H., Miyakado, T., Mabry, T. J. (1982) J. Nat. Prod., 45, 508.

[36] W. Donald Macrae and G. H. Tower (1984): Biological activities of lignans. Phytochemistry, 23, 1207

[37] R. silverstein and G. Bassler (1986): spectroscopic identification of Organic compounds. 2nd Ed. John Wiley & Sons. Inc., New York, London, Sydney

[38] F. Bouhlman, W. Kramp Gupta, R. King and H. Robinson (1981): Four guaianolides and other constituents from three Kaunia species. Phytochemistry

[39] Power, F., Browning, H. Jr. (1914) J. Chem. Soc., London, 105, 2280, in Becker, H., Reichling, J.(1981) Dtsch. Apoth. Ztg, 121, 1285.
[40] Sˇorm, P., Zekan, Z., Herout, V., Raskova, H. (1952) Chem. Listy, 46, 308.
[41] Kunde, R., Isaac, O. (1979) Planta Med., 37, 124.
[42] Carle, R. and Isaac, O. (1985) Dtsch. Apoth. Ztg., 125 Nr. 43/Suppl. 1, 2–8.
[43] Reichling, J., Becker, H., Exner, J., Dräger, P. D. (1979) Pharmaz. Ztg. 124, 1998.
[44] Elkiey, M. A., Darwish, M., Mustafa, M. A. (1963) Fac. Pharm. Cairo Univ., 2, 107, ref. in Becker, H., Reichling, J. (1981) Dtsch. Apoth. Ztg, 121, 1285.
[45] Greger, H. (1975) Plant. Syst. Evol., 124, 35.
[46] Lang, W., Schwandt, K. (1957) Dtsch. Apoth. Ztg., 97, 149.
[47] Hörhammer, L., Wagner, H., Salfner, B. (1963) Arzneim. Forsch., 13, 33.
[48] Tschirsch, K., Hölzl, J. (1992) PZ-Wissenschaft, 137, (5) 208–214.
[49] Redaelli, C., Formentini, L., Santaniello, E. (1979) Herba Hung., 18, 323.
[50] Wagner, H., Kirmayer, W. (1957) Naturwissenschaften, 44, 307.
[51] Exner, J., Reichling, J., Cole, T. H., Becker, H. (1981) Planta Med., 41, 198.
[52] Hänsel, R., Rimpler, H., Walther, K. (1966) Naturwissenschaften, 53, 19.
[53] Schilcher, H. (1985) Zur Biologie von Matricaria chamomilla, syn. "Chamomilla recutita (L.) Raus- chert," Research report 1968-1981, I Pharmakognosie and Phytochemie of the FU, Berlin.
[54] Kotov, A. G., Khvorost, P. P., Komissarenko, N. F. Khimiya Prirodnykh Soedinenii (1991), 853
[55] Janecke, H., Weiser, W. (1964) Planta Med., 12, 528.
[56] Janecke, H., Weiser, W. (1965) Pharmazie, 20, 580.
[57] Schilcher, H. (1987) Die Kamille — Handbuch für Arzte, Apotheker und andere Naturwissenschaftler. Wissenschaftl Verlagsgesellschaft, Stuttgart, Germany.
[58] Füller, E. (1992) Dissertation, University of Regensburg.
[59] Bayer, J., Katona, K., Tardos, L. (1958) Acta Pharm. Hung., 28, 164.
[60] Bayer, J., Katona, K., Tardos, L. (1958) Naturwiss., 45, 629.
[61] Schilcher, H. (1970) Planta Med., 18, 101-113.
[62] Streibel, M. (1980) Presentation, DFG Conference in Kiel, ref. in: Seifen, Öle, Wachse, 106, 503.
[63] Schilcher, H. (1987) Die Kamille — Handbuch für Ärzte, Apotheker und andere Wissenschaftler, Wissenschaftliche Verlagsgesellschaft, Stuttgart, Germany.
[64] Elena Darra , Safwat Abdel-Azeim , Anna Manara , Kazuo Shoji , Jean-Didier Mare´chal ,Sofia Mariotto , Elisabetta Cavalieri , Luigi Perbellini , Cosimo Pizza ,David Perahia , Massimo Crimi , Hisanori Suzuki , "Insight into the apoptosis-inducing action of a-bisabolol towards malignant tumor cells: Involvement of lipid rafts and Bid". 476 (2008) 113–123 Archives of Biochemistry and Biophysics
[65] J.H. Joo, G. Liao, J.B. Collins, S.F. Grissom, A.M. Jetten, Cancer Res. 67 (2007) 7929–7936.
[66] Adany, Cancer Lett. 79 (1994) 175–179. Rioja, FEBS Lett. 467 (2000) 291–295.
[67] Srivastava JK, Gupta S. Antiproliferative and apoptotic effects of chamomile extract in various human cancer cells. J. Agric. Food Chem. (2007) 55:9470- 9478.
[68] Deendayal Patel, Sanjeev Shukla and Sanjay Gupta, "Apigenin and cancer chemoprevention: Progress, potential and promise". International Journal of Oncology 30: 233-245, 2007
[69] Barton, H. (1959) Acta Biol. Med. Gem. 2, 555.

[70] Kazuaki Shimoniya, Toshio inoue, Yoshiaki Utsu, Shin Tokunaga, Takayoshi Masuoka, Asae Ohmori, and Chiaki Kamei, "Hypnotic Activities of Chamomile and Passiflora Extracts inSleep-Disturbed Rats". Biol. Pharm. Bull. 28(5) 808−810 (2005)

[71] Avallone R., Zanoli P., Puia G., Kleinschnitz M., Schreier P., Baraldi M., Biochem. Pharmacol. 59, 1387−1394 (2000).

[72] Viola H, Wasowski C 16. , Levi de Stein M, et al. Apigenin, a component of *Matricaria recutita* flowers, is a central benzodiazepine receptors-ligand with anxiolytic effects. Planta Med. 1995; 61:213-216.

[73] Gould L., Reddy C. V. R., Gomprecht R. F., J. Clin. Pharmacol., 13, 475−479 (1973).

[74] Della Loggia R., Tubaro A., Redaelli C., Riv. Neurol., 51, 297−310 (1981).

[75] Della Loggia, R.; Tubaro, A., Dri, P., Zilli, C., Del Negro, P. (1986) Plant Flavonoids in Biology and Medicine − Biochemical, Pharmacological and Structure-Activity Relationships, Alan R. Liss, Inc., pp. 481–484

[76] Carle, R., Gomaa, K. (1992) Drugs of Today 28, 559.

[77] Achterrath-Tuckermann, U., Kunde, R., Flaskamp, E., Isaac, O., Thiemer, K. (1980) Planta Med. 39, 38–50.

[78] Hava M., Janku J. (1957) Rev. Czech. Med. 3, 130

[79] Janku, J. (1981) Paper at 2nd Physiolog. Conf. Königgrätz, ref. in Becker, H., Reichling, J. (1981) Dtsch. Apoth. Ztg. 121, 1285.

[80] Della Loggia, R. (1985) Dtsch. Apoth. Ztg. 125, Suppl. I, 9.

[81] Hörhammer, L., Wagner, H., Salfner, B. (1963) Arzneim.-Forsch. 13, 33.

[82] Annuk H, Hirmo S, Turi E, et al. Effect on cell surface hydrophobicity and susceptibility of Helicobacter pylori to medicinal plant extracts. FEMS Microbiol Lett 1999;172:41-45.

[83] Shikov, A. N., Pozharitskaya, O. N., Makarov, V. G. et al. (1999) Method of allocation of biologically active substances from plant material. Patent Ru 214 1336 from Nov. 2, 1999.

[84] Turi M, Turi E, Koljalg S, Mikelsaar M. Influence of aqueous extracts of medicinal plants on surface hydrophobicity of Escherichia coli strains of different origin. APMIS 1997; 105:956-962.

[85] Berry M. The chamomiles. Pharm. J 1995; 254:191-193.

[86] Szabo-Szalontai, M., Verzár-Petri, G. (1976) 24. Jahres versammlung d. Ges. f. Arzneipflanzen forsch., Munich, Germany.

[87] Szalontai, M., Verzár-Petri, G., Florián, E., Gimpel, F. (1975) Dtsch. Apoth. Ztg. 115, 912.

[88] Szalontai, M., Verzár-Petri, G., Florián, E., Gimpel, F. (1975) Pharmaz. Ztg. 120, 982.

[89] Szalontai, M., Verzár-Petri, G., Florián, E. (1976) Acta Pharm.-Hung. 46, 232.

[90] Szalontai, M., Verzár-Petri, G., Florián, E. (1977) Parfümerie und Kosmetik 58, 121.

[91] Janmejai K. Srivastava, Mitali Pandey, Sanjay Gupta, "Chamomile, a novel and selective COX-2 inhibitor with anti-inflammatory activity". Life Sciences 85 (2009) 663–669

[92] Szelenyi, J., Isaac, O., Thiemer, K. (1979) Planta Med. 35, 218.

[93] Büchi, O. (1959) Arch. Int. Pharmacodyn. 123, 140.

[94] Zierz, P., Kiessling, W. (1953) Dtsch. Med. Wschr. 78, 1166.

[95] Zierz, P., Lehmann, A., Craemer, R. (1957) Hautarzt 8, 552.

[96] Uda, T. (1960) Nippon Yak. Zasshi 56, 1151; ref. in Chem. Abstr. 50, 4058 (1962).

[97] Kato, L., Gözsy, B. zit., Tur, W., Joss, B. (1959) Azulen im Lichte der medizinischen Weltliteratur, Flyer of the company Th. Geyer KG, Stuttgart, ref. in Thiemer, K., Stadtler, R., Isaac, O. (1973) Arzneim.-Forsch. 23, 756.

[98] Heubner, W., Grabe, E, (1933) Arch. Exp. Pathol. Pharmakol. 171, 329.

[99] Pommer, Ch. (1942) Arch. Exp. Pathol. Pharmakol. 199, 74.

[100] Ammon, H. P. T., Sabieraj, J., Kaul, R. (1996) Dtsch. Apoth. Ztg. 136, 1821

[101] Baumann, J., Wurm, G., Bruchhausen, F. (1980) Arch. Pharm. 313, 330.

[102] Della Loggia, R., Tubaro, A., Zilli, C. (1984) 32nd Annual Congress for Medicinal Plant Research, Antwerp, Abstracts L.16.

[103] Della Loggia, R.; Tubaro, A., Dri, P., Zilli, C., Del Negro, P. (1986) Plant Flavonoids in Biology and Medicine — Biochemical, Pharmacological and Structure-Activity Relationships, Alan R. Liss, Inc., pp. 481–484

[104] Wurm, G., Baumann, J., Geres, V. (1982) Dtsch. Apoth. Ztg. 122, 2062.

[105] Torrado S, Torrado S, Agis A, et al. Effect of dissolution profile and (-)-alpha-bisabolol on the gastrotoxicity of acetylsalicylic acid. Pharmazie 1995;50:141-143.

[106] Szelenyi I, Isaac O, Thiemer K. Pharmacological experiments with compounds of chamomile. III. Experimental studies of the ulcerprotective effect of chamomile (author's transl). Planta Med 1979; 35:218 227.

[107] Tomoya Yoshinari, Atsushi Yaguchi, Naoko Takahashi-Ando, Makoto Kimura, Haruo Takahashi, Takashi Nakajima, Yoshiko Sugita-Konishi, Hiromichi Nagasawa & Shohei Sakuda" Spiroethers ofGerman chamomile inhibit production ofa£atoxinG1 and trichothecenemycotoxin by inhibiting cytochromeP450 monooxygenases involved in their biosynthesis". FEMS Microbiol. let. 2008 Jul;284(2):184-90. E-pub 2008 May 19

[108] Atsushi Kato, Yuka Minoshima, Jo Yamamoto, Isao Adachi, Alison A Watson, and Robert J. Nash, "Protective Effects of Dietary Chamomile Tea on Diabetic Complications". J. Agric. Food Chem. 2008, 56, 8206–8211

[109] Cristina Lado, Ma´ ria Then, Ilona Varga, E´ va Szo¨ ke, and Kla´ra Szentmiha´ lyi, "Antioxidant Property of Volatile Oils Determined by the Ferric Reducing Ability". Z. Naturforsch. 59c, 354D358 (2004)

[110] Adel Gomaa,, Tahia Hashem, Mahmoud Mohamed, and Esraa Ashry, "*Matricaria chamomilla* Extract Inhibits Both Development of Morphine Dependence and Expression of Abstinence Syndrome in Rats". J. Pharmacol. Sci 92, 50 – 55 (2003)

[111] Atsushi Yamamoto, Ko Nakamura, Kazuhito Furukawa, Yukari Konishi, Takashi Ogino, Kunihiko Higashiura, Hisashi Yago, Kaoru Okamoto, and Masanori Osuka, "A New Nonpeptide Tachykinin NK1 Receptor Antagonist Isolated from the Plants of Compositae". Chem. Pharm. Bull. 50(1) 47−52 (2002)

[112] De la Motte S, Bose-O'Reilly S, Heinisch M, Harrison F. Double-blind comparison of an apple pectin-chamomile extracts preparation with placebo in children with diarrhea. Arzneimittel forschung 1997; 47:1247-1249.

[113] Weizman Z, Alkrinawi S, Goldfarb D, Bitran C. Efficacy of herbal tea preparation in infantile colic. J Pediatr 1993;122:650-652.

[114] Schmid, F. (1975) in Demling, L., Nasemann, T. (Eds.), Erfahrungstherapie — späte Rechtfertigung, Verlag G. Braun, Karlsruhe, Germany

[115] Weiss, R. F. (1987) Kneipp-Blätter, 1, 4.

[116] Schilcher, H. (1999) Phytotherapie in der Kinderheilkunde, 3rd ed., Wissenschaftliche Verlagsgesellschaft mbH, Stuttgart, Germany.

[117] Nasemann, T., Patzelt-Wenczler, R. (1991) Kamillosan im Spiegel der Literatur, pmi-Verlag Frankfurt/ Main.

[118] Carle, R., Isaac, O. (1987) Zschr.-f. Phytoth ., 8 , 67.

[119] Stechele, U. (1979) Expert report from a pediatric practice. Ref. in Nasemann, T., Patzelt-Wenczler, R. (Eds.) Kamillosan im Spiegel der Literatur, pmi-Verlag Frankfurt/Main (1991).

[120] Aertgeerts P., Albring M., Klaschka F. et al. Comparative testing of Kamillosan cream and steroidal (0.25% hydrocortisone, 0.75% fluocortin butyl ester) and non-steroidal (5% bufexamac) dermatologic agents in maintenance therapy of eczematous diseases. Z. Hautkr 1985;60:270-277.

[121] Born, W.: Personal communication to company Homburg (letter of August 6, 1980), ref. in T. Nasemann, R. Patzelt-Wenczler (Eds.), Kamillosan im Spiegel der Literatur , pmi-Verlag Frankfurt/ Main (1991).

[122] Contzen, H. (1975) in Demling, L., Nasemann, T. (Eds.), Erfahrungs therapie — späte Rechtfertigung; Verlag G. Braun, Karlsruhe, Germany.

[123] Glowania HJ, Raulin C, Swoboda M. Effect of chamomile on wound healing - a clinical double blind study. Z Hautkr 1987;62:1262,1267-1271.

[124] Gould L, Reddy CV, Gomprecht RF. Cardiac effectsof chamomile tea. J. Clin. Pharmacol. 1973;13:475 479.

[125] Fidler P, Loprinzi CL, O'Fallon JR, et al. Prospective evaluation of a chamomile mouthwash for prevention of 5-FU-induced oral mucositis. Cancer 1996;77:522-525.

[126] Carl W, Emrich LS. Management of oral mucositis during local radiation and systemic chemotherapy: a study of 98 patients. J Prosthet. Dent. 1991;66:361- 369.

[127] Maiche AG, Grohn P, Maki-Hokkonen H. Effect of chamomile cream and almond ointment on acute radiation skin reaction. Acta Oncol 1991; 30:395-396.

[128] Blumenberg, E.-W., Hoefer-Janker, H. (1972) Radiologie, 12, 209.

[129] Hinz, D. (1995) Therapiewoche,8, 478.

[130] Bruneton J. Pharmacognosy, phytochemistry, medicinal plants. Paris, Lavoisier, 1995.

7

Ximenia americana: Chemistry, Pharmacology and Biological Properties, a Review

Francisco José Queiroz Monte[1], Telma Leda Gomes de Lemos[1],
Mônica Regina Silva de Araújo[2] and Edilane de Sousa Gomes[1]
Programa de Pós-Graduação em Química Universidade Federal do Ceará, Fortaleza - Ceará
Depatamento de Química, Universidade Federal do Piauí, Teresina - Piauí,
Brasil

1. Introduction

The use of plants as medicinal agents to the treat of many diseases has been investigated for a long time since the antique civilizations. Several plants are used in traditional medicine against inflammatory diseases as well as various types of tumors on the base the potential of their chemical constituents. Although many compounds are extremely toxic, when we have the relation between the toxicity of a compound and its chemical pattern of substitution that can result in a more in-depth understanding of these compounds (Atta-ur-Rahman, 2005). Today, even after more than 200 years, the chemistry of natural products remains a challenge and an important field of research in several science areas (chemistry, biology, medicine, agronomy, botany and pharmacy). The reasons for it's large use are the considerable pharmacological potential observed in natural products, in the great development in the process of detection, isolation, purification and, especially, the advances in spectrometric techniques [infrared (IR), mass spectrometry (MS) and nuclear magnetic resonance (NMR ^{1}H and ^{13}C) for structural elucidation of new and complex compounds. These advances were outstanding in both NMR and MS spectrometry. The NMR allows the complete ^{1}H and ^{13}C NMR spectral assignments (chemical shifts and coupling constants) which serve to build a data base to support computer assisted structure elucidation. These data are also useful in the fuller understanding of the correlations between molecular conformation and biological activity of natural substances with biological importance (Loganathan *et al.*, 1990). Mass spectrometry has a huge application in chemistry, biochemistry, medicine, pharmacology, agriculture and food science. Although the mass spectrometric ionization techniques EI (electron impact) and CI (chemical ionization) required the analyte molecules to be present in the gas phase and were thus suitable only for volatile compounds, the development of several desorption ionization methods [FD (field desorption), FABMS (fast atom bombardment), ESIMS (electrospray), MALDI-MS (matrix assisted laser desorption ionization)] allowed the hight-precision mass spectrometric analysis of different classes of biomolecules.

The genus Ximenia belongs to the Olacaceae and comprises about 8 species (Brasileiro et al., 2008): Ximenia roiigi, Ximenia aegyptiaca, Ximenia parviflora, Ximenia coriaceae, Ximenia aculeata, Ximenia caffra, Ximenia americana and Ximenia aegyptica. X. caffra stands out for being used in Tanzania for the treatment of irregular menstruation, rheumatism and cancer (Chhabra & Viso, 1990) and, in Limpopo Province, South Africa, for treatment diarrhea (Mathabe, 2006). However, X. americana Linn. is the most common, being native to Australia and Asia where is commonly known as Yellow Plum or Sea Lemon. It is found mainly in tropical regions (Africa, India, New Zealand, Central America and south America), specially Africa and Brazil. The plant is characterized as a small tree spinose 3-4 feet tall, gray or reddish bark, with leaves small, simple, alternate, of bright green color and with a strong smell of almonds. The flowers are yellowish-white, curved and aromatic. Fruit are yellow-orange, aromatic, measuring 1.5 to 2.0 cm in diameter, surrounding a single seed and have a pleasant plum-like flavor (Matos, 2007). In Asia, the young leaves are consumed as a vegetable, however, the leaves also contain cyanide and need to be thoroughly cooked, and should not be eaten in large amounts.

X. americana, commonly called "ameixa do mato", "ameixa de espinho" and "ameixa da Bahia", is widely distributed in northeast Brazil. A tea obtained from its barks has been used in popular medicine as cicatrizing, adstringent and as an agent against excessive menstruation. As a powder, it treats stomach ulcers and the seeds are purgative (Braga, 1976; Pio-Correia, 1984). This specimen has been recently examined (Araújo et al., 2008,2009) and the stem ethanolic extract afforded steroids (stigmasterol and sitosterol), triterpenoids (betulinic acid, oleanolic acid, 28-O-(-D-glucopyranosyl) oleanolic acid, 3-oxo-oleanolic acid, 3β–hydroxycicloart-24(E)-ene-26-oic acid and sesquiterpenoids (furanoic and widdrane type). A large number of sesquiterpenes are constituents of essential oils of higher plants and seem to intervene in the pharmacological properties attributed to these volatile fractions (Bruneton, 1999). It has been clarified that the biological activities of the liverworths are due to terpenoids and lipophilic aromatic compounds (Atta-ur-Rahman, 1988). Steroids and triterpenes with therapeutic interest and manufacturing employment, are a group of secondary metabolites of outstanding importance (Bruneton, 1999). Considerable recent work strongly indicates the great potential of the triterpenoids as source of use medicinal (Mahato et al., 1992).

Investigations in the past 10 years showed that the constituents of X. americana have shown several biological activities such as, antimicrobial, antifungal, anticancer, antineoplastic, antitrypanosomal, antirheumatic, antioxidant, analgesic, moluscicide,   pesticidal, also having hepatic and heamatological effects.

In general, the compounds found in X. americana were saponins, glicosydes, flavonoids, tannins, phenolics, alkaloids, quinones and terpenoids types. In addition, the plant is potentially rich in fatty acids and glycerides and the seeds contain derivatives cyanide. The identified compounds did not demonstrate a representative pattern of each class. For example, the sesquiterpene were furanoic and widdrane while, triterpenes exhibited oleanane and cycloartane skeletal type. Concerning the fatty acids, in addition to common C16, C18 and C22, a distinctive feature is the presence of acetylenic, as well as, very long chain fatty acids.

We can see, from all the information summarized above, that work on plants of the genus Ximenia is justified, particularly Ximenia americana species, where systematic study is still not satisfactory, specially, relative to specific biological activity of their chemical constituents.

The present review compiles the published chemical and pharmacological information on the species X. *americana* and update important data reported in the last ten years in the scientific literature.

2. Biological activity

2.1 Antimicrobial and antifungal activities

To evaluate the scientific basis for the use of numerous plants species used to treat diseases of infectious origin, crude extracts of these plants were investigated. The antimicrobial activity of the extracts of the various parts of the investigated plants such as roots, leaves, seeds, stem barks and fruits, appears to be due to the presence of secondary metabolites such polyphenols, triterpenes, sterols, saponins, tannins, alkaloids, glycosides and polysaccharides (Geyid *et al.*, 2005; James *et al.*, 2007; Maikai *et al.*,2009; Ogunleye *et al.*, 2003).

X. *americana* is a plant used in traditional medicine for the treatment of malaria, leproutic ulcers and infectious diseases of mixed origin by natives in Ethiopia, Guinea, Sudan and in the Northern part of Nigeria (Geyid *et al.*, 2005; James *et al.*, 2007; Magassouba *et al.*, 2007; Maikai *et al.*, 2009; Ogunleye *et al.*, 2003; Omer & Elnima, 2003).

The crude extracts of X. *americana* show antimicrobial and antifungal activities. The crude aqueous, methanolic, ethanolic, butanolic and chloroform extracts from different parts (leaves, root, stem and stem bark) of the plant were subjected to phytochemical screening and from the test carried out, it was observed that the secondary metabolites contained were saponins, flavonoids, tannins, terpenoids, sterols, quinones, alkaloids, cyanogenetic glycosides, cardiac glycosides and carbohydrates in the form of sugars and soluble starch. The results of phytochemical screening of various parts solvent extracts of X. *americana* are presented in Table 1.

The MeOH extract from leaves of X. *americana* inhibited or retarded growth of *Neisseria gonorrhea* organism at dilution as low as 250 µg/ml. This same extract showed antifungal effect against *Candida albicans* and *Cryptococus neoformans* in concentration of 4000 µg/ml. Chemical screening conducted on the extract showed the presence of several secondary metabolites as tannins, sterols, terpenoids, flavonoids and saponins (Geyid *et al.*, 2005). The antimicrobial activities of ethanol extract of the leaves were evaluated against six common bacterial isolates (*Pseudomonas aeruginosa, Proteus vulgaris, Bacillus subtilis, Escherichia coli, Staphylococus aureus* and *Candida albicans*) and was active against all of them. The highest degree of activity was for *P. aeruginosa* (inhi bition zone: 20 mm), followed by *B. subtilis* and C. *albicans* (inhibition zone: 10 mm). Activity of the organic extract of the plant was comparable to that of commercially available penicillin disc (2 µg) which was more active against *P. aeruginosa* but less effective against S. *aureus*. The results of phytochemical analysis indicated the presence of saponins, flavonoids, tannins and cyanogenetic glycosides. Alkaloids and anthraquinones were not present (Ogunleye *et al.*, 2003). The root, stem bark and leaves aqueous and methanolic extracts of X. *americana* were tested against five bacteria and they inhibited the growth of *Staphylococus aureus* and *Klebsiella pneumoniae* while *Shigella flexineri* was inhibited by only methanolic leaves, aqueous bark and aqueous leaves extracts. *Salmonella typhi* and *Escherichia coli* were not affected by these extracts. The

Plant part	Solvent	Class of Compounds									Ref.
		Tannins	Steroids	Terpenes	Saponins	Flavonoids	Alcaloids	Cardiac	Glycosids	Quinones	
Leaves	MeOH	+		+	-	+	-	-		-	Geyid et al., 2005
Leaves	H₂O	+	-	-	+	+	-	+		-	Ogunleye et al., 2003
	EtOH	+	-	-	+	+	-	+		-	
Leaves	H₂O	+	-	-	+	+	-	+		+	James et al., 2007
	MeOH	+	-	-	+	+	-	+		-	
Stem bark	H₂O	+	-	-	+	+	-	+		+	
	MeOH	+	-	-	+	+	-	+		+	
Root	H₂O	+	-	-	+	+	-	+		+	
	MeOH										
Stem bark	BuOH	+	-	+	+	+	+	+		-	Maikai et al., 2009
	MeOH	+	-	+	+	+	+	+		+	
	H₂O	+	-	+	+	+	-	-		+	
Root	CHCl₃										Omer & Elnima, 2003)
	MeOH				+	+					
Stem	EtOH		+	+							Araújo et al., 2008,2009

+: present; -: absent; Ref.: references

Some extracts showed the presence of carbohydrates in the form of sugars and soluble starch (James *et al.*, 2007 & Ogunleye *et al.*, 2003); few extracts showed also the presence of cyanogenetic glycosides (Ogunleye *et al.*, 2003). Quinones are of the anthraquinone type; terpenes are sesquiterpenes and triterpenes type (Araújo *et al.*, 2008, 2009).

Table 1. Phytochemical screening of stem bark, leaves, root and stem extracts of X. *Americana*. (Placed on the table 1)

Minimum Inhibitory Concentration (MIC) was only evident for the methanolic extracts at 1.25×10^4 µgmL⁻¹ (1:4) against *Staphylococus aureus* while the Minimum Bactericidal Concentration (MBC) of the extracts was obtained at 2.50×10^{-4}µg mL⁻¹ (1:2) (James *et al.*, 2007). From the results, inhibitory activity of extracts (methanolic root) was more pronounced on *Klebsiella pneumonia* whereas it shows no activity against *Escherichia coli*, *Salmonella typhi* and *Shigella flexineri*. The methanolic root extract showed highly significant ($p < 0.05$) activity on *Klebsiella pneumonia* when compared with leaf extracts and methanolic bark extract. The phytochemical constituents present in the extracts were carbohydrates in the form of sugars and soluble starch (except for aqueous and leaves extracts), cardiac glycosides, saponins, tannins and flavonoids while alkaloids were absent in all the extracts. It was concluded that the extracts of methanolic roots, stem bark and leaves have bacteridal activities over the concentration of $2,5x10^4$ - $1,25x10^4$ μgmL^{-1} and that the presence of carbohydrates, glycosides, flavonoids and tannins in the diferent extracts are responsible for their antibacterial activity. The antimicrobial properties of the bark, leave, root and stem extracts of *Ximenia americana* were screened against *Bacillus subtilis*, *Staphyllococus aureus*, *Escherishia coli* and *Pseudomonas aeruginosa* (Table 2) using the cup-plate agar diffusion method and the minimum inhibitory concentration by agar dilution method (Omer *et al.*, 2003).

Part used	Solvent system	% Yield	Inhibition zone (mm)				MIC (mg/ml)			
			B.s	S.a	E.c	Ps.a	B.s	S.a	E.c	Ps.a
Bark	CHCl₃	1.1	13	12	11	15	N.D	N.D	N.D	N.D
	MeOH	21.1	23	30	19	22	0.31	0.62	19.79	19.79
	H₂O	8.9	18	18	16	14	0.40	1.62	3.24	1.62
Leaves	CHCl₃	10.7	13	14	-	12	N.D	N.D	N.D	N.D
	MeOH	26.6	23	22	-	25	1.55	0.77	9997	12.45
	H₂O	5.0	17	19	16	22	0.59	1.19	>25.5	19.11
Root	CHCl₃	2.2	15	13	12	13	N.D	N.D	N.D	N.D
	MeOH	3.7	15	21	19	15	3.27	6.54	>34.88	>34.48
	H₂O	5.7	13	13	-	-	2.68	10.74	28.65	28.65
Stem	CHCl₃	2.7	-	11	11	-	N.D	N.D	N.D	N.D
	MeOH	11.8	20	25	-	24	>72.75	3.41	>72.75	>72.75
	H₂O	2.7	17	17	13	13	5.12	5.12	>13.65	>13.65

B.s, *Bacillus subtilis*; S.a, *Staphyllococus aureus*; E.c, *Escherichia coli*; Ps.a, *Pseudomonas aeruginosa*; concentration of extracts 100 mg/ml, 0.1 ml/cup; inhibition zones are the mean of three replicates. MIC, minimum inhibitory concentration; N.D, not detected.

Table 2. Antibacterial activity of *Ximenia americana* extracts against standard organisms. (Placed on the table 2)

The methanolic extract was the most active one. The aqueous extract also exhibited high activity which justifies its traditional use. *Staphyllococus aureus* was the most susceptible bacterium among the tested organisms. The table 3 show the antibacterial activity of *Ximenia Americana* against the pharmaceuticals patterns.

Several other studies to determine the presence of antimicrobial activity in crude extracts of *Ximenia americana* were performed (Magassouba *et al.*, 2007; Maikai *et al.*, 2009). In all, the various extracts were found to have broad spectrum effect against standard organisms (*Escherichia coli*, *Pseudomonas aeruginosa*, *Staphylococus aureus*, *Proteus vulgaris*, *Candida albicans*, *Bacillus subtilis*, *Salmonella typhi* and *Shigella flexineri*) and supports the traditional usage of this plant as remedy in treatement of microbial infections.

In general, the antimicrobial activity of extracts of the various parts of the plants appears to be due to presence of secondary metabolites. In some experiments, was remarked that the

Reference drugs	Concentration µ/ml	MDIZ			
		B.s	S.a	E.c	Ps.a
Ampicillin	40	14	25	-	-
	20	13	22	-	-
	10	-	19	-	-
	5	-	18	-	-
Benzyl penicillin	40	-	37	-	-
	20	-	33	-	-
	10	-	28	-	-
	5	-	24	-	-
Cloxacillin	40	-	29	-	-
	20	-	27	-	-
	10	-	22	-	-
	5	-	18	-	-
Gentamicin	40	24	18	25	22
	20	22	16	17	15
	10	17	14	16	12
	5	15	13	11	-

Interpretation of sensitivity test results: Gram(+) bacteria*; Gram(-) bacteria **;
>18 mm (M.DIZ)= sensitive; >16 mm (M.DIZ)=sensitive;
14-18 mm (M.DIZ)= intermediate; 13-16 mm (M.DIZ)= intermediate;
<14 mm (M.DIZ)= resistant; and < 13mm (M.DIZ)= resistant.

Table 3. The activity of *Ximenia Americana* against the clinical isolates. (Placed on the table 3)

plants which accumulate polyphenols, tannins and unsaturated sterols/terpenes showed to inhibit or significantly retard growth of eight of the ten test organisms; the species, which constitute polyphenols and unsaturated sterols/terpenes; and polyphenols, tannins, unsaturated sterols/terpenes, saponins and glycosides inhibited six organisms each while, those with polyphenols, tannins, unsaturated sterols/terpenes, saponins; and alkaloids and unsaturated sterols/terpenes inhibited growth of five bacterial strains each (Geyid *et al.*, 2005). Cyanogenetic glycosides are reported to possess antimicrobial activity (Finnermore *et al.*, 1988). Tannins have been traditionally used for protection of inflamed surfaces of the mouth and treatment of catarrh, wounds, haemorrhoids and diarrhea and as antidote in heavy metal poisoning. They have the ability to inactivate microbial adhesions, enzymes, cell envelope transport proteins and also complex with polysaccharide (Maikai *et al.*, 2009; Scalbert, 1991; Ya *et al.*, 1988). Flavonoids are naturally occurring phenols, which posses numerous biological activities including anti-inflamatory, antiallegic, antibacterial, antifungal and vasoprotective effects and, also have been reported to complex with extracellular and soluble proteins and to complex with bacterial cell walls (Dixon *et al.*, 1983; Geyid *et al.*, 2005; Hostettman *et al.*, 1995; James *et al.*, 2007; Maikai *et al.*, 2009; Ogunleye *et al.*, 2003). Terpenoids have also been reported to be active against bacteria, the mechanism of action involve membrane disruption by the lipophilic compounds (Geyid *et al.*, 2005; James *et al.*, 2007; Maikai *et al.*, 2009; Ogunleye *et al.*, 2003). Although it is difficult to speculate on the mechanism of action of the constituents of the extracts on the basis of studies conducted to date, the antimicrobial activity of these extracts is due, no doubt, the presence of these secondary metabolites. In the case of extracts of *Ximenia americana*, probably, due the presence of tannins, flavonoids, triterpenes/steroids, saponins or cyanogenetic glycosides.

In summary, the results justified the use of *X. americana* as having antibacterial properties and support its use as agent in new drugs for therapy of infectious diseases caused by pathogens.

2.2 Pesticidal activity

Olecaceous seed oils are a rich source of acetylenic lipids and unsaturated fatty acids (Badami & Patil, 1981 & Sptizer *et al.*, 1997). Acetylenic metabolites show some biological activities including, insecticidal activity (Jacbson, 1971). *X. americana* was recorded to contain octadec-11-en-9-ynoic acid, named xymeninic acid as well as icosenoic-triacontenoic acids, all of which belong to the ω-9 series (Rezanka, & Sigler, 2007). Bioactivity-driven fractionation of the $CHCl_3$ extract of the root of *X. americana* using the Brine Shrimp Lethality Test (BST) and hatchability test with *Clavigralla tomentosicollis* eggs yielded two fractions (F006, soluble in petroleum ether and F005, soluble in 10% H_2O in MeOH) as the most actives (F005, BST LC_{50} 78 (129-48) μg/mL and F006, BST LC%$_{50}$ 76(121-49) μg/mL) (Fatope *et al.*, 2000). A combination of F005 and F006 was submitted to hatchability test (inhibition of hatching = 68 % of control) and successive BST-dircted fractionation on silica gel column and preparative TLC yielded oleanene palmitates (1), β-sitosterol (2) and C_{18} acetylenic fatty acids (3 and 4) as yellow oils.

The substance **4** suppressed the hatchability of *C. tomentosicollis* eggs at 92 % of control when tested at 4×10^{4} μg/mL (correcting for unhatched eggs in the control using Abbott's formula):

$$\% \text{ control} = [(\% \text{ unhatched of treated group - \% unhatched of untreated group})/ (100 - \% \text{ unhatched of untreated group})] \times 100$$

These acetylenic fatty acids show characteristic spectrometric data. The ^{13}C NMR spectrum of **3** displayed absorptions diagnostic of acetylenic carbons at δ_C 80.4 (C) and 80.1 (C) and of carboxylic carbon at δ_C 189.1 (C), in agreement with its IR spectrum which exhibited bands at 2200 and at 1713 cm[-1], characteristic of acetylenic and acid groups, respectively. Compound **3** had molecular formula$C_{18}H_{32}O_2$, as established by HREI-MS (*m/z* 280.2378 for [M+]) in combination with its ^{1}H and ^{13}C NMR spectra. From analysis spectral data compound **3** was thus established as octadeca-5-ynoic acid (tariric acid). Compound **4** had a mol wt 6 mass units less than that of **3** with molecular formula $C_{18}H_{26}O_2$ as revealed by HREI-MS (m/z 274.2021 for [M$^+$]) in combination with its ^{1}H and ^{13}CNMR spectra. The ^{13}C NMR spectrum of **4** displayed absorptions diagnostic of acetylenic carbons at δ_C 83.4 (C) and 74.1 (C) and of carboxylic carbon at 179.3 (C), in agreement with its IR spectrum which exhibited bands at 2232 and 1702 cm^{-1}, characteristic of acetylenic and acid groups, respectively. The ^{13}C RMN spectrum also exhibited six resonance at δ_C 148.2 (CH), 140.9 (CH), 136.9 (CH), 129.8 (CH), 109.3 3(CH) and 108.6 (CH), revealing the presence of three double bonds. From a detailed spectral analysis considering, especially, the multiplicity of signals and coupling constants in the ^{1}H NMR spectrum, as well as the presence of diagnostic peaks in the mass spectrum, compound **4** was thus established as 10Z,14E,16E-octadeca - 10,14,16-triene-12-ynoic acid, a ene-ene-yneene acetylenic fatty acid (Fatope *et al.*, 2000).

$$CH_3-(CH_2)_{11}C\equiv C-(CH_2)_3CO_2H \qquad CH_3CH=C_{16}HCH=C_{14}HC\equiv C_{12}CH=C_{10}H(CH_2)_8CO_2H$$

$$\textbf{3} \qquad\qquad\qquad\qquad\qquad\qquad\qquad \textbf{4}$$

In addition, *Ximenia* seed oil have been found to contain fatty acids with more than 22 carbon atoms (very long fatty acids) which are found only rarely in nature. Using liquid chromatography in combination with mass spectrometry was founded that *Ximenia* oil to contain fatty acids with chain length C_{34} and C_{36} (Rezanka & Sigler, 2007). Effectively, two very long chain unsaturated fatty acids C_{40} and C_{35} (**5** and **6**) were isolated (Saeed & Bashier, 2010) from *X. americana* seeds and fruits, respectively. The mass spectrum of the major component (**5**) showed a molecular ion at m/z 604 corresponding to the molecular formula $C_{40}H_{76}O_3$. The IR spectrum of **5** showed a broad absorption band at 3600-3200 cm^{-1} (OH) and the presence of strong absorption at 1742 cm^{-1} attributed to ester group. The base peak appeared at m/z 55 ($C_4H_7^+$) due to allylic bond cleavage and peaks at m/z 479 and 151 furnished from fragmentation in C_{28}-C_{29} and C_{26}-C_{27}, respectively. In addition, the peaks at m/z 31, 59, 73 and 74 (McLafferty rearrangement) were compatible with unit $CH_3OCO(CH_2)_3$-. The compound **5** was identified as methyl-14,14-dimethyl-18-hydroxyheptatracont-27,35-dienoate. The mass spectrum of **6** showed a molecular ion at 578, corresponding to the molecular formula $C_{35}H_{62}O_6$. The IR spectrum showed bands at 3500, 1731 and 1645 cm^{-1} corresponding to OH, C=O and C=C groups, respectively. The base peak appeared at m/z 73 ($C_3H_5O_2^+$) which is characteristic for the methyl ester, reinforced by additional peaks at m/z 31, 59 and 74 (McLafferty rearrangement). An peak at m/z 479 was due to M-$C_5H_7O_2$ and one at m/z 339 is due to the cleavage C_{13}-C_{14} while, those at m/z 126 and 265 were due to $C_7H_{10}O_2$ and M-$C_{17}H_{28}O_2$, respectively. The compound **6** was identified as dimethyl-5-Methyl-28,29-dihydroxydotriacont-3,14,26-triendioate.

$$[CH_3OCO(CH_2)_{12}C(CH_3)_2(CH_2)_3CHOH(CH_2)_8CH=CH(CH_2)_6CH=CHCH_3]$$

$$\textbf{5}$$

$$[CH_3OCOCH_2)CH=CHCH_3(CH_2)_8CH=CH(CH_2)_{10}CH=CH(CHOH)_2(CH_2)_2COOCH_3]$$

$$\textbf{6}$$

2.3 Analgesic activity

The aqueous extract of stem bark of *X. american* has analgesic properties that justify its use popular in countries such as Tanzania, Senegal, Zimbawe and Nigeria. The extract of *X.*

americana in doses containing 10 to 100 mg/kg P.C, inhibits contractions of the abdomen with analgesic effects comparable to those of phenylbutazone. In fact, at doses of 100 mg / kg P.C, phenylbutazone causes an inhibition of pain in 45.2±2%. The percentage of inhibition by extract of X. *ameriacana* is 61.1±% in the same concentration. These properties are probably due to the presence of flavonoids and saponins, detected in the extract (Soro *et al.*, 2009). The analgesic activity of the methanol extract of X. *americana* leaf was investigated in chemical models of nociception in mice. The extract at doses of 200, 400 and 600 mg/kg i.p. produced an inhibition of 54.13, 63.74, and 66.4% respectively, of the abdominal writhes induced by acetic acid in mice. In the formalin test, the administration of 200, 400 and 600 mg/kg i.p. had no effects in the first phase (0 to 5 min) but produced a dose dependent analgesic effect on the second phase (15 to 40 min) with inhibitions of the licking time of 29.3, 47.8 and 59.8%, respectively. These observations suggested that methanol extract of X. *americana* leaf possesses analgesic activity (Siddaiah *et al.*, 2009).

2.4 Antipyretic activity

The bark of stem of X. *americana* has been used in West Africa for the treatment of pain and fever. To verify this second property, the treatment of rats in hyperthermia with *Ximenia americana* stem bark aqueous and with beer yeast was compared to those obtained with lysine acetylsalicylate (Aspegic). The study showed an antipyretic action of the extract. Moreover, the toxicological study of the stem extract indicated a LD_{50} of 237.5 mg/kg P.C according to the classification of Diezi this plant is relatively toxic. The experiments show that the properties of X. *americana* could due to the presence of saponosides, as show by screening tests performed in this study. These results justified the use of X. *americana* in traditional cure of fever treatment (Soro *et al.*, 2009).

2.5 Antitrypanosomal activity

The in vitro antitrypanosomal activity of methanolic and aqueous extracts of stem bark of *Ximenia americana* was evaluated on Trypanosoma congolense. Blood obtained from a high infected mice with T. *congolense* (10(7) was incubated with methanolic and aqueous extracts at 20, 10 and 5 mg/ml and Diminal(R) (diminazene aceturate) at 200, 100 and 50 µg/ml in a 96 micro plate. The results revealed that methanol and aqueous extracts had activity at 20 and 40 mg/ml however, the methanolic extracts were more active than aqueous extracts at 10 and 5 mg/ml. Phytochemical screening of the methanolic and aqueous extracts of the bark showed that they both had flavonoids, anthraquinones, saponins, terpenes and tannins. The aqueous and methanolic extracts appears to show some potential activity against T. *congolense* (Maikai *et al.*, 2008).

2.6 Anticancer activity

Plants have been show to provide a useful source of natural products that are effective in the treatment of human neoplastic diseases. Information recorded from ancient civilizations has demonstrated the use of plants in search of treatment for various types of cancer (Hartwell, 1967-1971). An analysis of plant materials that had been studied at the National Cancer Institute (NCI), USA for discovering new anticancer drugs showed that if ethnopharmacological information had been used, the yield of plants harboring antineoplastic activity would have been significantly increased (Spjut & Perdue, 1976). The list of natural products stored for study as more effective drugs for the treatment of human cancers (NCI) were generated by searching for specific structural types (Steven & Russel, 1993). However, the presence of some large class cannot be ruled out. Examples of anticancer agents developed from higher plants are the antileukemic bis-indole alkaloids vinblastine and vincristine from the *Catharantus roseus* (Apocynaceae); diterpene taxol, used to treat breast cancer, lung cancer, and ovarian cancer and also used to treat AIDS-related (Kaposi's sarcoma) from *Taxus breviflora* (Taxaceae); pyrrolo[3,4,b]-quinoline alkaloid camptothecin (antileukemic) from *Camptotheca acuminate* (Nyssaceae) and pyridocarbazole alkaloid elipticine (antitumor) contained in *Ochrosia elliptica* (Apocynaceae). A large number of other active natural products with toxicity to cells in culture (Walker carcinosarcoma 256, mouse L-1210 leukemia, Ehrlich ascite tumor, sarcoma 180 and mouse P-388 leukemia cell lines) have been detected (Geran *et al.*, 1972 & Lee *et al.*, 1988).

	Cell line			
Tumor cell lines	IC_{10}[a] (ug/ml medium)	IC_{50}[b] (ug/ml medium)	IC_{90}[c] (ug/ml medium)	IC_{90}/IC_{10}[d] (ug/ml medium)
MCF7	0.6	1.7	10	16.7
BV173	0.4	1.8	7.0	17.5
CC531	0.8	3.3	12	15.0
U87-MG	1.0	9.0	100	100
K562	5.0	11	180	36
SKW-3	3.1	20	700	226
HEp2	5.0	21	100	20
NC1-H460	4.0	21	150	38
PC3	3.5	26	>1000	>300
MDA-MB231	5.0	33	100	20
HT29	8.0	40	350	44
U333	7.0	65	300	43
SAOS2	20	66	1000	50
LAMA84	10	90	600	60
HL60	30	90	1000	33
CML-T1	2.5	160	1000	400
AR230	17	170	700	41
Non tumor cell lines				
MCF10	35	>100	>100	>2.0
MDCK	12	27	60	5.0
N1H/3T3	2	33	>100	>50
PNT-2	2	20	>100	>50

[a]Inhibitory concentration 10 (concentration inhibiting the cell growth by 10%), as accessed by MTT assay;
[b]Inhibitory concentration 50 (concentration inhibiting the cell growth by 50%), as accessed by MTT assay.
[c]Inhibitory concentration 90 (concentration inhibiting the cell growth by 90%), as accessed by MTT assay.
[d]Ratio of IC_{90} and IC_{10} values.

Table 4. Antiproliferative activity of an aqueous extract from *X. americana* in 16 human and one rodent tumor cell lines and in 4 immortalized non-tumor cell lines.

The antineoplastic activity in vitro of various extracts from *Ximenia americana*, plant used in African traditional medicine for the treating cancer, was investigated (Voss *et al.*, 2006, 2006). The most active, aqueous extract was subjected to a detailed investigation in a panel of 17 tumor cell lines (Table 4) originating from human (16 lines) and rat (1 line), showing a averageI C_{50} of 49 mg raw powder/ml medium. The majority of cell lines (11 out of 17) were classified as sensitive (the sensitivity varied from 1.7 mg/ml in MCF7 breast cancer cells to 170 mg/ml in AR230 chronic-myeloid leukemia cells) and three of these (MCF7 breast cancer, BV173 CML and CC531 rat colon carcinoma) showed a particularly high sensitivity, with ratios lower than 0.1 of the average IC_{50}. The *in vivo* antitumor activity was determined in the CC531 coloretal rat model and significant anticancer activity was found following peroral administration, indicating a 95% reduced activity.

A comparison of the antineoplastic activity of the extract with three clinically used agents is given in Table 5. The cytotoxicity profiles of four cell lines are illustrated by the respective IC_{10}, IC_{50} and IC_{90} values, as well as by the corresponding IC_{90} to IC_{10} ratio, describing the slop of the concentration-effect curve. Most prominently, the ranking in sensitivity differed between the extract and the positive controls. In variance to the extract, which resulted in the lowest IC_{50} and IC_{90}/IC_{10} ratio in MCF7 cells, miltefosine and cisplatinum caused the lowest IC_{50} and IC_{90}/IC_{10} ratio in HEp2 cells. Similar to the extract, the lowest IC_{50} following gemcitabine exposure was seen in NCF7 cellls. However, this agent differed from all the others by its lack in effecting 90% growth inhibition, were the HEp2 cells; notably, the cells were most resistant to the agent. In contrast, SAOS2 cells were found to best most resistant to the extract as well as to miltefosine and cisplatinum.

Cell line	Treatment	IC_{50}	IC_{50}	IC_{90}	IC_{90}/IC_{10}
MCF7	Extract (µg/ml)	0.6	1.8	10	16.7
	Miltefosine (µM)	6.5	40	80	12.3
	Cisplatinum (µg/ml)	0.22	2.2	10	45
	Gemcitabine (µM)	0.001	0.012	>100	>10^5
U87-MG	Extract (µg/ml)	1.0	9.0	100	100
	Miltefosine (µM)	4.7	27	70	14.9
	Cisplatinum (µg/ml)	0.12	1.6	18	150
	Gemcitabine (µM)	0.002	0.014	>100	>5×10^4
HEp2	Extract (µg/ml)	5.0	21	100	20
	Miltefosine (µM)	1.2	2,8	8.0	6.7
	Cisplatinum (µg/ml)	0.09	0.4	1.4	15.6
	Gemcitabine (µM)	0.2	0.47	17	85
SAOS2	Extract (µg/ml)	20	66	1000	50
	Miltefosine (µM)	5.0	40	120	24
	Cisplatinum (µg/ml)	0.11	3.1	10	91
	Gemcitabine (µM)	0.007	0.034	>100	>10^4

Table 5. Cytotoxicity profiles of the extract and three standard antineoplastic agents in a subpanel of the cell lines

In order to define the substance class of the active component(s) (Voss *et al.*, 2006) experiments were carried out on physicochemical properties. In the process, lipids and lipophilic plant secondary metabolites could be excluded, since the biological activity was only extracted by strongly polar solvents. Large amounts of tannins were identified in the aqueous extract. However, extracts prepared in methanol or 70% acetone, both solvents known to efficiently extract tannins from plant materials, had only a low (methanol) or no (70% acetone) cytotoxic activity. Molecules smaller than 10 kDa were excluded by ultrafiltration. Out of the known class of plant cell macromolecules, DNA and RNA were not found in the aqueous extract and digestion experiments with DNase or RNase had not effect biological activity. However, proteins and polysaccharides were shown to be present in the aqueous extracts and could not be further separated by physicochemical methods. Digestion experiments with trypsin and proteinase K hinted at a protein being responsible for the cytotoxic activity.

A well-defined family of cytotoxic plant proteins is that of the type II ribosome-inactiving proteins (RIPs). These proteins with molecular weight of about 60 kDa, consist of two polypeptide chain, termed A- and B- chain, with an MW of about 30 kDa each, being held together by disulphide bridge. Cumulative evidences (cytotoxic effects, MW, two-chain structure of the proteins in the affinity-purified fraction and one mass-spectrometrically sequenced tryptic peptides) strongly suggests that the active components of the plant material are so far unknown proteins belonging to the type II RIP family.

By a combination of preextraction, extraction, ion exchange and affinity chromatography, a mixture of two cytotoxic proteins was isolated. The eluted peptides were analyzed by electro-spray ionization mass spectrometry (MS/MS). The MS/MS mass spectrum is a method in which a first analyzer isolates a precursor ion which then undergoes a fragmentation yielding a product ions and neutral fragments. A second spectrometer analyzes the product ions. MS/MS applications are plentiful in the study of fragmentation mechanisms, observation of ion-molecule reactions, applications to high-selectivity and high-sensitivity analysis and determination of elementary compositions. Thus, it is a rapid selective analysis method for the components of a complex mixture and macromolecules in biological fluids. The homology of the translated protein sequence from isolated peptides to known type II RIP precursor protein sequence demonstrates that the new protein termed "riproximin" is a so far unknown member of this class. In conclusion, from biological activity of each of the two proteins as well as from MS/MS sequence analysis, showing the presence of two B-chain and two A-chain in the mixture, the *X. americana* extract analyzed contains a mixture of two new proteins, riproximin, belongs to the family of type II ribosome-inactivating proteins.

Two sesquiterpenes (7 and 8) isolated from the EtOH extract of the stems of *X. americana* did not inhibit the growth of HL-60 (human leukemia), HTC-8 (human colon) and MDA-MB-435 (human breast cancer) cell lines.

The compounds **7** and **8** were recently isolated and their structures were elucidated on the basis of spectral analysis (IV, MS and NMR) and the complete assignment of the ^1H and ^{13}C NMR signals were achieved by 1D(^1H, ^{13}C and DEPT) and 2D (^1H - ^1H COSY, ^1H - ^{13}C HMQC, ^1H-^{13}C HMBC and ^1H - ^1H NOESY) NMR experiments. The sesquiterpene **7**, isolated as a white powder, has molecular formula $C_{15}H_{20}O_4$ deduced from its EIMS (M^{+} 264) in combination with its ^1H and ^{13}C NMR spectra. The ^1H and ^{13}C NMR spectra combined with distortionless enhancement by polarization transfer (DEPT) technique exhibited signals that allowed characterize the three isoprene units (C-1, C-2, C-3, C-4 and C-13; C-8, C-9, C-10, C-11 and C-12; C-5, C-6, C-7, C-14 and C-15) of **7**. Thus, the ^{13}C NMR spectra exhibited signals for six sp^2 carbons [olefinic bond: C-2 (δ_C 128.9), C-3 (δ_C 141.7) and furan ring: C-9 (δ_C 127.9), C-10 (δ_C 147.1), C-11 (δ_C 144.4), C-12 (δ_C 108.9)], two carbonyl [conjugated ketone, C-8 (δ_C 195.3) and conjugated carboxylic acid, C-1 (δ_C 173.1)]), three methylene [C-4 (δ_C 41.2), C-6 (δ_C 36.5) and C-7 (δ_C 35.9), three methyl [C-13 (δ_C 12.4), C-14 (δ_C 25.9) C-15 (δ_C 25.9) and one quaternary carbon [C-5 (δ_C 34.3)]. One conjugated ketone (δ_C 195.3) was also evident from the absorption at 1682 cm^{-1} in the IR spectrum. In the HMBC spectrum, obvious long-range connectivities between the methylene group 2H-7 (δ_H 2.71, dd, 7.9, 6.0 Hz) and C-8 (δ_C 195.57) and between the methylene group 2H-4 (δ_H 2.20, d, 7.7 Hz) and C-5 (δ_C 34.56) allowed the assembly of the molecule and show it to consist of a furanoid sesquiterpene. Others diagnostic ^1H-^1H COSY, ^1H-^{13}C HMQC and ^1H-^{13}C HMBC correlations permitted to assign all the hydrogen and carbon atoms. The sesquiterpene, **8** isolated as a white solid, has molecular formula $C_{15}H_{22}O_2$ deduced from its EIMS (M^{+} 234) in combination with its ^1H and ^{13}C NMR spectra. The ^1H and ^{13}C NMR spectra combined with distortionless enhancement by polarization transfer (DEPT) technique exhibited signals that allowed characterize the three isoprene units (C-1, C-2, C-3, C-11 and C-12; C-4, C-5, C-6, C-13 and C-14; C-7, C-8, C-9, C-10 and C-15) of **8**. The ^{13}C NMR spectra exhibited signals for four sp^2 carbons [three substituted, C-8 (δ_C 132.34) and C-9 (δ_C 145.01) and disubstituted, C-1 (δ_C 154.71) and C-12 (δ_C 111.63) bonds; one conjugated carboxylic acid, C-15 (δ_C 173.71), besides signals to five methylene, two methyne, one quaternary and two methyl carbons. The possibility of himachalano type structure was eliminated based on the interpretation of spin-spin interactions revealed by ^1H-^1H COSY spectrum, which clearly showed the presence of cross peaks corresponding to the couplings of two atoms of hydrogen 2H-6 [δ_H 1.68 (m) and 1.50 (m)] with H-5 hydrogen [δ_H 1.81 (m)] and with the two hydrogen atoms 2H-7 (δ_H 2.45 and 2.35) besides interaction of H-5 (δ_H 1.81) with H-11 (δ_H 2.50, q). This sequence does not appear in the skeleton type himachalano. The *trans* configuration fusion ring was supported by correlations observed in NOESY NMR spectrum, that exhibited the presence of nOes indicating that the hydrogens 3H-13 (δ_H 1.01, s), H-5 (δ_H 1.81) and H-3ax (δ_H 1.58, t, 10.8 Hz) are oriented on the same side (á) of the molecule, while the hydrogens 3H-14 has the same orientation (â) that the hydrogens H-11 (δ_H 2.50, q), H-6ax (δ_H 1.50) and H-3eq (δ_H 1.74, dd, 10.8 , 8.9). Others diagnostic ^1H-^1H COSY, ^1H ^{13}C C HMQC and ^1H ^{13}C ^{13}C HMBC correlations permitted to assign all the hydrogen and carbon atoms.

2.7 Others activities

2.7.1 Antiviral effect

The stem bark MeOH extract of *X. americana* as well as several others plant species used by the Maasai pastoralis of East Africa showed antiviral effect against measles virus *in vitro* by plaque reduction neutralization assay. Potentially active constituents from extracts of all the plants include polyphenols, alkaloids, tannins, sterols, terpenes, saponins and glycosides, between others (Parker *et al.*, 2007).

2.7.2 Hepatic and heamatological effects

A study (James *et al.*, 2008) was conducted from the leaves, stem bark and root aqueous extract of *X. americana* with albino rats. The results of this work shows that the extracts significantly (P<0.05) increasing the level of serum alanine transaminase (ALT) and aspartate transaminase (AST), results indicative of hepatocellular damage. The result also shows that the root has the ability to impair albumin synthesis as observed by the decrease of level of serum albumin. The weight of the animal showed a significant (P<0.05) reduction on administering the leaves extract as compared to the control and the others extracts. This reduction might be due to poor intake and utilization of food by the animals in the leaves extract group. The significantly (P<0.05) higher content of hydrogen cyanide, saponins, and oxalates in the root extracts indicates that the root extracts may be more toxic. Hydrogen cyanide is known to cause gastrointestinal inflammation and inhibition of cellular respiration. Saponins are known to have haemolytic properties and the ability to reduce body cholesterol by preventing its reabsorption. The high saponin content in the root may lead to gastroenteritis manifested by diarrhea. Oxalates have been known to cause irreversible oxalate nefrosis when ingested in large doses. Thus, there is need to isolate the specific component(s) responsible for the toxicity in the root extract in order to standardized the preparation for maximum therapeutic benefit.

2.7.3 Toxicity

The stem bark of *X. americana* was evaluated for its phytochemical constituents and acute toxicity effect on the Swiss albino mice (Maikai *et al.*, 2008). The results from the extracts administered intraperitoneally/orally at doses of 10, 100 and 1000 mg/kg body weight revealed no death with doses up 5000 mg/kg body weight. Post mortem, hematological and histopathological examination did not show any significant (P<0.05) weight changes. Phytochemical screening of the aqueous extract stem bark revealed the presence of cardiac glycosides, flavonoids, saponins and tannins. The results suggested that the aqueous extract is not acutely toxic to the mice.

2.7.4 Food composition and cosmetic use

Glyceride blends containing ximenynic acid (9) (found in *X. americana*) are useful for the preparation of food compositions or food supplements, including margarine, chocolate, ice cream, mayonnaises, cheese, dry soups, drinks, cereal bars and sauces and snack bars. The blend provides a composition providing health benefits consisting of insulin resistance, or related disorders such as diabetes, delaying the onset of symptoms related to development of Alzheimer's disease, improving memory function, lowering blood lipid levels, anticancer effects or skin antiageing effects (Koenen *et al.*, 2004). Food *X. americana* flowers are a replacement for orange blossoms with similar fragrance and soothing cosmetic properties (Paolo, 1979).

$$CH_3(CH_2)_5CH \overset{E}{=\!=\!=} C \equiv C(CH_2)_7CO_2H$$

9

3. Others constituents isolated from *X. americana*

Besides the substances mentioned in the text of this chapter, several other originated from *Ximenia americana* were isolated.

Isoprenoids

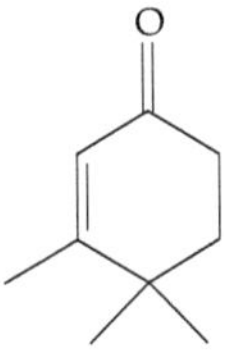

10

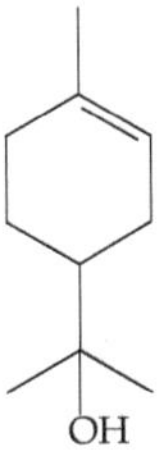

11

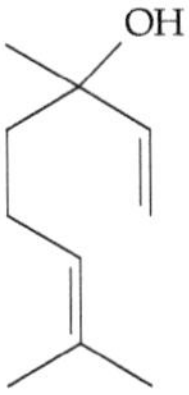

12

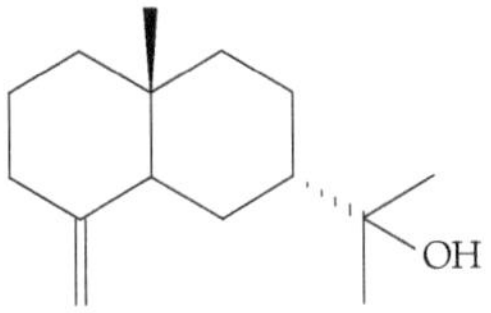

13

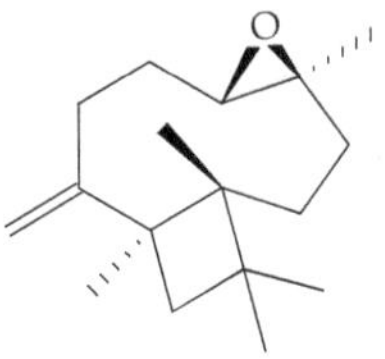

14

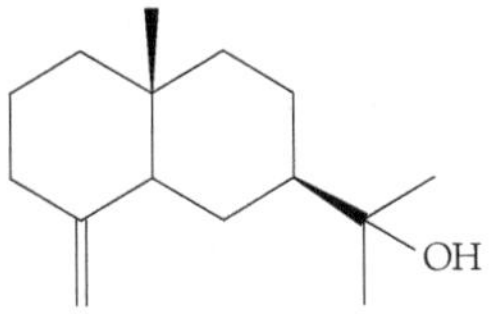

15

Fatty acids

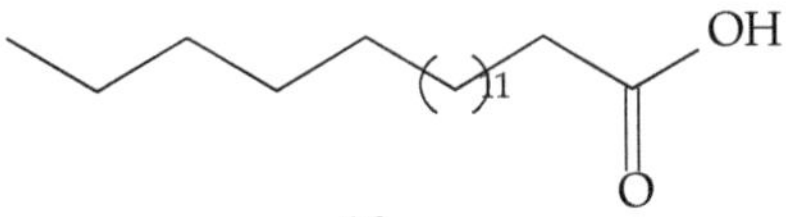

16

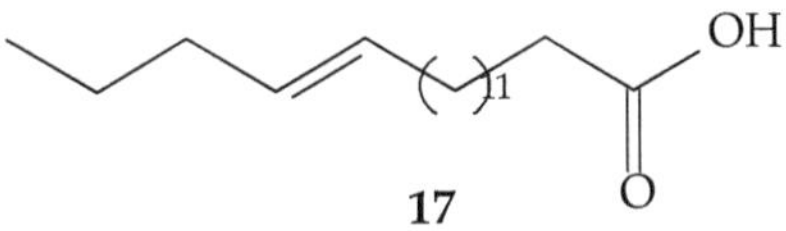

17

Triterpenes

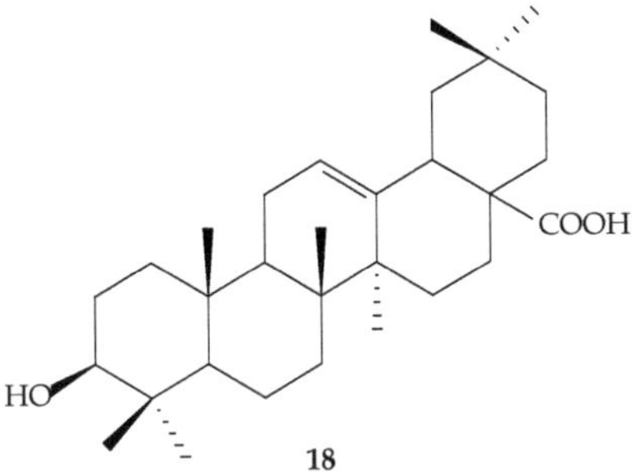

18

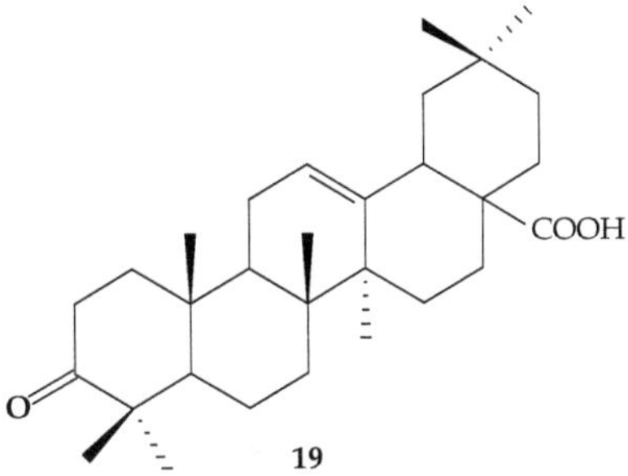

19

20

21

22

23

Steroids

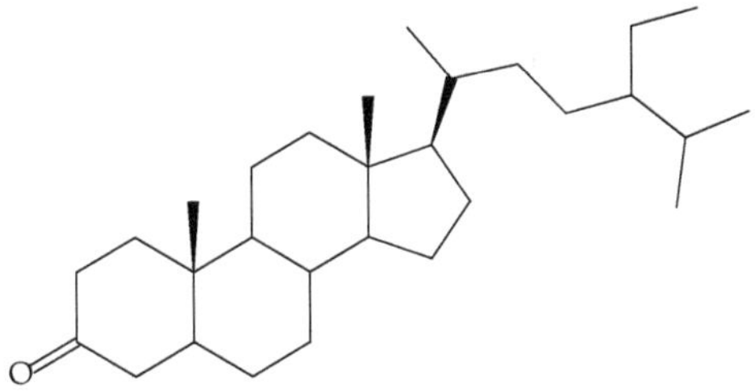

24

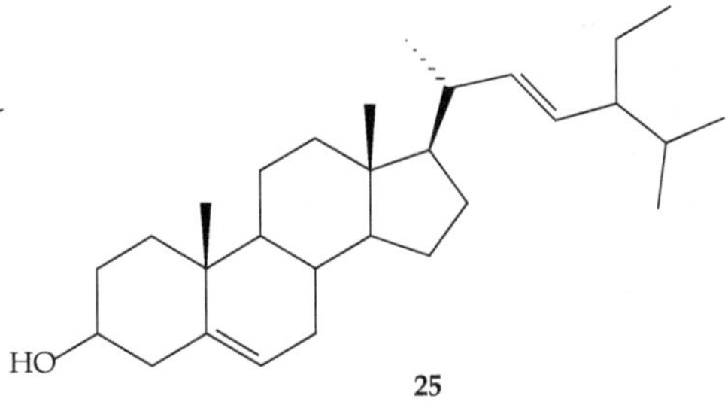

25

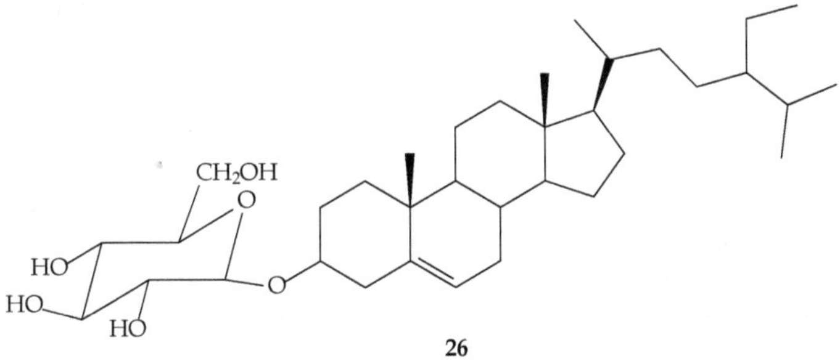

26

4. Summary/conclusion/future directions

From an extensive literature review was observed that the *Ximenia americana* is widely used as a popular alternative remedy in certain regions of some countries of the Africa (Guinea, Ethiopia, Nigeria, Sudan) and in the Brazil. The plant, used by their crude extracts, especially, aqueous and methanolic, showed several biological activities such as antimicrobial, antifungal, anticancer, antitrypanosomal, antirheumatic, antioxidant, analgesic, moluscicide, pesticidal, antipyretic, antifugal, among others. There are several papers in the literature confirming these activities. The crude extracts consist of complex mixture of compounds called secondary metabolites produced by plants, which include, mainly, flavonoids, saponins, alkaloids, quinones, terpenoids, phenols, glycosides and sterols.

Many plants have a prolonged and uneventful use that may serve as indirect evidence to their efficacy. However, in the absence of objective proof of efficacy and without the knowledge of the constituents responsible for the physiological actions, the validity of the remedies is questionable and its use restricted. It generally was observed that the more the constituents in a given species, the more diverse the micro-organisms it acts upon. The difference of activity appears to be directly related to the qualitative and/or quantitative diversity of the compounds that are being accumulated by the plants investigated.

However, detailed studies on the toxicity of extracts revealed through phytochemical screening showed that many constituents chemicals can affect the animal positively or negatively as a result of prolong usage. Thus, was founded that tannins and anthraquinones are thought to have both proxidant and antioxidant effects on the body. While the antioxidant protects, the proxidant damage the tissues and organs. Also, was observed that the presence of tannins and other compounds interferes with absorption of nutrients such proteins and minerals resulting in weight loss. The extracts contained the presence of saponins has been reported to produce free radicals and hydrogen peroxide during its oxidation to semiquinone in the body, is thought to damage the cells of the body. The results of several studies conducted so far have produced a scientific basis that can justify the use of *Ximenia americana* in medicine. As we see the many works on *X. americana* show its effectiveness in treating various diseases. In all studies, were highlighted the participation and importance of secondary metabolites produced by them. However, there are still many details to be clarified. As mentioned above, in general, it was observed that the more the constituents in a given species, the more diverse the micro-organisms it acts upon. Moreover, the activity of plant extracts seems to be related to quality and quantity of metabolites present, possibly due to the possibility of synergism while, different types of metabolites appear to be related to specific biologic actions. In this context it is important to point out that the norisoprenoid isophorane (10), shown to be carcinogenic agent (Mevy *et al.*, 2006), was identified in the leaves of *X. americana*, which would conflict with its use in treating cancer. The last report about compounds isolated from *X. americana* up to date were the sesquiternes 7 and 8, triterpenoids 18-22 and steroids 24-26, all from ethanol extract of stems (Araújo *et al.*, 2008, 2009). Some of them have not yet been exhaustively investigated from the point of view of biological activity.

Future studies should be performed using chromatographic methods such as HPLC (high performance liquid chromatography) and LC-MS (Liquid chromatography coupled to mass spectroscopy) to obtain the chromatographic profile of the chemical composition of the extracts. Then carry out guided study (biological activity) in order to isolate and identify the pure constituents. Finally, as reported, many compounds may exhibit both carcinogenic and anticarcinogenic effects but it is not excluded that the occurrence of compounds other than volatile constituents may act in the anticarcinogenic process. Consequently, these results encourage further investigations to extracts and identify the active chemical compounds responsible for the specific biological activity in order to standardized the plant preparation for maximum therapeutic benefit.

5. References

Araújo, M. R. S.; Assunção, J. C. C., Dantas, I. N. F., Costa-Lotufo, L. V. & Monte, F. J. Q. (2008). Chemical Constituents of *Ximenia americana*. *Natural Products Communications*, Vol. 3, No. 6, pp. 857-860, ISSN 1934-578X

Araújo, M. R. S.; Monte, F. J. Q. & Braz-Filho, R. (2009). A New Sesquiterpene from *Ximenia americana* Linn. *Helvetica Chimica Acta*, Vol. 92, pp. 127-129, ISSN 0018-019X.

Atta-ur-Rahman. (1988). Studies *in Natural Products Chemistry, Structure Elucidation*, Vol.32, Elsevier, New York, U.S.A.

Atta-ur-Rahman (Elsevier) (2005). *Studies in Natural Products, Bioactive Natural Products (Part L), Vol. 32*, Atta-ur-Rahamn, Karachi, Pakistan , ISBN 9780444521712.

Badami, R. C. & Patil, K. B. (1981). Structure and Ocurrence of Unusual Fatty Acids in Minor Seed Oils. *Progress in l Lipid Research*, Vol. 19, pp. 119-153, ISSN 01637827.

Braga, R. (3ª Ed). (1976). *Plantas do Nordeste, especialmente do Ceará*, Escola Superior de Agricultura, Mossoró, Brasil.

Brasileiro, M. T.; Egito, M. A. & Lima, J. R.; Randau, K. P.; Pereira G. C.; Neto, P. J. R. (2008). *Ximenia americana* L: botânica, química e farmacologia no interesse da tecnologia farmacêutica. *Revista Brasileira Farmacognosia*, 89, 2, pp. 164-167, ISSN 0370-372X.

Bruneton, J. (3ª Ed) (1999). *Pharmacognosie, phytochimie, plantes médicinales*, Tec & Doc Ed., Angers, France.

Chhabra S. C.; Viso, F. C., (1990). A Survey of the Medicinal Plants Eastern Tanzania for Alkaloids, Flavonoids, Saponins and Tannins. *Fitoterapia*, Vol. 61, No. 4, pp. 307-316, ISSN 2367326X.

Dixon, R. A.; Dey, P. M. & Lamb, C. J. (1983). Phytoalexins: enzymology and molecular bilogy. *Advance Enzymology*, Vol. 55, pp. 1-69.

Fatope, M. O.; Adoum, O. A. & Takeda, Y. (2000). C_{18} Acetylenic Fatty Acids of *Ximenia americana* with Potential Pesticidal Activity. *Journal of Agricultural and Food Chemistry*, Vol. 48, pp. 1872-1874, ISSN 00218561.

Finnermore, H. J. M. Cooper, M. B. Stanlet, J. H. Cobcroff & L. J. Harris, (1988). Journal of the Indian chemical Society, Vol. 57, pp. 162-169 ISSN 0019-4522.

Geran, R. T.; Greenberg, M. N.; MacDonald, A. M.; Schumacher, A. M. & Abbot, B. J. (1972). Protocols for screening chemical agents and natural products against animal tumors and other biological systems. *Cancer Chemotherapy Reports*, Vol. 3. p. 1, ISSN 00690112.

Geyid, A.; Abebe, D.; Debella, A.; Makonnen, Z.; Aberra, F.; Teka, F.; Kebede, T.; Urga, K.; Yersaw, K.; Biza, T.; Mariam, B. H. & Guta, M. (2005). Screening of medicinal plants of Ethiopia for their anti-microbial properties and chemical profiles. *Journal of Ethnopharmacology*, Vol. 97, pp. 421-427, ISSN 0378-8741.

Hartwell, J. L. (1967; 1968; 1969; 1970; 1971). Plants used against cancer. *Loydia*, Vol. 30 p. 379; Vol. 31, p. 71; Vol. 32, p. 71, 153, 247; Vol. 33, p. 98, 288; Vol. 34, p. 103, 204, 310, 386.

Hostettman, K.; Marston, A. J.; Wolfender, L & Miallard, M. (1995). *Screening for flavonoids and related compounds in medicinal plants by LC-UV-MS and subsequent isolation of bioctive compounds*, Akademiiai, Kiaho, Budapest, Hungry.

Jacbson, M. (1971). *Naturally Occurring Insecticides*, M. Crosby. D. G. Eds.: Dekker, New York, U.S.A.

James, D. B.; Abu, E. A.; Wurochekke, A. U. & Orgi, G. N. (2007). Phytochemical and Antimicrobial Investigation of the Aqueous and Methanolic Extracts of *Ximenia americana*. Journal of *Medical Science*, Vol. 7, No. 2, (15th february 2007), pp. 284-288, ISSN 20721625.

James, D. B.; Owolabi, A. O.; Ibiyeye, H.; Magaji, J. & Ikugiyi, Y. A. (2008). Assessment of the hepatic effects , heamatological effect and some phytochemical constituents of

Ximenia Americana (Leaves, stem and root) extracts. *African Journal of Biotechnology*, Vol. 7, No. 23, (December, 2008), pp. 4274-4278, ISSN 1684-5315.

Koenen, C.; Schmid, U.; Rogers, J.; Peilow, A.; Bosley, J.; Eggink, M. & Stam, W. (2004). Blend used in preparing, food composition, e. g. margarine, comprises ximenynic acid originating from natural source and fatty acids or glycerides. *Derwent Innovations Index*, patent No. EP1402787-A1, (June 2004), U.S.A., 4p.

Loganathan, D.; Trivedi, G. K. & Chary, K. V. R. (1990). A Two Dimensional NMR Strategy for the Complete ^{1}H Chemical Shift Assignment of Extended Proton Spin Systems in Triterpenoids. *Magnetic Resonance in Chemistry*, 28, 11, (July 1990), pp. 925-930, ISSN 1097-458X.

Magassouba, F. B.; Diallo, A.; Kouyaté, M.; Mara, F.; Mara, O.; Bangoura, O.; Camara, A.; Traoré, S.; Diallo, A. K.; Zaoro, M.; Lamah, K.; Diallo, S.; Camara, G.; Kéita, A.; Camara, M. K.; Barry, R.; Kéita, S.; Oularé, K.; Barry, M. S.; Donzo, M.; Camara, K.; Toté, K.;. Vanden Berghe, D.; Totté, J.; Pieters, L.; Vlietinck, A. J. & Baldé, A. M. (2007). Ethnobotanical survey and antibacterial activity of some plants used in Guinean traditional medicine. *Journal of Ethnopharmacology*, Vol. 114, pp. 44-53, ISSN 0378-8741.

Mahato, S. B.; Nandy, A. K. & Roy, G. (1992). Triterpenoids. *Phytochemistry*, Vol. 31, pp. 2199-2249, ISSN 0031-9422.

Maikai, V. A.; Kobo, P. I. & Adaudi, A. O. (2008). Acute toxicity studies of aqueous stem bark extract of *Ximenia Americana*. *African Journal of Biotechnology*, Vol. 7, No. 10, (May, 2008), pp. 1600-1603, ISSN 1684-5315.

Maikai, V. A.; Maikai, B. V. & Kobo, P. I. (2009). Antimicrobial Properties of Stem Bark Extracts of *Ximenia americana*. *Journal of Agricultural Science.*, Vol.1, No. 2, (December 2009), pp. 30-34. ISSN 00218596.

Maikai, V. A.; Nok, J. A.; Adaudi, A. O. & Alawa, C. B. I. (2008). In vitro antitrypanosomal activity of aqueous and methanolic crude extracts of stem bark of *Ximenia americana* on *Trypanosoma congolense*. *Journal of Medicinal Plants*, Vol. 2, No. 3, pp. 55-58, ISSN 16840240.

Mathabe, M. C.; Nikova, R. V.; Lall, N. & Nyazema, N. Z. (2006). Antibacterial activities of medicinal plants used for the treatment of diarrhoea in Limpopo province, South Africa. *Journal of Ethnopharmacology*, 105, pp. 286-293, ISSN 0378-8741.

Matos, F. J. A. (2007). *Plantas medicinais: guia de seleção e emprego de plantas usadas em fitoterapia no Nordeste do Brasil*, Imprensa Universitária, Fortaleza, Brasil.

Mevy, J-P.; Bessiere, J-M.; Greff, S.; Zombre, G. & Viano, J. (2006). Composition of the volatile oil from leaves of *Ximenia americana* L. *Biochemical Systematics and Ecology*, Vol. 34, pp. 549-553, ISSN 0305-1978.

Ogunleye, D. S.; Ibitoye & Trop,S. F. (2003). Studies of antimicrobial activity and chemical constituents of *Ximenia americana*. *Journal of Pharmmaceutical Research*, Vol. 2, No. 2, (December 2003), pp. 239-241, ISSN 00223549.

Omer, M. E. F. A. & Elnima, E. I. (2003). Antimicrobial activiy of *Ximenia americana*. *Fitoterapia*, Vol. 74, pp. 122-126, ISSN 0367326X.

Paolo, R. (1979). Cosmetic use of the oil and flowers of *Ximenia americana*. *Rivista Italiana Essenze*, Vol. 61, No. 5, pp. 190-193, ISSN 0391-4658.

Parker, M. E.; Chabot, S.; Ward, B. J. & Johns, T. (2007). Traditional dietary additives of the Maasai are antiviral against the measles virus. *Journal of Ethnopharmacology*, Vol. 114, pp. 146-152, ISSN 0378-8741.

Pio-Correia, M. (1984). *Dicionário de Plantas Úteis do Brasil e das Éxoticas Cultivadas*, Imprensa Nacional, Rio de Janeiro, Brasil.

Rezanka, T & Sigler, K. (2007). Identification of very long chain unsaturated fatty acids from *Ximenia* oil by atmospheric pressure chemical ionization liquid chromatography-mass spectroscopy. *Phytochemistry*,Vol. 68, pp. 925-934, ISSN 00319422.

Saeed, A. E. M. & Bashier, R. S. M. (2010). Physico-chemical analysis of *Ximenia americana* L. oil and structure elucidation of some chemical constituents of its seed oil and fruit pulp. *Journal of Pharmacognosy and Phytotherapy*, Vol. 2, No. 4, pp. 49-55. ISSN 21412502.

Scalbert, A. (1991). Antimicrobial properties of tannins. *Phytochemisty*, Vol. 30, pp. 3875-3883, ISSN 00319422.

Siddaiah, M.; Jayavcera, K. N.; Mallikarjuna, R. P.; Ravindra, R. K.; Yasodha, K. Y. & Narender, R. G. (2009). Phytochemical screening and analgesic activity of methanolic extract of *Ximenia americana. Journal of Pharmacy and Chemistry*, Vol. 3, No. 1, pp. 23-25, ISSN 0973-9874.

Soro, T. Y.; Traore, F. ; Datte, J. Y. & Nene-Bi, A. S. (2009). Antipyretic activity of aqueous extract of *Ximenia americana. Phytoterapie*, Vol. 7, No. 6, pp. 297-303, ISSN 1624-8597.

Soro, T. Y.; Traore, F. & Sakande, J. (2009). Activité analgésique de l' extrait aqueux de *Ximenia americana* (Linné) (Olacaceae). *Comptes Rendus Biologies*, Vol. 332, pp. 371-377, ISSN 16310691.

Spjut, R. W. & Perdue Jr., R. E. (1976). Plant folklore: a tool for predicting sources of antitumor activity ?. *Cancer Treatiment Reports*, Vol. 60, pp. 979-985.

Sptizer, V.; Tomberg, W. & Aichholz, R. (1997). Analysis of Seed Oil of *Heisteria silvanii* (Olacaceae) – A rich Source of Novel C_{18} Acetylenic Fatty Acid. *Lipids*, Vol. 32, pp. 1189-1200, ISSN 00244201.

Steven, M. C. & Russel, J. M. (1993). *Bioactive Natural Products*, CRC Press, ISBN 0-8493-4372-0, Boca Raton, U. S. A.

Tassou, C. C.; Drosinos, E. H. &. Nychas, G. J. E. (1995). Effects of essential oils from mint (*Mentha piperita*) on *Salmonella enteitidis* and *Listeria monocytogenes* in model Food systems at 4° and 10°C. *Journal of Applied Bacteriology*, Vol. 78, pp. 593-600, ISSN 00218847.

Taylor, R. S.L.; Edet, F. Manandhar, N. P. & Towers, G. H. N. (1996). Antimicrobial activities of southern Nepalase medicinal plants. *Journal of Ethnopharmacology*, Vol. 50, pp. 97-102, ISSN 0378-8741.

Voss, C.; Eyol, E. & Berger, M. R. (2006). Identification of potent anticancer activity in *Ximenia americana* aqueous extracts used by African traditional medicine. *Toxicology and Applied Pharmacology*, Vol. 211, pp. 177-178, ISSN 0041-008X.

Voss, C.; Eyol, E.; Frank, M.; von der Lieth, Claus-W & Berger, M. R. (2006). Identification and characterization of riproximin, a new type II ribosome-inactivating protein with antineoplastic activity from *Ximenia americana*. *Toxicology and Applied Pharmacology*, Vol. 20, pp. 334-345, ISSN 0041008X.

Ya, C.; Gaffney, S. H.; Lilley, T. H. & Haslam. E. (R. W. Heminway and J. J. Karchesy Ed). (1988). *Carbohydrate-polyphenol complexation*, Plenum Press, New York, U.S.A.

8

Phytochemicals and Their Pharmacological Aspects of *Acanthopanax koreanum*

Young Ho Kim, Jeong Ah Kim and Nguyen Xuan Nhiem
Chungnam National University,
South Korea

1. Introduction

Botanical medicines have been applied for the treatment of various human diseases with thousands of years of history all over the world. In some Asian and African countries, 80 % of population depends on traditional medicine in primary health care. On the other hand, in many developed countries, 70 % to 80 % of the population has used some forms of alternative or complementary medicine. The long tradition of using plants for medicine, supplemented by pharmaceutical research, has resulted in many plant-based Western medicines. Traditional medicine has provided Western medicine with over 40 % of all pharmaceuticals (Samuelsson & Bohlin, 2004). In the past decades, therefore, research has been focused on scientific evaluation of traditional drugs of plant origin.

Acanthopanax species (Araliaceae) are widely distributed in Asia, Malaysia, Polynesia, Europe, North Africa and the America. There are about 40 species of *Acanthopanax* to be found in over the world. *Acanthopanax* species have traditionally been used as a tonic and sedative as well as in the treatment of rheumatism, and diabetes. *A. koreanum* Nakai is an indigenous plant prevalently distributed throughout South Korea. It is deciduous shrub with upright to slightly arching stems, small, fresh green, trilobed to palmately divided leaves and several axillary as well as terminal round clusters of decorative, bluish black berries in late summer and autumn. Extensive investigation of chemical components in *A. koreanum* has been reported by many researchers in the worldwide. Several types of compounds have been isolated from this plant. Major active constituents are reported as lupanes and their glycosides, diterpenes, monoterpenes, lignans, phenylpropanoids, flavonoids from whole parts of *A. koreanum*. Of these, lupane triterpenes were reported as major components of leaves and *ent*-kauranes are main components of the roots of *A. koreanum*. They showed significant biological effects by several bioassay systems such as 1) anti-inflammatory activities: inhibit lipopolysaccharide (LPS)-stimulated TNF-α, IL-6, and IL-12 p40 productions in bone marrow-derived dendritic cells, decrease the expression of inducible nitric oxide synthase (iNOS) and cyclooxygenase-2 (COX-2) proteins, and reduce iNOS and COX-2 mRNA in a dose-dependent pattern, 2) anticancer, and 3) anti-osteoporosis by effects on the differentiation of osteoblastic MC3T3-E1 cells. The desired target of this chapter is to introduce explanations of structures and pharmacological activities of novel compounds, which have been isolated and identified from *A. koreanum* since 1985. Those studies have reported and focused on bioactivities of unambiguous compounds from *A. koreanum*, therefore we discuss new pharmacological findings on these compounds.

The depth and breadth of research involving this plant has been organized into easily accessible and comparable information. Using Chemical Abstracts, Scifinder Scholar, and BIOSIS databases, relevant research papers were selected by based on pertinence and specificity to ethnopharmacology and phytochemistry, as well as readability. This collection was then carefully reviewed, extracted, and corroborated with available characterization data from other sources.

2. Phytochemistry and pharmacology of *A. koreanum*

2.1 Lupane aglycones

Impressic acid (1) was isolated for the first time from *Schefflera impressa* by (Srivastava, 1992) and it was found in the roots (Cai et al., 2004b) and the leaves (Kim et al., 2010) of *A. koreaum*. Impressic acid exhibited potently NFAT inhibitory activity with IC_{50} value of 12.6 µM. In the studies of (Kim et al., 2010), impressic acid (1) and (20*R*)-3α-hydroxy-29-dimethoxylupan-23,28-dioic acid (4) showed significantly anti-inflammatory activities by inhibiting TNF-α, IL-6, and IL-12 p40 productions in bone marrow-derived dendritic cells with LPS-stimulated. Furthermore, impressic acid was found to inhibit TNF-α-induced NF-κB activity by inhibiting the induction of COX-2 and iNOS in HepG2 cells. Impressic acid also up-regulated the transcriptional activity of PPAR by elevating the expression of PPARγ1, PPARγ2, and SREBF-2, and by suppressing the expression of Insig-2 (Kim et al., 2011). One new norlupane, 3α,11α-dihydroxy-20,23-dioxo-30-norlupane-28-oic acid (2) as well as two known lupane aglycones, impressic acid (1), 3α,11α-dihydroxy-lup-20(29)-en-23-al-28-oic acid (3) were isolated and determined by (Park et al., 2010). They were evaluated for the differentiation of osteoblastic MC3T3-E1 cells. Among of them, compound 1 significantly increased osteoblastic cell growth and differentiation as assessed by MTT assay and collagen content. Compound 2 significantly increased the growth of MC3T3-E1 cells and caused a significant elevation of osteoblastic cell differentiation as assessed by the alkaline phosphatase activity (Park et al., 2010). Other compounds, 3α,11α-dihydroxy-lup-20(29)-en-23-al-28-oic acid, 3α-hydroxylup-20(29)-en-23,28-dioic acid (5), and 3α,11α,23-trihydroxy-lup-20(29)-en-28-oic acid (6) were also isolated from steamed leaves (Kim et al., 2010). However, they showed weak anti-inflammatory activity. 3α-Hydroxylup-20(29)-en-23,28-dioic acid (5) possessed broader antiviral activity against respiratory syncytial, influenza (H1N1), coxsackie B3, and herpes simplex virus type 1 viruses with IC_{50} values of 6.2, 25.0, 12.5, and 18.8 µg/mL, respectively (Li et al., 2007).

2.2 Lupane-triterpene glycosides

Up to date, eighteen lupane-type triterpene glycosides have been isolated from this plant and almost of them from the leaves of *A. koreanum*. They are main saponin components of the leaves of *A. koreanum*. The first lupane triterpene glycoside, acantrifoside A (1) was isolated from both *A. koreanum* and *A. trifoliatus* in a year of 1998 by (Yook et al., 1998). And then, two new saponins, acankoreoside A (10) and acankoreoside B (11) were isolated from the leaves of this plant (Chang et al., 1998). Our group reported seven new lupane-type triterpene glycosides, acankoreosides I-O. Their biological activities were evaluated for

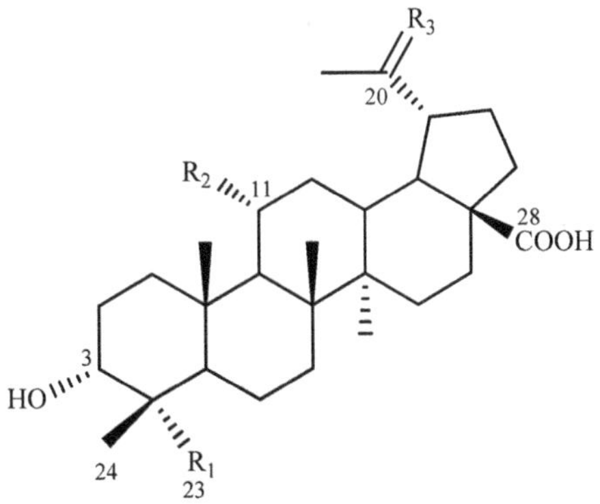

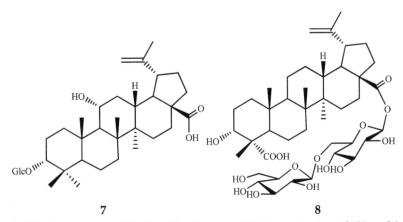

Name	Parts	R_1	R_2	R_3	Reference
Impressic acid (1)	leaves roots	CH_3	OH	CH_2	(Cai et al., 2004b)
3α,11α-Dihydroxy-20,23-dioxo-30-norlupane-28-oic acid (2)	leaves	CHO	OH	=O	(Park et al., 2010)
3α,11α-Dihydroxy-lup-20(29)-en-23-al-28-oic acid (3)	leaves	CHO	OH	CH_2	(Park et al., 2010)
(20R)-3α-Hydroxy-29-dimethoxylupan-23,28-dioic acid (4)	steamed leaves	COOH	H	$CH(OCH_3)_2$	(Kim et al., 2010)
3α-Hydroxylup-20(29)-en-23,28-dioic acid (5)	steamed leaves	COOH	H	CH_2	(Kim et al., 2010)
3α,11α,23-Trihydroxy-lup-20(29)-en-28-oic acid (6)	steamed leaves	CH_2OH	OH	CH_2	(Kim et al., 2010)

Fig. 1. Structures of main lupane-type triterpenes isolated from *Acanthopanax koreanum*

Fig. 2. 3-*O*-β-D-glucopyranosyl 3α,11α-dihydroxylup-20(29)-en-28-oic acid (7) and 3α-hydroxylup-20(29)-en-23,28-oic acid 28-*O*-[β-D-Glucopyranosyl-(1→6)-β-D-Glucopyranosyl] ester (8) (Kim et al., 2010)

cytotoxic activities including A549 (lung), HL-60 (acute promyelocytic leukemia), MCF-7 (breast), U937 (leukemia) cancer cell lines; immune enhancement activity (INF-γ and IL-2 release in spleen cells); anti-inflammatory (inhibitory TNF-α, IL-6, and IL-12 p40 productions in bone marrow-derived dendritic cells with LPS-stimulated, and RAW 264.7). Searching for anticancer activities from natural compounds, several acankoreosides showed significantly cytotoxic activities in various cancer cell lines (A549, HL-60, MCF-7, and U937). The effects of three new lupane glycosides, acankoreosides F-H (**13**, **14**, and **21**) on the LPS-induced production of nitric oxide and prostaglandin E_2 were evaluated in RAW 264.7 macrophages. Among of them, acankoreoside F (**13**) showed the most potent inhibitory PGE_2 (59.0 %) and NO (42.0 %) production at concentration of 200.0 µM. Furthermore, eleven lupane triterpene glycosides from *A. koreanum*, including three new compounds acankoreoside M-O (**16**, **24**, and **25**) were evaluated for Con A-induced splenolytic production of IL-2 and IFN-γ. The results indicated that acankoreosides A (**10**), D (**12**), L (**24**), and acantrifoside A (**9**)

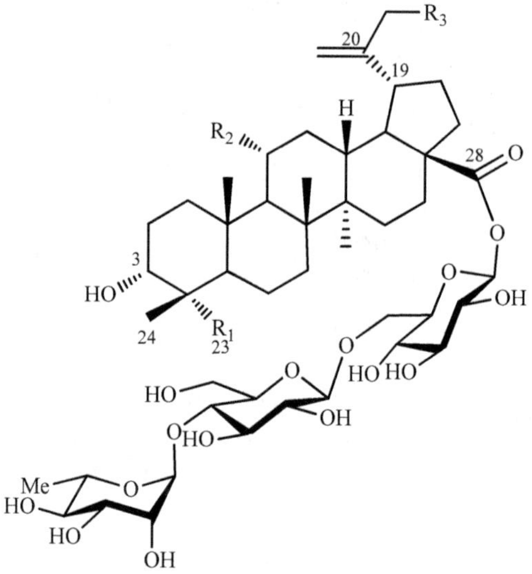

Names	Parts	R_1	R_2	R_3	Ref.
Acantrifoside A (**9**)	leaves	CH₃	OH	H	(Yook et al., 1998)
Acankoreoside A (**10**)	leaves, roots	COOH	H	H	(Chang et al., 1998) (Cai et al., 2004b)
Acankoreoside B (**11**)	leaves	CH₂OH	OH	H	(Chang et al., 1998)
Acankoreoside D (**12**)	leaves	CHO	OH	H	(Chang et al., 1999)
Acankoreoside F (**13**)	leaves	COOH	H	OH	(Choi et al., 2008)
Acankoreoside G (**14**)	leaves	CHO	H	OH	(Choi et al., 2008)
Acankoreoside I (**15**)	leaves	CHO	OH	OH	(Nhiem et al., 2009)
Acankoreoside M (**16**)	leaves	COOH	OH	OH	(Nhiem et al., 2010b)
3-Epibetulinic acid 28-O-glc-glc-rha (**17**)	leaves, roots	CH₃	H	H	(Cai et al., 2004b)

Fig. 3. Structures of lupane-type triterpene glycosides from *A. koreanum*

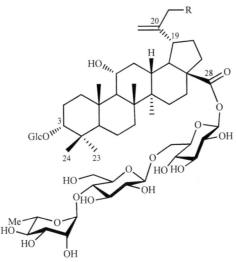

Name	Part	R	Reference
Acankoreoside C (18)	leaves	H	(Chang et al., 1999)
Acankoreoside N (19)	leaves	OH	(Nhiem et al., 2010b)

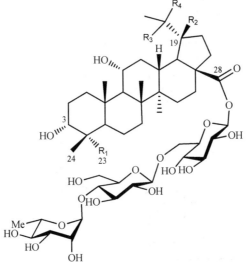

Name	Part	R₁	R₂	R₃	R₄	Reference
Acankoreoside E (20)	leaves	COOH	H	H	CHO	(Park et al., 2005)
Acankoreoside H (21)	leaves	CHO	H	H	COOH	(Choi et al., 2008)
Acankoreoside J (22)	leaves	COOH	H	=O	-	(Nhiem et al., 2010a)
Acankoreoside K (23)	leaves	COOH	H	OH	Me	(Nhiem et al., 2010a)
Acankoreoside L (24)	leaves	COOH	H	OH	CH₂OH	(Nhiem et al., 2010a)
Acankoreoside O (25)	leaves	COOH	OH	H	CH₃	(Nhiem et al., 2010b)

Fig. 3. Structures of lupane-type triterpene glycosides from *A. koreanum* (continued)

significantly increased both IL-2 and IFN-γ. The structure-activity relationship of these compounds was also discussed. Moreover, lupane aglycones and lupane glycosides were assayed for LPS-stimulated pro-inflammatory cytokine production. These results suggested lupane aglycone inhibited pro-inflammatory cytokine production stronger than lupane glycosides (Kim et al., 2010). This was further confirmed by the study of (Cai et al., 2004b).

2.3 Pimarane-type diterpenes

A number of pimarane-type diterpenes have been isolated and associated with significant biological activity. There are seven pimarane-type diterpenes from *A. koreanum*. All of them were isolated from the roots. Acanthoic acid was presented in roots and leaves of this plant, and was one of compounds having potent anti-inflammatory activity. Acanthoic acid, a pimarane diterpene ((-)-pimara-9(11),15-dien-19-oic acid), was isolated for the first time from *A. koreanum* in a year of 1988 by (Kim et al., 1988b) and was proved with high content of this plant. Acanthoic acid has widely exhibited of biological activities. In study of (Kang et al., 1996), acanthoic acid has potent anti-inflammatory effects by reducing the production of proinflammatory cytokines such as IL-1 and TNF-α. It was also effective in supressing experimental silicosis and cirrhosis. Furthermore, acanthoic acid was found to suppress TNF-α gene expression (Kang et al., 1998) and TNF-α-induced IL-8 production in a dose-dependent manner. Acanthoic acid also inhibited TNF-α-induced MAPKs activation, IκB degradation, NF-κB nuclear translocation, and NF-κB/DNA binding activity (Kim et al., 2004). Furthermore, acanthoic acid significantly inhibited production of both TNF-α and tryptase in trypsin-stimulated human leukemic mast cell-1 at concentrations of 10 and 100 µg/mL with a dose-dependent manner. Acanthoic acid inhibited ERK phosphorylation and NF-κB activation induced by trypsin treatment without blocking of trypsin activity even though 100 µg/mL. These results suggested that acanthoic acid may inhibit the production of inflammatory mediators through inhibition of ERK phosphorylation and NF-κB activation pathway in human mast cells (Kang et al., 2006).

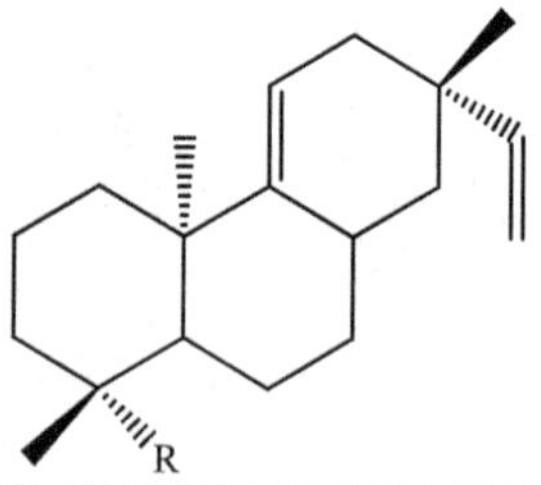

Name	Part	R	Reference
(-)-Pimara-9(11),15-dien-19-ol (**26**)	root barks	CH_2OH	(Kim et al., 1988b)
Acanthoic acid (**27**)	roots, leaves	COOH	(Kim et al., 1988b)
(-)-Pimara-9(11),15-dien-19-ol 19-acetate (**28**)	root barks	CH_2OAc	(Kim et al., 1988b)
(-)-Pimara-9(11),15-diene (**29**)	root barks	CH_3	(Kim et al., 1988b)

Fig. 4. Structures of pimarane-type diterpenes from *A. koreanum*

The hepatoprotective effects of acanthoic acid were evaluated in a D-galactosamine/ lipopolysaccharide-induced fulminant hepatic failure mouse model. The effects were likely associated with a significant decrease in serum TNF-α levels, which are correlated not only with those of alanine aminotransferase and aspartate aminotransferase but also with the reduced number of apoptotic hepatocytes in the liver as confirmed using the terminal deoxynucleotidyl transferase-mediated (dUTP) nick end-labeling method and DNA fragmentation assay (Nan et al., 2008). The protective effect of acanthoic acid was investigated in acetaminophen-induced hepatic toxicity. These results indicated that acanthoic acid protected liver tissue from oxidative stress elicites by acetaminophen-induced liver damage (Wu et al., 2010). Acanthoic acid markedly suppressed the protein expression of TNF-α, COX-2, NF-κB and chymase as well as the mRNA expression of TNF-α and COX-2 (Kang et al., 2010).

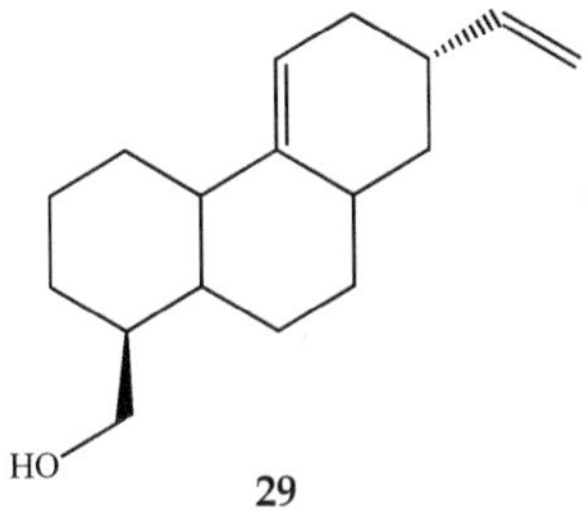

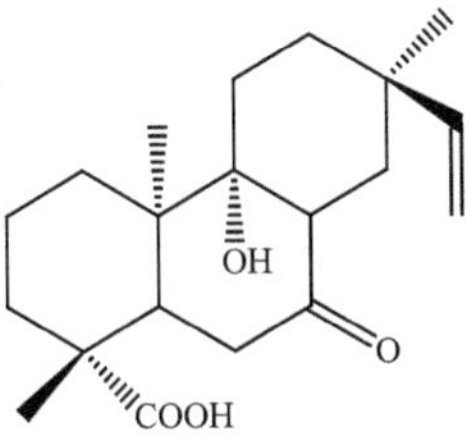

Isopimara-9(11),15-dien-19-ol (29)	roots	(Chung & Kim, 1986)
Acanthokoreoic acid A (30)	roots	(Cai et al., 2003a)

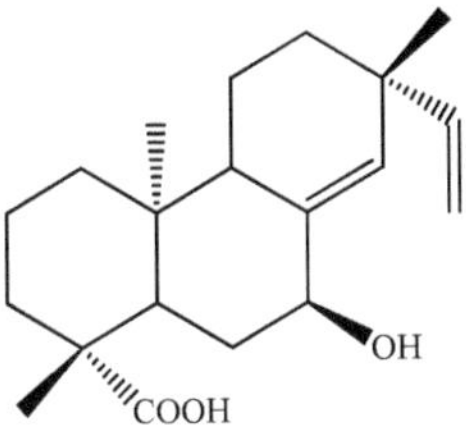

7β-Hydroxy-*ent*-pimara-8(14),15-dien-19-oic acid (31)	roots	(Cai et al., 2004a)
Sumogaside (32)	roots	(Cai et al., 2004a)

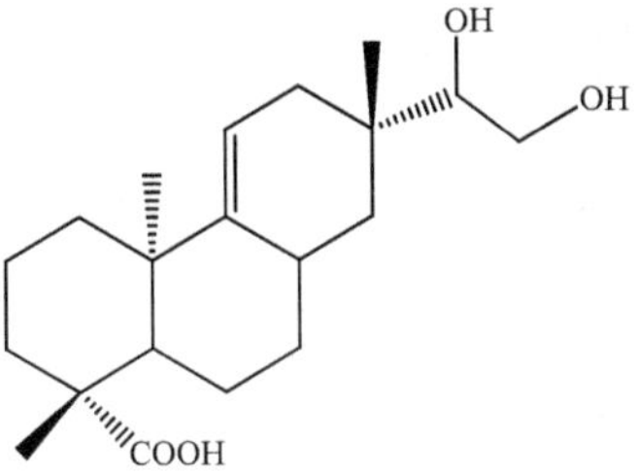

Fig. 4. Structures of pimarane-type diterpenes from *A. koreanum* (continued)

In study of (Cai et al., 2003a), a new compound, acanthokoreoside acid A (30) as well as acanthoic acid (27), (-)-pimara-9(11),15-dien-19-ol (26), and sumogaside (32) were isolated from CH₂Cl₂ fraction of *A. koreanum* roots. They were evaluated for inhibitory activity on IL-8 secretion in TNF-α-stimulated HT-29 and TNF-α secretion in trypsin-stimulated HMC-1. In the TNF- α-stimulated HT-29, acanthoic acid and sumogaside significantly inhibited IL-8 secretion at concentrations of 1, 10, and 100 μM and at concentrations of 10 and 100 μM, respectively.

2.4 *ent*-Kaurane-type diterpenes

ent-Kaurane, a tetracyclic diterpene, has been proven to excert various biological activities like cytotoxicity, anti-inflammation, and so on. From the roots of *A. koreanum*, (Kim et al., 1988b) and (Cai et al., 2003b) isolated six *ent*-kaurane-type diterpenes, including *ent*-kaur-16-en-19-oic acid (**33**), 16α-hydroxy-*ent*-kauran-19-oic acid (**34**), paniculoside IV (**35**), 16αH,17-isovaleryloxy-*ent*-kauran-19-oic acid (**36**), 16α-hydroxy-17-isovaleryloxy-*ent*-kauran-19-oic acid (**37**), and 16α,17-dihydroxy-*ent*-kauran-19-oic acid (**38**). (Cai et al., 2003b) evaluated five *ent*-kauranes for TNF-α secretion from HMC-1, a trypsin-stimulated human leukemic mast cell line. The results indicated that 16αH,17-isovaleryloxy-*ent*-kauran-19-oic acid (**36**) exhibited potently an inhibitory activity with IC$_{50}$ value of 16.2 μM. Furthermore, these compounds were assayed for their inhibitory effect against NFAR transcription factor and 16α-hydroxy-17-isovaleryloxy-*ent*-kauran-19-oic acid (**37**) was found to significantly inhibit NFAT transcription factor with IC$_{50}$ of 6.7 μM (Cai et al., 2004a). The authors also found that remain compounds containing a hydroxyl group at C-16 or a glycoside at C-4 showed no activity.

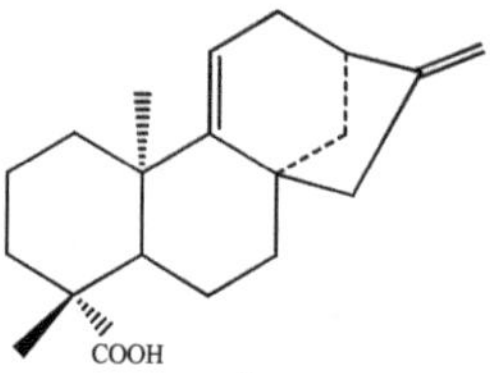

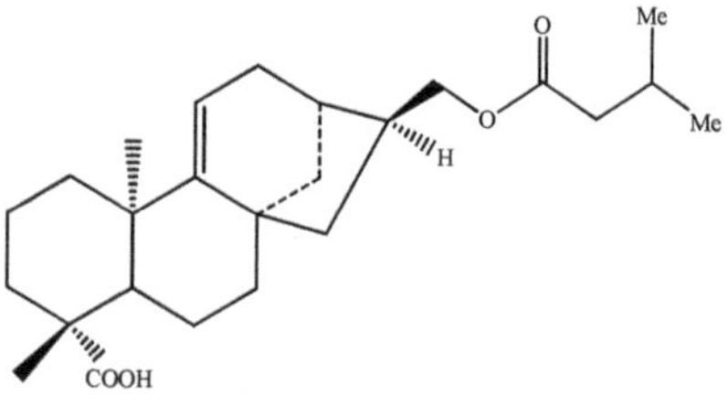

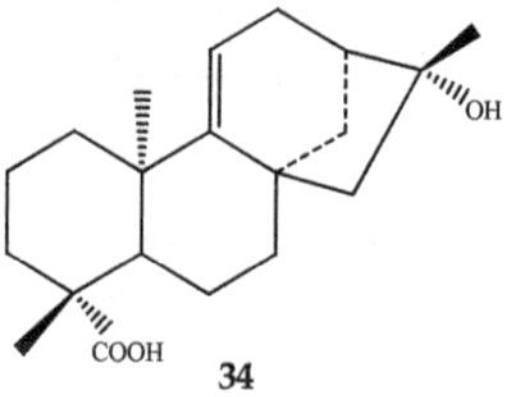

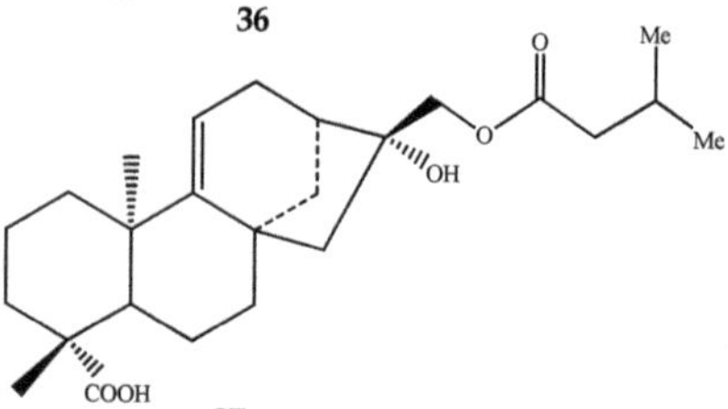

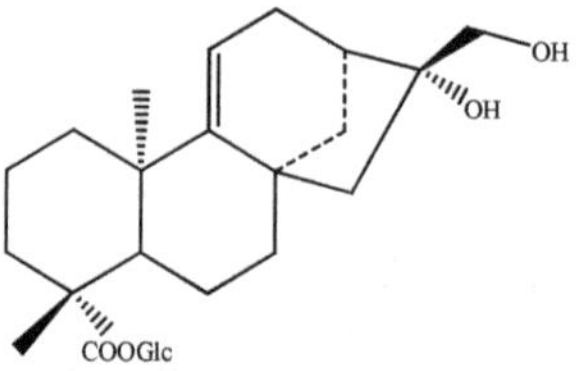

Name	Part	Reference
ent-Kaur-16-en-19-oic acid (**33**)	roots	(Kim et al., 1988b)
16α-Hydroxy-ent-kauran-19-oic acid (**34**)	roots	(Cai et al., 2003b)
Paniculoside IV (**35**)	roots	(Cai et al., 2003b)
16αH,17-Isovaleryloxy-*ent*-kauran-19-oic acid (**36**)	roots	(Cai et al., 2003b)
16α-Hydroxy-17-isovaleryloxy-*ent*-kauran-19-oic acid (**37**)	roots	(Cai et al., 2003b)
16α,17-Dihydroxy-*ent*-kauran-19-oic acid (**38**)	roots	(Kim et al., 1988b)

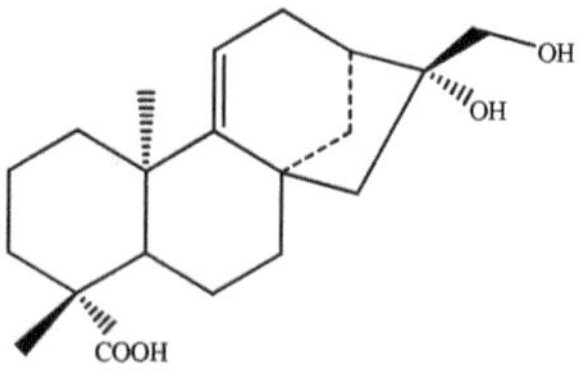

Fig. 5. Structures of *ent*-kaurane-type diterpenes from *A. koreanum*

2.5 Other class compounds

Two lignans were found from the roots of A. *koreanum*. Those were acanthoside D (**39**) (Hahn et al., 1985) and ariensin (**40**) (Kim et al., 1988a). Beside these lignans, the first

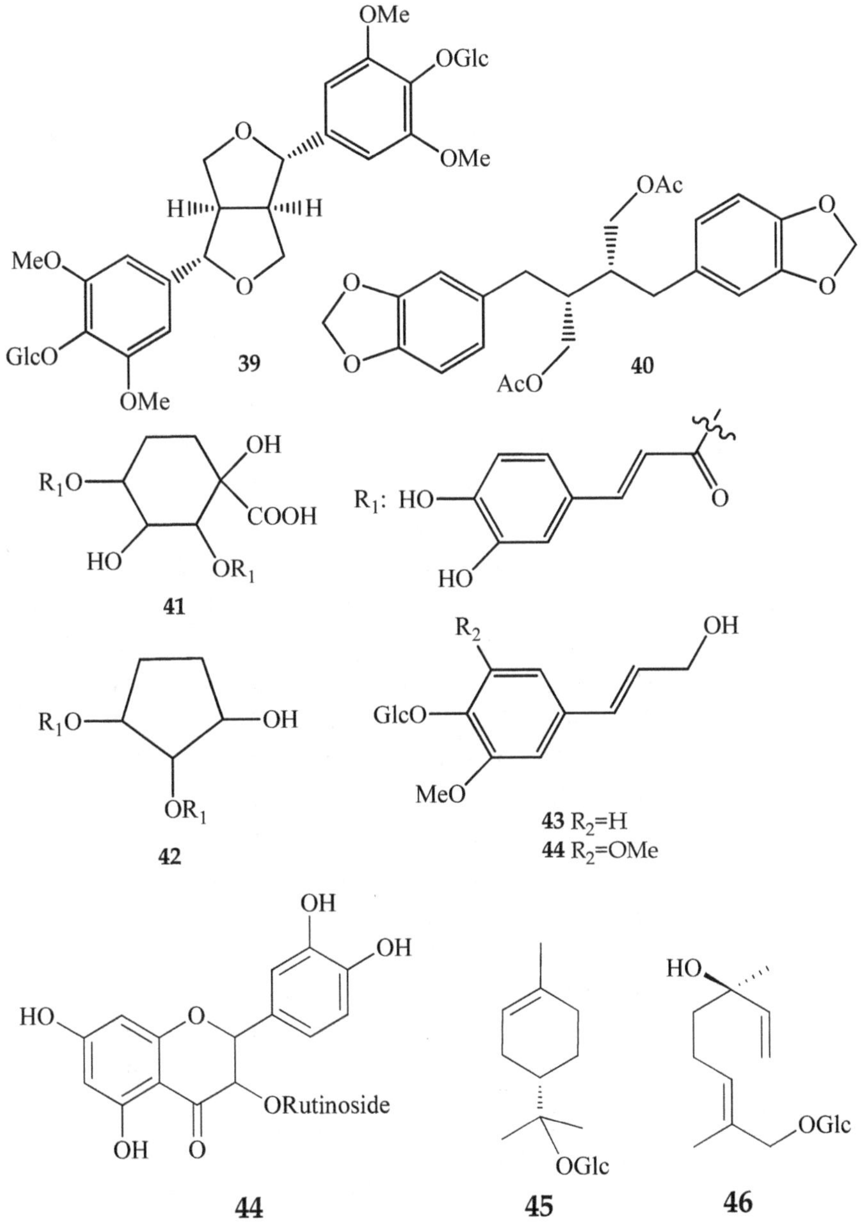

Fig. 6. Structures of compounds isolated from A. *Koreanum*

Pos.	1	2	3	4	5	6	7	8	9	10	11	12
1	35.8	35.7	35.1	32.8	32.6	35.9	36.2	33.1	36.2	33.1	35.9	34.9
2	26.8	26.9	25.5	26.0	25.9	27.1	21.9	26.2	26.9	26.2	27.1	26.8
3	74.8	73.7	75.8	72.8	72.7	75.9	81.5	71.5	75.3	73.0	75.7	72.7
4	38.4	53.5	37.7	51.8	51.7	41.2	37.9	51.9	38.5	52.8	41.1	52.6
5	49.4	44.4	48.8	44.7	44.8	43.9	50.6	45.3	49.6	45.0	43.8	43.9
6	19.2	21.8	19.3	21.6	21.0	18.3	18.4	21.7	18.6	21.8	18.3	21.0
7	36.0	35.7	35.4	23.8	34.5	35.6	35.7	34.6	35.7	34.6	35.4	35.2
8	42.7	43.2	42.2	41.6	41.5	42.8	42.7	41.8	42.8	42.8	42.7	42.4
9	55.9	56.2	55.6	50.7	50.8	56.2	55.9	51.0	56.2	51.2	55.6	55.6
10	39.8	39.6	39.1	38.2	37.2	39.6	39.7	37.4	39.9	37.6	39.6	38.7
11	69.8	70.7	70.4	21.1	21.5	69.9	69.9	20.9	69.8	21.2	69.8	69.4
12	38.4	39.4	37.7	27.7	25.8	38.4	38.3	26.0	38.3	26.0	38.3	37.8
13	37.5	37.5	37.2	28.6	38.4	37.6	37.7	38.4	37.4	38.4	37.4	37.0
14	42.9	44.1	42.6	43.0	42.7	42.8	42.9	42.9	43.0	43.0	42.9	43.0
15	29.9	30.6	29.5	30.2	30.0	30.1	30.2	30.1	30.0	30.1	30.0	29.6
16	32.8	32.7	32.0	34.7	32.8	32.8	32.9	32.2	32.3	32.4	32.2	31.9
17	56.5	57.1	56.2	56.7	56.4	56.5	56.6	57.0	56.9	57.7	56.9	56.6
18	47.5	50.0	46.6	49.1	49.5	49.4	49.4	49.8	49.5	49.7	49.4	49.1
19	49.4	52.5	48.6	43.7	47.5	47.5	47.5	47.4	47.2	47.5	47.1	46.8
20	151.0	215.0	149.7	37.6	151.1	150.8	150.9	150.9	150.4	151.0	150.4	150.1
21	31.0	29.4	30.5	24.6	30.9	31.2	31.3	30.8	30.9	30.9	30.9	30.6
22	37.5	37.7	36.8	37.2	37.3	37.4	37.4	36.9	36.8	37.2	36.7	36.4
23	29.6	210.9	28.7	178.9	179.6	71.9	29.9	181.3	29.8	179.0	71.9	209.7
24	22.7	15.1	22.2	17.8	17.7	18.3	23.0	18.1	22.9	18.0	18.3	14.6
25	18.0	17.2	17.3	16.6	16.5	17.0	16.8	16.8	16.9	16.8	17.1	16.5
26	17.4	17.8	16.2	16.6	16.5	17.7	17.6	16.7	17.7	16.6	17.7	17.4
27	14.4	15.0	14.6	14.5	14.6	14.8	14.8	14.8	14.8	14.8	14.8	14.4
28	179.2	179.4	181.5	179.4	178.6	178.8	178.9	175.0	175.0	175.9	175.0	174.6
29	110.0	30.0	110.2	107.8	109.7	110.0	110.1	110.0	110.2	110.0	110.0	109.9
30	19.2		17.9	16.4	19.2	19.5	19.6	19.4	19.5	19.3	19.5	19.2
Solv.	a	a	b	a	a	a	a	a	a	a	a	a

[a] recorded in pyridine-d_5, [b] recorded in methanol-d_4.

Note: NMR data were obtained from **1**: (Srivastava, 1992); **2**, **3** (Park et al., 2010); **4**, **8**: (Kim et al., 2010); **5**, **6**, **10**, **11**: (Chang et al., 1998); **7**, **12**: (Chang et al., 1999)

Table 1. ^{13}C-NMR data of lupane aglycone moieties

Pos.	13	14	15	16	17	18	19	20	21	22	23	24	25
1	33.2	33.1	35.9	35.5	36.5	36.1	36.7	33.3	33.1	34.0	34.2	33.9	34.5
2	26.1	26.7	27.0	26.4	26.6	21.8	19.2	26.1	26.7	26.1	26.1	26.1	26.1
3	72.8	73.0	73.8	73.8	73.5	81.3	82.4	72.7	73.0	73.4	73.3	73.6	73.3
4	51.8	52.5	53.7	53.0	40.3	37.8	38.5	51.7	52.5	52.2	52.1	52.3	52.1
5	45.4	44.0	44.5	45.4	49.9	50.5	51.0	45.6	44.0	46.6	46.9	46.2	47.4
6	21.7	20.9	22.0	22.6	19.2	18.4	22.2	21.7	21.1	22.2	22.2	22.3	22.2
7	34.5	34.1	36.2	36.1	36.3	35.4	36.4	34.6	34.1	35.1	35.5	35.3	35.5
8	41.8	41.8	41.6	43.5	43.4	42.6	43.5	41.7	41.8	42.5	43.0	42.6	43.1
9	51.0	50.6	56.3	56.7	50.2	55.8	56.3	50.6	50.2	51.9	52.0	51.7	52.0
10	37.4	36.9	38.2	40.0	38.3	39.6	40.4	37.4	36.9	38.2	38.1	38.1	38.2
11	21.0	21.0	71.1	71.1	24.2	69.7	71.2	20.9	20.8	22.0	22.4	22.0	22.2
12	27.1	27.0	38.3	39.4	26.5	38.1	39.5	26.9	26.9	28.5	29.8	28.3	26.1
13	38.3	38.3	39.5	38.2	38.2	37.3	38.3	38.2	38.2	38.6	39.5	39.4	39.1
14	42.8	42.8	44.3	44.3	43.8	42.9	44.0	43.0	43.0	43.6	44.5	44.0	44.3
15	30.2	30.1	30.8	30.8	31.6	30.0	30.9	30.0	30.0	30.9	31.2	30.9	30.9
16	32.2	32.1	32.8	32.9	32.8	32.2	32.9	32.0	32.1	32.4	33.1	32.9	34.5
17	57.0	56.9	57.9	57.9	57.9	56.8	58.0	57.0	57.3	58.0	60.1	58.0	59.4
18	50.2	50.2	50.9	50.9	50.1	49.4	51.0	48.5	48.9	50.8	49.5	49.7	50.4
19	43.2	43.2	43.7	43.7	48.2	47.1	43.8	37.3	40.6	52.8	45.7	39.3	85.4
20	156.5	156.5	155.9	155.9	151.3	150.4	156.0	50.1	42.1	215.4	76.1	39.5	36.8
21	32.7	32.7	33.5	33.6	30.6	30.8	33.6	24.6	25.0	29.3	28.8	24.38	34.5
22	36.8	36.7	37.3	37.4	37.5	36.7	37.4	37.4	37.3	37.6	37.5	38.3	37.2
23	181.2	209.8	211.2	180.6	29.5	29.8	29.8	181.8	209.9	183.4	184.2	181.8	185.2
24	18.2	14.6	15.2	18.2	23.0	23.0	23.3	18.3	14.6	18.3	18.4	18.2	18.6
25	16.8	16.4	17.2	17.5	17.8	16.8	17.3	16.8	16.3	17.2	17.4	17.2	17.4
26	16.7	16.5	18.3	18.1	17.0	17.6	18.0	16.6	16.5	16.9	17.2	17.0	17.1
27	14.9	14.8	15.1	15.1	14.9	14.7	15.2	14.7	14.9	15.2	15.6	15.1	15.5
28	175.1	175.0	176.3	176.3	176.2	174.8	176.4	175.0	174.9	176.2	177.0	176.4	176.7
29	106.1	106.1	107.7	107.7	110.8	110.1	107.6	204.6	180.0	29.9	71.2	8.9	21.9
30	64.3	64.3	65.5	65.5	19.6	19.6	65.6	7.0	10.0		19.6	110.3	27.0
Solv.	a	a	b	b	b	a	b	a	a	b	b	b	b

[a] recorded in pyridine-d_5, [b] recorded in methanol-d_4.

Note: NMR data were obtained from **13, 14, 21:** (Choi et al., 2008); **15:** (Nhiem et al., 2009) (Cai et al., 2004b), **16, 19, 25:** (Nhiem et al., 2010b); **17:** (Cai et al., 2004b); **18:** (Chang et al., 1999), **20:** (Park et al., 2005); **21:** (Choi et al., 2008); **22, 23, 24:** (Nhiem et al., 2010a).

Table 1. ^{13}C-NMR data of lupane aglycone moieties (continued)

phenylpropanoid, syrinoside (**44**) were isolated from the roots of *A. koreanum* by (Hahn et al., 1985) and then was ariensin (**43**) (Kim et al., 1988a). In study antioxidant activity of chemical components from the leaves of this plant, (Nhiem et al., 2011) isolated one new phenylpropanoid named acanthopanic acid and one known 1,2-O-dicaffeoylcyclopenta-3-ol. These compounds showed significantly antioxidant activity by the intracellular ROS radical scavenging DCF-DA assay with IC_{50} values of 3.8 and 2.9 μM, respectively. Until now, only rutin (**45**), a quercetin glycoside was isolated from this plant with large amount. Rutin is used in many countries as medication for blood vessel protection and are ingredients of numerous multivitamin preparations and herbal remedies. Rutin has various biological activities that are beneficial to human health such as antioxidant effect (Nhiem et al., 2011), protective effect against hepatotoxicity, and anti-inflammatory effect. On the other hand, from the leaves of *A. koreanum*, two monoterpenoids, 4S)-α-terpineol O-β-D glucopyranoside (**46**) (Nhiem et al., 2011) and betulabuside B (**47**) (Park et al., 2010) were isolated. From fruits, citric, maleic succinic, malonic, furmaric, and malic acid were isolated (Shin & Kim, 1985).

3. NMR data of lupane aglycones

Lupane triterpenes are a class of the most compounds isolated from the leaves and roots of *A. koreanum*, which were determined that this type of compounds are main chemical components of this plant.

Structure of lupanes were elucidated with ¹H-NMR, ¹³C-NMR, DEPT (distortionless enhancement by polarization transfer), COSY (¹H-¹H shift correlation spectroscopy), TOCSY (total correlation spectroscopy), HMBC (heteronuclear multiple bond correlation), HSQC (heteronuclear single quantum coherence), NOESY (nuclear overhauser enhancement spectroscopy, and ROESY (rotating frame overhause effect spectroscopy). Proton coupling networks of sugar moieties were indicated with ¹H-NMR, COSY, HMBC and HSQC. Herein, we suggest statistical results of ¹³C-NMR data of lupane-type triterpene aglycones and their derivatives in comparison with data of references (Table 1).

Observed the isolated compounds from *A. koreanum*, we found that there are four main classes including lupane triterpenoids, pimarane diterpenoids, *ent*-kaurane diterpenoids, and lignans. Among of them, lupane triterpenes were isolated as numerous of compounds with high yield. These lupanes often contain hydroxyl group at C-3, carboxyl at C-28. In some compounds, hydroxyl, aldehydic, carboxylic groups were at C-11, C-23, and C-30, glycoside was at C-28 and rarely at C-3.

From Table 1, we summarized all ¹³C-NMR characteristics of lupane aglycones as follows:

1. When hydroxyl group at C-3, chemical shift of C-3 was about 73.0 ppm and configuration of hydroxyl group at C-3 is α orientation. When glycosidation is at C-3, chemical shift of C-3 moved to down field with $δ_C$ of 81.0 ppm.
2. Free carboxylic group at C-28 were confirmed by chemical shift about 178.0~180.0 ppm. When sugar moiety was at C-28, chemical shift of C-28 is 174.6~176.3 ppm, decreased about 2.5-3.8 ppm.

3. When 23-methyl group was replaced with aldehydic group, chemical shifts of C-23 and C-4 moved to down field from 28.0-28.8 to 209.0-210.0, 37.5-39.5 to 54.9-56.3 ppm, respectively. When 23-methy group was replaced with carboxylic group, chemical shifts of C-23 and C-4 changed from 28.5 to 178.0, 37.8 to 53.0 respectively, and when 23-methyl group was replaced with CH_2OH, chemical shift of C-23 had a large change from 28.0 to 71.5 ppm; chemical shift of C-4 had small change about 2.0ppm.

4. When 30-methyl group was replaced with CH_2OH, the chemical shifts of C-20 and C-30 downshifted from 151.0 to 156.5, from 19.5 to 64.5 ppm, respectively; chemical shifts of C-19 and C-29 upshifted from 47.5 to 43.0, from 110.0 to 106.0 ppm, respectively.

5. When hydroxyl group was at C-11, chemical shift of C-11 downshifted from 21.1 to 71.0 ppm. Furthermore, configuration of hydroxyl group at this position is α.

4. Conclusion

This chapter is intended to serve as a reference tool for people in all fields of ethnopharmacology and natural products chemistry. The pharmacological studies on *A. koreanum* indicated the immense potential possibility of this plant in the treatment of conditions such as inflammation, rheumatism, diabetes, cardiovascular, and virus. However, the diverse pharmacological activities of solvent extracts and phytochemicals of *A. koreanum* have only been tested in *in vitro* assay using laboratory animals, and obtained too unclearly and ambiguously for the case of human beings to be conducted on enough. However, these gaps in the studies demand to be bridged in order to exploit medicinal potential of the entire plant of *A. koreanum*. It is still clear that *A. koreanum* is massively and widespreadly consumed, and also contiuously studied expecting clinical treatment of various diseases for the future in Korea as well as in the world. From these viewpoints, impressic acid and acanthoic acid, major components of *A. koreanum* are good candidates for further studies in clinical trials, and the development of products derived from *A. koreanum* can be an important part of our biodiversity to respect and sustain for coming generation.

5. References

Fact sheet N⁰ 134: Traditional medicine. World Health Organization. December 2008.

Cai, X. F.; Shen, G.; Dat, N. T.; Kang, O. H.; Kim, J. A.; Lee, Y. M.; Lee, J. J., & Kim, Y. H. (2003a). Inhibitory effect of TNF-α and IL-8 secretion by pimarane-type diterpenoids from *Acanthopanax koreanum*. Chemical & Pharmaceutical Bulletin, Vol.51, No.5, pp. 605-607, ISSN 0009-2363

Cai, X. F.; Shen, G.; Dat, N. T.; Kang, O. H.; Lee, Y. M.; Lee, J. J., & Kim, Y. H. (2003b). Inhibitory effect of kaurane type diterpenoids from *Acanthopanax koreanum* on TNF-α secretion from trypsin-stimulated HMC-1 cells. Archives of Pharmacal Research, Vol.26, No.9, pp. 731-734, ISSN 0253-6269

Cai, X. F.; Lee, I. S.; Dat, N. T.; Shen, G., & Kim, Y. H. (2004a). Diterpenoids with inhibitory activity against NFAT transcription factor from *Acanthopanax koreanum* Phytotherapy Research, Vol.18, No.8, pp. 677-680, ISSN 0951-418X

Cai, X. F.; Lee, I. S.; Shen, G.; Dat, N. T.; Lee, J. J., & Kim, Y. H. (2004b). Triterpenoids from *Acanthopanax koreanum* root and their inhibitory activities on NFAT transcription. Archives of Pharmacal Research, Vol.27, No.8, pp. 825-828, ISSN 0253-6269

Chang, S. Y.; Yook, C. S., & Nohara, T. (1998). Two new lupane-triterpene glycosides from leaves of *Acanthopanax koreanum*. Chemical & Pharmaceutical Bulletin, Vol.46, No.1, pp. 163-165, ISSN 0009-2363

Chang, S. Y.; Yook, C. S., & Nohara, T. (1999). Lupane-triterpene glycosides from leaves of *Acanthopanax koreanum*. Phytochemistry, Vol.50, No.8, pp. 1369-1374, ISSN 0031-9422

Choi, H. S.; Kim, H. J.; Nam, S. G.; Kim, I. S.; Lee, K. T.; Yook, C. S., & Lee, Y. S. (2008). Lupane glycosides from the leaves of *Acanthopanax koreanum*. Chemical & Pharmaceutical Bulletin, Vol.56, No.11, pp. 1613–1616, ISSN 0009-2363

Chung, B. S. & Kim, Y. H. (1986). Studies on the constituents of *Acanthopanax koreanum*. Saengyak Hakhoechi, Vol.17, No.1, pp. 62-66, ISSN 0253-3073

Hahn, D.-R.; Kim, C. J., & Kim, J. H. (1985). A study on the chemical constituents of *Acanthopanax koreanum* Nakai and its pharmacological activities. Yakhak Hoechi Vol.29, No.6, pp. 357-361, ISSN 0513-4234

Kang, H. S.; Kim, Y. H.; Lee, C. S.; Lee, J. J.; Choi, I., & Pyun, K. H. (1996). Suppression of interleukin-1 and tumor necrosis factor-α. production by acanthoic acid, (-)-pimara-9(11),15-dien-19-oic acid, and its antifibrotic effects in vivo. Cellular Immunology, Vol.170, No.2, pp. 212-221, ISSN 0008-8749

Kang, H. S.; Song, H. K.; Lee, J. J.; Pyun, K. H., & Choi, I. (1998). Effects of acanthoic acid on TNF-a gene expression and haptoglobin synthesis. Mediators of Inflammation, Vol.7, No.4, pp. 257-259, ISSN 0962-9351

Kang, O.-H.; Choi, Y. A.; Park, H. J.; Kang, C. S.; Song, B. S.; Choi, S. C.; Nah, Y. H.; Yun, K. J.; Cai, X. F.; Kim, Y. H.; Bae, K., & Lee, Y. M. (2006). Inhibition of trypsin-induced mast cell activation by acanthoic acid. Journal of Ethnopharmacology, Vol.105, No.3, pp. 326-331, ISSN 0378-8741

Kang, O. H.; Kim, D. K.; Cai, X. F.; Kim, Y. H., & Lee, Y. M. (2010). Attenuation of experimental murine colitis by acanthoic acid from *Acanthopanax koreanum*. Archives of Pharmacal Research, Vol.33, No.1, pp. 87-93, ISSN 0253-6269

Kim, J. A.; Kim, D. K.; Tae, J.; Kang, O. H.; Choi, Y. A.; Choi, S. C.; Kim, T. H.; Nah, Y. H.; Choi, S. J.; Kim, Y. H.; Bae, K. H., & Lee, Y. M. (2004). Acanthoic acid inhibits IL-8 production via MAPKs and NF-kappaB in a TNF-a-stimulated human intestinal epithelial cell line. Clinica Chimica Acta, Vol. 342, No.1-2, pp. 193-202, ISSN 0009-8981

Kim, J. A.; Yang, S. Y.; Koo, J.-E.; Koh, Y. S., & Kim, Y. H. (2010). Lupane-type triterpenoids from the steamed leaves of *Acanthopanax koreanum* and their inhibitory effects on the LPS-stimulated pro-inflammatory cytokine production in bone marrow-derived dendritic cells. Bioorganic & Medicinal Chemistry Letters, Vol.20, No.22, pp. 6703-6707, ISSN 0960-894X

Kim, J. A.; Yang, S. Y.; Song, S. B., & Kim, Y. H. (2011). Effects of impressic acid from *Acanthopanax koreanum* on NFκB and PPARγ activities. Archives of Pharmacal Research, Vol.34, No.8, pp. 1347-1351, ISSN 0253-6269

Kim, Y. H.; Chung, B. S.; Ko, Y. S., & Han, H. J. (1988a). Studies on the chemical constituents of *Acanthopanax koreanum*. (II). Archives of Pharmacal Research, Vol.11, No.2, pp. 159-162, ISSN 0253-6269

Kim, Y. H.; Chung, B. S., & Sankawa, U. (1988b). Pimaradiene diterpenes from *Acanthopanax koreanum*. Journal of Natural Products, Vol.51, No.6, pp. 1080-1083, ISSN 163-3864

Li, Y.; Jiang, R.; Ooi, L. S. M.; But, P. P. H., &Ooi, V. E. C. (2007). Antiviral triterpenoids from the medicinal plant *Schefflera heptaphylla*. Phytotherapy Research, Vol.21, No.5, pp. 466-470, ISSN 0951-418X

Nan, J. X.; Jin, X. J.; Lian, L. H.; Cai, X. F.; Jiang, Y. Z.; Jin, H. R., & Lee, J. J. (2008). A diterpenoid acanthoic acid from *Acanthopanax koreanum* protects against D-galactosamine/lipopolysaccharide-induced fulminant hepatic failure in mice. Biological & Pharmaceutical Bulletin, Vol.31, No.4, pp. 738-742, ISSN 0918-6158

Nhiem, N. X.; Tung, N. H.; Kiem, P. V.; Minh, C. V.; Ding, Y.; Hyun, J. H.; Kang, H. K., & Kim, Y. H. (2009). Lupane triterpene glycosides from leave of *Acanthopanax koreanum* and their cytotoxic activity. Chemical & Pharmaceutical Bulletin, Vol.57, No.9, pp. 986-989, ISSN 0009-2363

Nhiem, N. X.; Kiem, P. V.; Minh, C. V.; Ha, D. T.; Tai, B. H.; Yen, P. H.; Tung, N. H.; Hyun, J. H.; Kang, H. K., & Kim, Y. H. (2010a). Lupane-type triterpene glycosides from the leaves of *Acanthopanax koreanum* and their in vitro cytotoxicity. Planta Medica, Vol.76, No.2, pp. 189-194, ISSN 0032-0943

Nhiem, N. X.; Kiem, P. V.; Minh, C. V.; Tai, B. H.; Tung, N. H.; Ha, D. T.; Soung, K. S.; Kim, J. H.; Ahn, J. Y.; Lee, Y. M., & Kim, Y. H. (2010b). Structure-activity relationship of lupane-triterpene glycosides from *Acanthopanax koreanum* on spleen lymphocyte IL-2 and INF-γ. Bioorganic & Medicinal Chemistry Letters, No.20, pp. 4927-4931, ISSN 0960-894X

Nhiem, N. X.; Kim, K. C.; Kim, A.-D.; Hyun, J. W.; Kang, H. K.; Kiem, P. V.; Minh, C. V.; Thu, V. K.; Tai, B. H.; Kim, J. A., & Kim, Y. H. (2011). Phenylpropanoids from the leaves of *Acanthopanax koreanum* and their antioxidant activity. Journal of Asian Natural Products Research Vol.13, No.1, pp. 56-61, ISSN 1028-6020

Park, S. H.; Nhiem, N. X.; Kiem, P. V.; Choi, E. M.; Kim, J. A., & Kim, Y. H. (2010). A new norlupane triterpene from the leaves of *Acanthopanax koreanum* increases the differentiation of osteoblastic MC3T3-e1 cells. Archives of Pharmacal Research, Vol.33, No.1, pp. 75-80, ISSN 0253-6269

Park, S. Y.; Choi, H. S.; Yook, C. S., & Nohara, T. (2005). A new lupane glycoside from the leaves of *Acanthopanax koreanum*. Chemical & Pharmaceutical Bulletin, Vol.51, No.1, pp. 97-99, ISSN 0009-2363

Samuelsson, G. & Bohlin, L. (2004). Drugs of natural origin: A textbook of pharmacognosy. 5 Ed.; Swedish Pharmaceutical Press, ISBN 9197431842, Stockkholm, Sweden

Shin, E. T. & Kim, C. S. (1985). Composition of fatty acid and organic acid in Acanthopanax. Han'guk Sikp'um Kwahakhoechi, Vol.17, No.5, pp. 403-405, ISSN 0367-6293

Srivastava, S. K. (1992). A new triterpenic acid from *Schefflera impressa*. Journal of Natural Products, Vol.55, No.3, pp. 298-302, ISSN 0163-3864

Wu, Y. L.; Jiang, Y. Z.; Jin, X. J.; Lan, L. H.; Piao, J. Y.; Wan, Y.; Jin, H. R.; Lee, J. J., & Nan, J. X. (2010). Acanthoic acid, a diterpene in *Acanthopanax koreanum*, protects acetaminophen-induced hapatic toxicity in mice. Phytomedicine, Vol.17, No.6, pp. 475-479, ISSN 0944-7113

Yook, C. S.; Kim, I. H.; Hahn, D. R.; Nohara, T., & Chang, S. Y. (1998). A lupane-triterpene glycoside from leaves of two Acanthopanax. Phytochemistry, Vol.49, No.3, pp. 839-843, ISSN 0031-9422

Bioavailability of Phytochemicals

Indah Epriliati[1] and Irine R. Ginjom[2]
[1]Widya Mandala Catholic University,
[2]Swinburne University of Technology, Sarawak Campus,
[1]Indonesia
[2]Malaysia

1. Introduction

Phytochemicals are increasingly accepted as health promoting, maintaining, and repairing agents in cells, tissues, or the whole human body. Phytochemicals are compounds obtained from plants that exert particular health effects; generally, they are not necessarily basic nutrients (minerals, vitamins, carbohydrates, proteins or lipids), medicines or toxins. The phytochemicals that are frequently associated with human health are phenolics, carotenoids, organic acids, and several miscellaneous bioactive compounds such as saponin and sterols. The contributions of phytochemicals in public health cover various issues world-widely and thus it is seen by researchers, industries, general society, and policy makers as a new tool to manage public health. Ironically, the roles of phytochemicals in health are poorly understood, which warrant the needs for validation as well as scientific database on safety issues and mechanisms of the functions. Even though various genetic-base studies propose mechanisms and health interventions of phytochemicals (Noe et al., 2004), many findings are inconclusive. Hence, the emerging health potentials of phytochemicals are inconclusive; and internationally it has been the reason for new policies/regulations in food trading. This is partly due to limited understanding on phytochemical bioavailability by which the health benefits depend on. Moreover, transport mechanisms for phytochemicals delivery into the target sites, phytochemical metabolisms by the human body, and biomarkers exerting the health benefits are also poorly understood. These complexities call for a new framework on how and to what extent dietary phytochemicals should be recommended in order to reach biologically-safe active dosages.

In the human body, bioavailability is defined as substances obtained from ingested materials that reach circulatory system for further delivery into designated tissues so that the beneficial compounds are biologically available for exerting healthy functions. The normal routes of dietary phytochemicals thus include ingestion, digestions, and transport across gastrointestinal epithelium prior to circulatory vessels. The epithelium in the gastrointestinal tract is a polarized enterocyte cell having two different sides facing luminal hollow (Apical side) and blood capillaries (Basolateral side) where each side is equipped with different transport facilities and barriers. The epithelial cells are critical for bioavailability of target compounds either as entrance gates or as metabolizing machines which release different compounds from the parent molecules. These make further complexing bioavailability routes because the metabolisms and transport processes are also involved in the orchestrated physiological regulations maintaining homeostasis states of the human body. However, bioavailability of phytochemicals by which the health benefits depend on are not well understood; consequently, it is difficult to be measured.

The difficulties in studies of bioavailability are mainly due to the complexities involved in the biological system, i.e. (a) variation in food materials and the human subjects or surrogate models which are not always representative; (b) complex interactions amongst huge chemicals/food components during postharvest, storage, processing, digestion, and absorption that may alter health benefits; and (c) mechanism pathways. In this paper, fundamental aspects of phytochemical bioavailability are reviewed.

2. Digestibility of phytochemicals

It is known that major phytochemicals are located inside vacuoles of plant cells; and several phenolics form complexes with fibres in the cell wall. These natural existences make the phytochemicals poorly accessed by enzymes or hardly released out from the plant matrices during digestion. Most cell wall materials are indigestible by human enzymic systems. Moreover, it is also poorly permeable for important molecules such as phytochemicals. Therefore, digestibility of the phytochemicals is of great interest, in particular, to reveal how the phytochemicals can affect human health and fight or prevent diseases if the phytochemicals are strongly contained in the food matrices.

2.1 Digestion: principles of human gastrointestinal tract

The digestion compartments in human consist of mouth, gastric, small intestine, and colon (Figure 1). Each has slightly different digestion performances depending on age and gender as listed in Table 1. In the gastrointestinal tract, net nutriome[1] is released as a result of orchestrated secretions, enzymic activities, and physical-mechanical actions of peristaltic movements. The nutriomes will diffuse out from the food particles to chyme solutions. The levels of nutriome in this stage are called availability or accessibility of the components. However, bio-/chemical degradations of the molecules can take place. Hence, digestibility will also provide metabolites/derivatives. Nevertheless, availability and accessibility parameters can only account for intact molecules but not the metabolites.

Architecture and material of the plant tissues is generally unfavourable for activities of enzymic system in the human gastrointestinal tract. As a consequence, limited cell contents of the ingested food materials are released into chyme solution in the gastrointestinal tract. Natural pores and plasmodesmatas may not play predominant roles in diffusion of the nutriome. Nevertheless, according to Stolle-Smits et al. (2009), natural matrices of tomato, mango, apple, and kiwi undergo galactan solubilisation during ripening stage; thus the release of nutriome can be altered. However, processing and chemical compositions of the food matrices themselves may change physicochemical environments of the chyme for nutriome mass transfer. The most recent finding indicates that ingested foods are necessarily designed such that the diffusion of the nutriome favours nutriome absorption by epithelial cells; even for phenolics, it requires lipid-complex called phytosome (Kidd & Head, 2005) to penetrate gut lining and to enter the circulatory system.

---

[1] Nutriome is a term referring to all beneficial food components

Digestion sites	Infant	Adults	Elderly	Female	Male
Mouth	Improper chewing, imperfect salivary enzymes	Chewing, complete salivary enzymes	Improper chewing, may be with incomplete salivary enzymes	Chewing	Chewing
Gastric	Acid & pepsin digestion	Acid & pepsin digestion	Acid & pepsin digestion	Acid & pepsin digestion	Acid & pepsin digestion
Small intestine	Immature system	Complete tissues and enzymes	Complete tissues and enzymes	Hormonal related digestive secretion, undisturbed by reproductive cycles	Hormonal related digestive secretion, disturbed by reproductive organ cycles
Large intestine	Predominant Bifido bacteria	Lossing Bifido bacteria	Lossing Bifido bacteria	Lossing Bifido bacteria	Lossing Bifido bacteria

Table 1. Summary of digestion characteristics of infant, adult and elderly, female and male

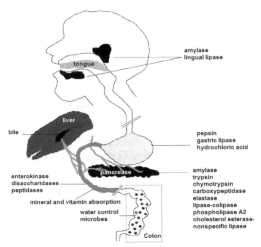

Fig. 1. Principles of human digestion system adapted and modified from Johnson (2001)

2.4 Effects of digestion on phytochemicals

Cell wall materials significantly modulate digestion of plant foods. Nunan et al. (1998) state that in grape berry during its development of the berry fruits the Na_2CO_3-soluble fraction increases before veraison but decreases as the berries softened. It implies that the Na_2CO_3 soluble fraction is the cell wall component which is responsible for firmness and strength. Epriliati (2008) observe that ripe mango, tomato, and papaya behave differently when Na_2CO_3 is added into *in vitro* digestion model mimicking small intestine where not all aggregated boli from human *in vivo* chewing can be broken down. The diverse resistances of plant cell wall material amongst plant species during digestion may be partly due to Na_2CO_3 soluble fractions. It is more likely that mango and tomato have different levels of Na_2CO_3 soluble fractions which result in diverse *in vitro* digestion effects compared to papaya. Furthermore, processing will affect the way nutriome being released. Meanwhile, heating of the filtered fresh-juices (tomato, mango, and papaya) results in formation of clumpy substances (Epriliati, 2008). Similar clumps are also found as remnant of pectin gel used for taste masking agent of paracetamol and ambroxol (Miyazaki et al., 2005). These imply that consumption of fresh and processed various fruits, rich in pectin, can yield a wide range of phytochemical bioavailability depending on their cell wall material compositions. Furthermore, pasteurisation may render phytochemical release from the clumpy substances.

Phenolics. There are two main routes for digestion of dietary phenolics; i.e. digestion along the gastrointestinal tract and digestion inside the enterocytes. This can happen because hydrolase enzymes, i.e. lactase phlorizin hydrolase are available in intestinal lumen, brush border, and enterocyte (Williamson, 2004). Metabolisms that take place along the gastrointestinal tract are mainly aiming at deglycosilation of glycoside form of dietary phenolics. This deglycosilation is also carried out by microbiota in the colon.

Inside the enterocyte, dietary phenolic glucuronidation of the aglycone form are catalyzed by UGT[2]. Meanwhile, the glycone forms are hydrolyzed and conjugated. The conjugated forms from both glycone and aglycone dietary phenolics are either effluxed into intestinal lumen or translocated into the portal blood vessel. The circulated conjugates of dietary phenolics in plasma can be absorbed by liver and hepatocytes will metabolize them further. For instance, the hepatocyte converts flavonoids into glucuronidated and sulphated forms, which are polar rendering to dissolve in water easier and then be excreted in urine or bile. The pivotal roles of liver indicate that these conjugations are apparently one of physiological needs in the body, for example for bile synthesis in mammalians.

All compounds in wine, which are free from cell wall materials, show clearer responses during gastrointestinal digestion. Flavonol and proanthocyanidin interact with protein in the salivary secretion. However, catechin interacts stronger than epicatechin indicating that molecular characteristics play an important role in this interaction (de Freitas & Mateus 2001). Flavonols and proanthocyanidins remain intact but they may also be broken down when pH is sufficiently low in the stomach. Phenolics stability is strongly affected by pH as studied by Ginjom (2009). For example, syringic and *p*-coumaric acids are stable at pH 2-9 for 24 h. Generally, pH higher than 7.4 is unfavourable for phenolics and the effects of high pH are worsened by lengthy exposures. The number of -OH groups in benzene ring of simple phenolics can also be critical clues for phenolic stability. High pH results in unstable quinones which are oxidized further into diketones and other degradation products. In contrast, the stability of polyphenols such as quercetin, malvidin-3-glucoside, and resveratrol which have more than one benzene ring does not solely depend on their -OH groups. Quercetin is unstable during gastric and pancreatic digestions because quercetin is easily degraded at high pH, yet it is stable at pH 2 and pH 5.5 (Ginjom, 2009). In contrast, *trans*-resveratrol is stable at pH 1-7. Catechin isomers also show different stability at high

---

[2] UDP glucuronosyltransferase

pH as detected by Ginjom (2009). Similarly, (+)-catechin is stable in *in vitro* digestion up to pH 7.4 at 37 °C for 8 h different from that of (-)-catechin (Friedman & Jurgen, 2000 and Donovan et al., 2006). Overall, phenolics in wine do not undergo significant changes during gastric digestion.

In red wine, anthocyanidin is important component of phenolics. Anthocyanin availability is reduced by 32% after pancreatic digestion compared to that of gastric digestion and undigested sample (Ginjom, 2009). Pancreatic environment, however, decreases monomeric anthocyanin more severely (58.75%) than polymeric anthocyanins (17.72%). Pancreatic condition in the intestine modifies molecular structures of peonidin-3-glucoside, malvidin-3-glucoside, and malvidin glucoside pyruvate as indicated by the changes in their retention time during HPLC/UPLC analyses, although it is unclear why this can happen. However, during *in vitro* digestion, Ginjom (2009) speculates that the losses of monomer are related to their polymerization during the pancreatic digestion. Although non-anthocyanins are insignificantly affected by gastric digestion, pancreatic digestion severely reduces them by ca 88% (equivalent to 22% of total phenolics in red wine). On the other hand, flavan-catechin is speculated to polymerize with anthocyanins or tannin forming precipitates during pancreatic digestion; consequently, they either being eliminated during sample preparation or disposed in aqueous fractions.

Phenolics in tomato products are released into digest solutions more during *in vitro* gastric digestion than during pancreatic digestion and the highest release is from tomato juice (Epriliati, 2008). The main phenolics in tomato are caffeic, catechin, rutin, chlorogenic acid, and coumaric acids. More phenolics are obtained from tomato juice than those from dried and fresh tomato indicating the natural barrier of cell wall has been eliminated. Noticeable changes of phenolic compounds due to processing and digestion are found but the new compounds are not able to be identified. Rutin and catechin are consistently found in fresh, juiced, and dried products. Meanwhile, no *p*-coumaric is found in fresh product whereas *p*-coumaric gradually appears in juiced and in dried products. In contrast, chlorogenic acid is present in fresh products but it gradually disappears in juiced and dried products. This could be caused the different extractability due to different matrices of the products or by chemical changes due to processing and digestion environments (Epriliati, 2008). Gastric digestion does not affect phenolic compounds. However, the phenolic levels are significantly reduced in consecutive gastric-intestinal digestion. Apparently, tomato pectin neither gels nor traps phenolic compounds at lower pH. Altering pH from gastric to intestine may obstruct the molecular phenolic stability.

Similarly, there are different phenolics released from mango during *in vitro* digestion. The phenomena consistently support the possibilities of impermeable pectin where more phenolics are released in a consecutive gastric-intestinal digestion when aggregated boli can be broken down with the addition of $Na_2CO_3/NaHCO_3$ (Epriliati, 2008). Recently, phenolics in gastrointestinal tract markedly behave in a similar way to that of carotenoids incorporated in chylomicrons, thus, all emulsified phytochemical compounds are called phytosome[3] (Kidd & Head, 2005). Therefore, the presence of pancreatic juices and bile extract improve phenolics release during consecutive gastric-intestinal digestions of mango.

---

[3] Phytosome is a term for vehicles in which phytochemical compounds are bound

Carotenoids. About 50% of extractable carotenoids dominated by lycopene and β-carotene in tomato, mango, and papaya products are released to digest solution in a non-lipidic digestion model (Epriliati, 2008). The release of carotenoids increases significantly in intestinal digestion where bile extract and pancreatic secretions exist. Consecutive gastric-intestinal digestions do not help with higher release of carotenoids. This is more likely due to insufficient emulsifier-water ratios to provide emulsification of carotenoids which are fat soluble. It is concluded that mango, tomato, and papaya carotenoids are released better in intestinal digestion where the model is without addition of oil (Epriliati, 2008).

Organic acids. Pectin content in tomato hinders organic acid release thus the total organic acids in *in vitro* gastric digest solution is lower than that of consecutive gastric-pancreatic digestion. This is evidenced by the changes in pH from highly acidic gastric pH to higher small intestinal pH (~6), that causes disaggregation of boli during *in vitro* digestion. For all types of mango samples, organic acid including ascorbic acid (Vitamin C) is released better during gastric digestion. Apparently, the pectinous materials in mango do not trap organic acids (Epriliati, 2008).

3. Absorption of phytochemicals

Currently, there is no well-established molecular form of absorbed substances in the gastrointestinal tract, i.e. whether they are absorbed intact or as metabolites. On the other hand, it is well known that lifestyle, behavior, diets, and basal metabolism of the subjects are more important affecting factors than age, gender, body weight, and plasma volume (Manners et al., 2003) in bioavailability determination. Therefore, standardized experimental conditions controlling such critical factors of absorption *in vivo* and *in vitro* is a must despite individual human variability.

3.1 Absorptive tissue structures

The main absorptive tissue is the small intestine. In human 81% of the total intestinal lengths is by small intestine and 19% is large intestine. The stretched length of jejunum is around 30.78% of the intestinal lengths. The transit time along human small and large intestine is 3-4 h and 2-4 d, respectively (Vermeulen, 2009). Principles of the intestinal absorptive structures are depicted in Figure 2. A single enterocyte has microvilli and each microvillus has glycocalyx. Such structure considerably increases contact surface areas with luminal contents. Each microvillus also contains a complex structure providing various facilities for uptake/influx and efflux molecules, signalling ports, cytoplasm, and lipid matrix. The glycocalyx and microvilli are the areas where the human body depends on for collecting nutriomes but rejecting hazardous compounds including microbes.

Each enterocyte attaches onto adjacent cells through tight, adherence and gap junctions. Cellular transport from intestinal lumen to portal blood vessel occurs in two ways: paracellular and transcellular. The paracellular entrances for hazards are tightly controlled by those three types of junctions. Molecular weight cut off limits the hazardous substances crossing through both enterocyte lining cells and tight junction. The enterocytes collect compounds that reach apical side. The compounds then traverse into basolateral side where they end up in capillary vessel for circulation into the whole human body.

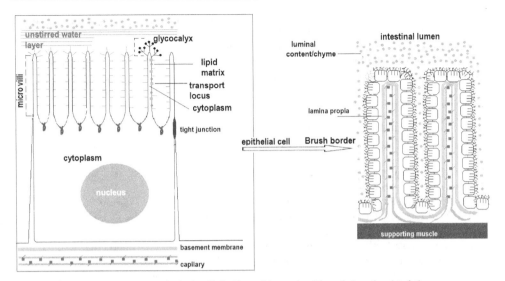

Fig. 2. Absorption tissue: epithelial cell (left) and intestinal brush border (right)

Other barrier in intestine is mucus. Most absorptive tissues comprise of epithelial cells which protect the human body from hazardous components in ingested foods. The epithelial cells are critical gate for human body. Due to its critical roles, the epithelial cells along gastrointestinal tract are covered with mucus secreted by goblet cells making an unstirred water layers so that the coarse particles are not abrasive towards the epithelial cells.

3.2 Transport mechanisms

Epithelial cell membrane is an important part of transport facility. It controls and selectively takes up molecules required for living or treats hazardous molecules. The fate of its work is not well understood despite studies finding many facilities and signaling processes available for regulating transport molecules. The transport modes include passive and active mechanisms. Passive transport is transcellular or paracellular transports and cynocitosis. Active transports are characterized by the use of protein transporters: channels/pump, binding protein transport, and formation of vehicles that is mainly emulsion system incorporating oil soluble compounds, such as chylomicrons. The transporter is able to promote transmembrane movement without hydrolyzing ATP (Johnson, 2001). They are categorized as uniporter (single compound moving down along the electrochemical gradients) and symporter (two molecules at the same time moving in one direction) or antiporter (two molecules at the same time moving in opposite directions).

Several transporters act as cellular efflux port for flavonoids: P-glycoproteins, multidrug resistance associated proteins, and breast cancer resistance protein (Johnson, 2001). They generally have loose substrate specificity and also involve in regulating non-nutritional compounds. Several findings point out glucose transporters which allow quercetin glucoside to be absorbed intact besides its aglycone forms. They are SGLT1[4] (SLC5A1[5]),

---

[4] Sodium dependent glucose transporter

GLUT2[6] (SLC2A2), MCT[7], OAT[8], and OATP[9]. However, results from the *in vitro* cell culture-based experiments are contradictive. Recently, bilitranslocase transport was introduced (Passamonti et al., 2009), that suggests the existence of a uniporter for flavonoids which is assumed to be an analogue of phthalien due to their similar molecular structures. The bilitranslocase is distributed in goblet and parietal cells in gastric, in apical jejunum of rat intestine, and in basolateral site of proximal tubular cell in kidney. However, further research is required for better understanding.

Briefly, bilitranslocase description indicates that target molecules interact with bilitranslocase through hydrogen bonds (hydrophilic properties of the active site); thus, nonionic inhibitors would not interact with it electrostatically. However, a negative charge is found to play an important role for electrogenic movement along the translocation pathway. These are observed through structural analysis (Passamonti et al., 2009). Similarly, the competitiveness of the target compounds can be explained by characteristics of C_4 in C-ring flavon building block where the target molecules are inactively competitive if the sugar moiety is in non-planar position; otherwise, the molecules will be actively competitive. Taking an example of quercetin-3-glucoside, the C_4 carbonyl forces 3-glucosyl moiety is perpendicular to the plane of flavonol aglycone resulting in a non-planar molecule. In contrast, its best competitor cyanidin-3-glucoside has a co-planar sugar moiety to the aglycone. Similarly, comparison of myricetin and delphinidin behave noncompetitively and competitively, respectively. Consequently, noncompetitor and competitor can be in one target molecule if its molecular structure has quinoidal, anionic tautomer, and neutral phenolics. They simultaneously can bind both the noncompetitive and competitive sites of bilitranslocase. Inconclusive role of bilitranslocation is compounded further by noninhibitor responses of other flavonoids, for instance flavonol (+)-catechin and isoflavones—genistin, genistein, daidzin, daidzein, and puerarin (Passamonti et al., 2009).

Bilitranslocase sheds a light for phenolics bioavailability and transport studies. The most striking relevance is that phenolics bioavailabilty is not delivered to blood circulation; instead, it is delivered through lymphatic system. This corrects understanding of hydrophobic nature of phytochemicals. The presence of bilitranslocase also clarifies disappearance of flavonoids in apical side but no basolateral level obtained in Ginjom (2009) and Epriliati (2008), despite GLUT2, MRP[10], organic cation, and amino acid/peptide transporters are available in basolateral domain. This specificity is promising for explaining the diverse bioavailability studies of phytochemicals.

3.3 Phytochemical absorption

There are two groups of nutriome: water soluble and less polar-solvent soluble. The water soluble components diffuse out from the food particles into chyme, traverse across the epithelial lining cells along the brush borders, and enter the portal blood circulation. On the other hand, the lipid soluble nutriome will be emulsified by bile salts and lipidic

---

[5] Solute carrier
[6] Glucose transporter
[7] Monocarboxylate transporter
[8] Organic anion transporter
[9] Organic anion transporting polypeptide
[10] Multidrug resistance-associated protein

components of diets immediately after diffusing out from the food particles. The emulsion acts as vehicles moving along the intestinal lumen. Contacting with the epithelial brush border and unstirred water layer on the top of the epithelial lining cells, rearrangement of vehicle emulsion take place which eventually releases the lipid soluble compounds into the cells. These compounds then traverse across the epithelium cells and end up in the lymph circulation. Nevertheless, many studies show losses material balances during transport across the epithelial lining gut. Moreover, the proportion of traversing compounds which are both water soluble and lipid soluble nutriomes that survive intact entering the circulatory system is not well understood. Similarly, proportion of metabolized nutriome used up by the epithelial cells as energy source is unclear.

Phenolics. Many studies support evidences that aglycone polyphenols are not only absorbed in the small intestine but also in the large intestine after microbial digestions. The steps may involve hydrolysis of sugar moiety by intestinal enzymes.

In the human small intestine and stomach, 95% of caffeic acid is absorbed while 62% of its ester form (called chlorogenic acid) is reduced. All are absorbed intact, except chlorogenic acid which mostly enters the human body from colon. Proanthocyanidins are pH sensitive thus it is likely to be broken down in stomach so that they may be readily absorbable. Meanwhile, catechin and epicatechin is poorly absorbed in the small intestine (≤20%) in a dose dependent manner. However, enterocytes can act differently; for instance, in intestinal jejunum it metabolizes flavanols into glucuronidated conjugates whereas in ileum it translocates flavanols intact. In the large bowel, most microflora metabolize flavonols and proanthocyanidins; for example, catechin metabolites include (-)-5[3'4'5'-trihydroxyphenyl]-γ-valerolactone; (-)-5[3'4'-dihydroxy phenyl]-γ-valerolactone; 3-hydroxyphenylpropionic acid; 3-hydroxybenzoic acid; or 3-hydroxyhippuric acid (Ginjom, 2009).

With a new bilitranslocase transport mechanism it is likely that the determinations of bioavailability of phytochemicals are necessarily being revised. pH and temperature are necessarily taken into account in order to avoid underestimation/overestimation regarding its stability. Several issues include absorption of quercetin and anthocyanin, glycone and aglycone forms, and conjugation/glucuronidation of phytochemicals as well as the presence of alcohol. Quercetin absorption varies from one food source to another. Its absorption from wine is enhanced by alcohol presence. Resident time of quercetin expressed as half-life clearance is 11-28 h (Manach et al., 2005). A very low level of intact anthocyanins is found in plasma after administration of anthocyanins. Resveratrol is absorbed well in the small intestine and being glucuronidated. Consumption of red wine would provide a good level of resveratrol bioavailability can be questioned whether this is because of alcohol presence.

Flavonoid is one of the group molecules with molecular weights >500 Da and has bioavailability level of <1%. Such molecules are unlikely to be transported through passive diffusion pathways. Further study found that influx membrane transporters cannot recognize flavonoid (signalling) whereas the efflux transporters do. Consequently, potential of flavonoids to be expelled is higher than that of influxed into the cells (Johnson, 2001).

In determination of phytochemical bioavailability, researchers should not limit their detection for ingested molecular forms only based on reported presence in the diets. It has been proven that at plasma levels many phytochemicals have been conserved by digestion and by hepatic activity. Fitting the mass balance of ingested phytochemical is challenging.

For instance, total metabolites in plasma levels are found reaching 4 mmol/L when intake is 50 mg aglycone equivalent whereas urinary excretion levels are 0.3-43% of the ingested doses, depending on polyphenol types. Flavonol such as quercetin in broccoli is rarely found as free quercetin. Human who consume 21-100 mg/d of quercetin show exclusive form of methyl, sulphate, or glucuronic acid conjugates totally amounted to maximum 1-5 μmol/L aglycone equivalent (Moreno et al., 2006). However, several phytochemicals are found intact, especially those which are absorbed easily. The ranks of phytochemical absorption is gallic acid and isoflavones > catechins and flavanones, quercetin glucoside > proanthocyanidins, galloylated tea catechins, and anthocyanins (Moreno et al., 2006).

Carotenoids. Carotenoids of mango, tomato, and papaya in caco-2 absorption model are not detected (Epriliati, 2008) in spite of *in vivo* data indicates that carotenoid plasma level increase after consumption of carotenoid-rich foods. Processing altered matrices of ingested food system and more likely degraded carotenoids which caused variation in bioavailability of carotenoids. A comparative study of organic and inorganic carrot found that apparently organic farming practices do not affect bioavailability of carotenoids in carrot consumption. Ingestion of total carotenoids of 24.3±1.4 mg organic carrot and 23.2±2.5 mg inorganic carrot results in 700 nmol/L β-carotene and 350 nmol/L α-carotene, and 150 nmol/L lutein after 2 weeks interventions (Stracke et al., 2009).

Organic acids. Organic acid provides organic anion important for metal binding and counteracting acidosis as well as preventing chronic diseases (Sabboh et al., 2011). Particular organic acids are apparently absorbed into plasma. Most organic acids in tomato, mango, and papaya products are absorbed in *in vitro* caco-2 model but they are not found in the basolateral sides (Epriliati, 2008). On the other hand, citric acid and oxalic from banana and sweet potato are consistently found to be absorbed and translocated into basolateral sides in *in vitro* caco-2 model (Sabboh et al., 2011). The absorbed organic acids are much lower compared to the original levels in food materials, thus, the retained organic acids in particles may be useful for controlling pH in colonic fermentation because selection of microbes in the large bowel is important.

Miscellaneous. Phytosterol could be absorbed at very low level using the same transport facilities for cholesterol due to structural similarities. It needs emulsion vehicle to diffuse in the aqueous lumen system, crossing the lipid membrane, and, finally, entering circulatory system. This requires evaluation because absorption is closely connected to which mechanisms are involved in health function, which is still debatable (Kang et al., 2010).

Triterpenoids citrus limonin glucoside is one of metabolites in citrus plant. Generally, it is water soluble; yet few aglycone forms of liminoids are insoluble. According to Manners et al. (2003) liminoid metabolites are found in human after ingestion of citrus juice containing limonin glucoside which may undergo epimerization from limonin glucoside to epilimonin (m/z 471.2). This may be from reaction pathways of hydrolization of glucoside moiety followed by lactonization. Although low level of limonin is ingested, it is eventually available in plasma after 6 h (Manners et al., 2003). During the first 3 h the higher ingestion level of limonin results in more significant changes in plasma epilimonin levels, regardless of age and gender. However, after 6 h, all volunteers show increased levels of plasma epilimonins at any ingestion levels of 0.25 g/200 mL-2 g/200 mL that is equivalent to 7 glasses of natural juices. The authors conclude that ingestion of limonin glucoside produces epimer limonin at C_{17}. It is clear that the human body does not necessarily control levels of plasma limonin and its absorption in the gut whereas limonin glucoside enters blood plasma through GLUT pathways, but it is necessarily hydrolyzed and lactonized. If it is absorbed through GLUT pathways without being metabolized, it should enter blood plasma at the same rate with sugars. The problem is that variation of individuals cannot be ignored since by the time it shows accumulation or decrease of detected limonin levels. The consequence of this accumulation is also not understood. Overall, limonin aglycone form is apparently safer than that of limonin glucosides; therefore, the high level of limonin glucoside form is controlled. Based on transit time of chyme in the gut, 6 h will be long enough to bring the chyme completely passing the small intestine. Therefore, lower level of ingestion results in limonin absorption after microbial glucoside hydrolisis in bowel. These speculations remain to be elucidated.

Interactions involve in various phytochemicals and nutrient transports. Since phytochemical are generally reactive molecules they can interact with various compounds in the chyme and this will affect phytochemical bioavailability and vice versa. Phytochemicals that interact with vitamin E include lignans, curcumin, anthocyanins, phenolic acid and catechin, as well as cereal alkylresorcinol (Frank, 2004). Interaction of vitamin E and plant lignans significantly increases vitamin E bioavailability as much as 900% in plasma level; 1,350% in liver; and 1,556% in lung using rat model. On the other hand, using human and rat model tocopherol-ω-hydrolase activity is effectively inhibited by sesamin[11]. Sesamin also reduces degradation of γ-tocopherol and urinary secretion so that it increases γ-tocopherol level in plasma. However, not all lignans show similar effects. For instance, sesamin or flaxseed lignan secoisolariciresinol diglucoside, either its monomer or oligomers decrease tocopherol by 50%. Experiment using rat model indicates that flaxseed lignan decreases α and γ tocopherol availability in a dose dependent manner. However, it presence increases lipid peroxidation. The majority of flaxseed lignan is converted into mammalian lignan allowing them to be absorbed (Frank, 2004).

In contrast, the effect of curcumin studied using rat model on α tocopherol bioavailability is less apparent when compared to flaxseed or sesame lignans where it is only detected in lung. In fact, curcumin is absorbed, metabolized, and secreted as glucuronidated metabolites. Similarly, the effect of anthocyanins on tocopherol bioavailability is neglected. Using the same rat model, it is found that caffeic acid increases γ-tocopherol in the liver and it is also converted into its metabolites 5-caffeoylquinic acid which in turn increases the levels of α-tocopherol in lung. However, when ingested as 5-caffeoylquinic acid, it is metabolized into caffeic acid and quinic acid; and caffeic acid is absorbed and found in plasma both in human and rat models. In contrast, ferulic acid is found to form complexes with albumin in blood plasma and LDL; hence, it does not affect tocopherol bioavailability. Interestingly, (+)-catechin and (-)-catechin isomers similarly improve α-tocopherol bioavailability in plasma and liver (Frank, 2004). There is a slight difference regarding their effects on γ-tocopherol where 2R,3R-isomer(-)-epicatechin enhances γ-tocopherol bioavailability whereas 2R,3R-(+)-catechin has no effect on it. The differences between γ– and α– tocopherol is estimated due to (i) antioxidant activity of catechin isomers on a tocopherol and (ii) different effects of the isomers on cytochrome P450 enzymes such as

---

[11] Lignan exists in sesamin

CYP1A1, CYP1A2, CYP2B1, AND CYP3A4 as well as CYP4F2. Alkylresorcinols in outer layer of wheat and rye is also absorbed and metabolized. Its presence improves γ-tocopherol in liver and lung but not α-tocopherol observed in rat. The various effects on tocopherol isomers are unclear although molecular differences of alkylresorcinol and tocopherol is known.

Addition of citric acid affects iron uptake. In reverse, citrate reduction improves iron bioavailability (Glahn et al., 1998). Iron bioavailability is also influenced by purple and brown pigments in rice; apparently, the pigment behaves similarly to tannin, phenolic, anthocyanin, or phytic acid (Glahn et al., 2002).

Interactions amongst carotenoids (Kostic et al., 1995; van den Berg, 1999) show that β-carotene inhibits lutein uptake. These interactions perhaps also occurred at the micelle formation and transport levels, or their combination (van het Hof et al., 2000). Similarly, β-carotene shows competitive inhibition to lycopene transport (Johnson, 1998). Meanwhile, carotenoids can interact with proteins and pectin decreasing absorption the carotenoids (Williams, 1998). Moreover, the cathecol structure in the B–ring of flavonols and 2,6-di-*tert*-butyl-4-mehtylphenol inhibits the dioxygenase enzyme and conversion of β-carotene (Nagao et al., 2000; Nagao, 2004). On the other hand, metabolites of bio-oxidation may act as pro-oxidants in the body (Nagao, 2004). Konishi found that tea phenolics inhibit other dietary phenolics (Konishi et al., 2003).

Among several fruits and vegetables, papaya and tomato consumption are found to be benefecial in hypolipidemic diet components, with similar mechanisms observed during *in vivo* experiments using rats (Kumar et al., 1997). Here, soluble and insoluble fibers can bind bile acids, thus influencing micelle formation and absorption of lipophilic substances by the brush border. Lignin and guar gum are apparently better bile binders than cellulose, which is relatively inert. Interaction also occurs between fiber and intestinal mucin, which probably alters absorption and nutrient diffusion from bulk lumen content (Vahouny & Cassidy, 1985). Moreover, fiber bound health promoters include lycopene in tomato peel (Awad et al., 2002) and antioxidants in mango peel (Larrauri et al., 1996), where the antioxidants found in mango peel, pulp and seed include gallotannins (Berardini et al., 2004). Consumption of fiber-rich food products can reduce minerals and vitamin (Schneeman & Gallaher, 1985). Generally, those authors agree that pectin and cellulose play important roles, especially in reducing the activity of digestive enzymes, or hormones such as insulin (Schneeman & Gallaher, 1985; Vahouny & Cassidy, 1985).

4. Kinetics simulation of phytochemical bioavailability

Kinetics is a study observing changes of the phytochemicals after ingestion including elimination period. To understand kinetics of phytochemicals after ingestion, kinetics simulation is frequently carried out. The limitations of simulations should be acknowledged in interpreting the results. Moreover, bioavailability closely relates to absorption and metabolism, yet there are limited understanding of bioavailability markers. Furthermore, the markers need validating, i.e. the molecular forms selected as bioavailability markers are necessarily those which actually cause health effects.

Affecting factors of phenolic bioavailability include matrix of food sources, processing condition during food preparations, chemical compositions, and molecular physicochemical properties of the target molecules. Molecular forms of phenolics such as glycone or aglycone definitely make diverse variations on bioavailability levels. In addition to these factors, individual gastrointestinal tract of the human also affects bioavailability. Gastrointestinal pH, level of secretions, microbiota, and age have been established as crucial factors affecting digestion and absorption of phytochemicals. Equally, the role of interactions amongst food components and their interactions with gastrointestinal secretions contribute significant effects in determining bioavailability of phytochemicals.

Tannin-protein interactions occur starting from mouth and food systems. The interaction depends on size, conformation, and charges of proteins; molecular size, flexibility, and water solubility of phenolics; and environmental conditions such as pH. Proteins with higher molecular weights or loose conformational structures or rich in proline/hydrophobic amino acids, increase its potential to be precipitated by tannin. On the other hand, flavonols (three orthohydroxyl groups on the B-ring) has higher affinity to protein compared to those with two orthohydroxyl groups. Similarly, the affinity increases with increasing galloylation degrees. The order of flavonols affinity is (-)-epigallocatechin gallate >(-)-gallocatechin gallate >(-)-epicatechin gallate >(-)epigallocatechin or (-)-epicatechin or (+)-catechin (Ginjom, 2009). Interestingly, tannin also plays pivotal roles in its capability to act as health protective antioxidant.

4.1 *In vitro* model of digestion and transport

Effects of *in vitro* digestion on wine phytochemicals are significant during pancreatic digestion step, especially for nonpolar compounds. Therefore, water solubility level is crucial in generating an appropriate *in vitro* digestion model. In contrast, acid does not significantly affect the phytocemical components in wine.

In vitro model for absorption using a monolayer cell culture can help bioavailability determinations with human surrogates; however, the results should be carefully considered. More importantly, the results cannot be liberately generalized for human system biology. Yun et al. (2004) propose a constant to equalize *in vitro* measurement using caco-2 monolayer with human *in vivo* measurement for iron. Furthermore, there are critical factors in utilizing such *in vitro* model for a bioavailability study that should be carefully considered. For instance, the original composition of digest containing bile salts decreases TEER (transepithelial electrical resistance) indicating serious detrimental effect on the cell monolayer integrity. In addition, alcohol content in wine also affects the monolayer integrity so that alcohol removal is required although alcohol enhances phenolic absorption. This is unrealistic wine samples. Furthermore, the delicate properties of the monolayers may result from lacking of mucus/unstirred water layer protecting the epithelium. The development of an appropriate and standardized *in vitro* model needed to be persued continuously.

4.2 Kinetics of phytochemical bioavailability

Kinetics study of phytochemicals is scarce. Several experiments are reviewed below to understand phytochemical kinetics after ingestion.

Quercetin. Quercetin is more likely to be absorbed quickly in the human gut after ingestion, e.g. quercetin-3-glucoside from blackcurrant juice is 4 h or pure quercetin glucoside capsule is ca 30 min. Quercetin-3-rutinoside takes longer time to reach peak plasma levels compared to the two previously mentioned, i.e. after 5-10 h. Short- and long- term studies show kinetics absorption of quercetin is quick and easy; and there are no interactions with other food components. Moreover, bioavailable quercetin can be obtained from normal diet regardless of whether it contains the berries or not. Therefore, it is proposed that fasting quercetin bioavailability is used as a biomarker of high fruit and vegetable intakes for all plant based foods (Erlund et al., 2006).

Soyasaponin. Soyasaponin has a very low bioavailability when investigated using *in vivo* experiments involving animals and human (Kang et al., 2010). However, it is also found that possible metabolites of soyasaponin are detected in *in vitro* and *in vivo* studies, although it is found several days after ingestion (Kang et al., 2010). The metabolites include soyasapogenol B, which is secreted into faeces in human *in vivo* experiments. However, the metabolism is more likely due to microbiota in the colon which is supported by *in vitro* data using fresh faecal microbiota. *In vitro* data show sequential metabolism of sapogenin by the microbiota as follows: soyasaponin I after 48 h incubation at 37 °C, and it is converted into soyasaponin III after 24 h and disappeared at 48 h where the predicted final metabolite is soyasapogenol B. These sequential metabolisms take place through sugar hydrolysis which results in the formation of more hydrophobic metabolites and smaller molecules (Kang et al., 2010).

Lignan. Low lignan bioavailability is recovered in plasma in human after ingestion of lignans (Kang et al., 2010). It is interesting that lignan is easily absorbed into plasma after ingestion. The available information is for secoisolariciresinol diglucoside and its aglycone secoisolariciresinol and matairesinol. Based on the studies, at least 40% of ingested lignans are metabolized by intestinal bacteria and these metabolites can be detected in the plasma. Metabolites of lignans appearing in the human plasma after ingestion follows the sequences: (i) at 14.8±5.1 h enterodiol is maximally found in plasma, (ii) at 19.7±6.2 h enterolactone is maximally bioavailable, and (iii) at 8-10 h enterolignans is bioavailable. Resident time of lignan metabolites in plasma is 20.6±5.9 h for enterodiol and 35.8±10.6 h for enterolactone, respectively (Kang et al., 2010).

Phytosterol. Low phytosterol bioavailability is observed in human plasma after ingestion. Definite small amount (0.6-7.5%) of phytosterol is transported through gut epithelial cells *in vivo*. Chemically, phytosterol is similar to cholesterol; yet cholesterol is absorbed at much higher levels than phytosterol. This is because of side chain differences, i.e. ethyl/methyl group in C_{24} which increases hydrophobicity but reduces absorption; and the presence of $\Delta 5$ double bond. The similarity of absorption mechanism of phytosterol and cholesterol is that (i) they need to be in emulsion system and (ii) to be facilitated by Niemann-Pick C1 like 1 (NPC1L1) protein. Surprisingly, it is just recently acknowledged that many of bioactive compounds need to be in emulsion system to make them more bioavailable (Kang et al., 2010).

Phytate. Phytate bioavailability is low in human plasma levels after ingestion. Plasma myo-[inositol-2-H^3(N)]hexakisphosphate in human after ingestion is dose-dependent and it only reaches 3-5 times higher than that of diet poor in myo-[inositol-2-H^3(N)]hexakisphosphate. Further study using rat found that absorbed phytate is quickly distributed into tissues such as brain, kidneys, liver, and bone in its original dietary molecular forms. The highest level is in brain reaching 10 times compared to average of tissues (Kang et al., 2010). This is beyond conventional nutrition believes that phytic acid and phytate is not traversed across lipid bilayer.

Sulfur compounds. Bioavailability of isothiocyanates is better than glucosinolate in the human gut. In spite of different cruciferous origins and types, isothiocyanate is always found in plasma and its metabolites in urine is consistently found as dicarbamate or mercapturic acid. It is important to note that not all glucosinolates behave similarly. Generally, heated or cooked glucosinolate is less bioavailable (1.8-43%) than raw (8.2-113); and it is quickly absorbed in the gut and quickly excreted in urine (24 h). The exceptions are from pak choi (butenyl and pentenyl isothiocyanates, 8%), garden cress (benzyl isothiocyanate, 14%), and water cress (phenylethyl isothicyanate, 50%) compared to 100% isothiocyanate. Critical factors of the study remain: (i) individual variations (different microflora in the bowel, metabolism, and chewing ability), (ii) natural cruciferous matrices so that strongly entrapped glycosinolate in the cells will be hardly released during chewing, and (iii) types of glucosinolates (Vermeulen, 2009).

Vegetable consumption during lunchtime shows a general lag phase for excretion of mercapturic acid at 4 h after ingestion (Vermeulen, 2009). The sulfocompounds (isothiocyanate) in the body is conjugated. Raw vegetable consumption results in a fast excretion whereas cooked vegetable has longer resident time of conjugated form. Elimination for half-life of the compound is 2-4 h, which is longer than that of other study (1.8 h) (Ye et al., 2002), with excretion rate of 0.18-0.33 h^{-1} by assuming the first order reaction.

Food source of sulfur compounds is a determinant factor in absorption in addition to processing and physiological conditions. Sulforaphane content in raw and cooked broccoli is 9.92 and 61.4 μmole/kg, respectively; and 37 and 3.4 % of them are recovered in urine in the form of sulforaphane mercapturic acids. On the other hand, 54% of benzyl isothicyanate from garden cress is found in urine but phenylethyl isothicyanate from watercress after chewing is 47%. When cooked watercress is administered, only 1.2-7.3% of glucosinolates is recovered; this is much lower than sulforaphane (17.2-77.7%). Monitoring dithiocarbamate in urine shows 12% recovery from boiled broccoli sprout. The recovery increased to 80% when the boiled broccoli sprout is treated with myrosinase. About 68% of allyl isothiocyanate from mustard is excreted in urine as mercapturic acid while sinigrin is present at 15% and 37% from cooked and raw cabbage[12], respectively (Vermeulen, 2009). Generally, the routes of metabolisms in the human body vary depending on the target molecules and food sources. Glucoraphanin and sulforaphane from cooked and raw broccoli peak for maximum 6 and 1.6 h, respectively (Vermeulen, 2009). The half-life clearance of sulforaphane in the human body from the aforementioned vegetables is 4.6 and 3.8 h, respectively. These are different from half-life time of mercapturic acid which is 2.4 and 2.6 h, respectively. Further investigations using human subjects show inconclusive results that particular polymorphism S-glutathione transferase (GST M1, T1 and P1) and N-acetyl transferase (NAT2) gene affect the variations (Vermeulen, 2009). It is important to view these phenomena under the holistic affecting factors.

---

[12] Data is calculated from : First order kinetics

k_a: intercept and slope with a residual method; k: natural log of plasma amounts plotted against time; k_e: natural log of absolute excreted amounts vs time; area under curve (concentration vs time) extrapolated using trapezoid method; lag phase is determined from empiric curve obtained; base line is not used

Phenolics. Generally, the least absorbed polyphenols are proanthocyanidins, galloylated tea catechins, and anthocyanins (Epriliati, 2008 and Ginjom, 2009).

Caffeine. Using pharmacological principles, absorption simulations of pure compound in intestine is mimicked by caco-2 monolayers. During the simulated transit method (model A), unchanged caffeine was transported across epithelial cells (Figure 3). This indicates that caffeine is directly transported to the basolateral compartment without damaging the tight junctions. This transport is selectively occurring in the apical to basolateral direction over the bioassay time (240 min). The apical caffeine levels from simulation of transit method even after 120 min (Figure 3, top panel) are higher than that of semi dynamic apical solution method (B model) (Figure 3, middle panel). Caffeine was transported by the enterocytes in the apical to basolateral direction apparently without an equilibrium state being generated. Uptake of caffeine was rapid and basolateral secretion possibly required a certain amount of caffeine intracellularly is retained. When a high gradient concentration was maintained, continuous basolateral secretion of caffeine took place at a constant rate. As a result, the final level of basolateral caffeine was higher than the apical levels, even when it was subjected to a 22 h bioassay (C model) (Figure 3, bottom panel). The transport mechanism of caffeine may be a simple passive diffusion. However, another study shows caffeine can also be transported by the transcellular route (Mao, 2007). In addition, caffeine is found interacts with glucose uptake sensitivity (Pizziol, 1998).

Catechin. The simulation transit method of catechin indicates that it is retained in the apical compartment at about one-third of the initial amount (86.8 nmol) and remains at about the same level throughout the experiment (Figure 4, top panel). However, basolateral compartment analysis did not indicate equal amount of translocated catechin. In contrast, most basolateral samples contain very little catechin. In the static apical solution method (Figures 4, middle and bottom panels), apical catechin was reduced to 39 nmol after 22 h, but there were no indication of transported catechin in the basolateral compartment. In the present study, there may have been some metabolism of catechin based on apical losses which require further study to identify possible metabolites of catechin.

Lycopene. Lycopene is neither transported (Figure 5) nor chemically changed during bioassay using all three bioassay methods for all time periods. Its hydrophobicity and unfavorable molecular geometry apparently prevents lycopene from passing through monolayers via either paracellular or transcellular routes. This was confirmed by the decrease of TEER values for all monolayers, which is not accompanied by lycopene translocation into the basolateral compartment from the apical solutions. In the present study, the apical lycopene do not show disappearance in the transit model (Figure 5, top panel). Instead, lycopene shows apical accumulations with renewal solutions. Similar results are obtained from the semi dynamic model (Figure 5, middle panel) and confirmed in the 22 h static model (Figure 5, bottom panel). Lycopene absorption has been shown to be affected by the presence of other carotenoids, the lipid status, and plasma antioxidant capacity (Bohm & Bitsch, 1999). However, another study found that lycopene plasma levels after consumption of cherry tomatoes are insignificantly different from the plasma base line (Bugianesi et al., 2004). Further absorption from micelles has been shown to be slow (e.g. lycopene absorbed by LNCaP and Hs888Lu cells took approximately 10 h; Xu et al., 1999). This suggests that epithelial cells may have specific mechanisms that are not micelle dependent.

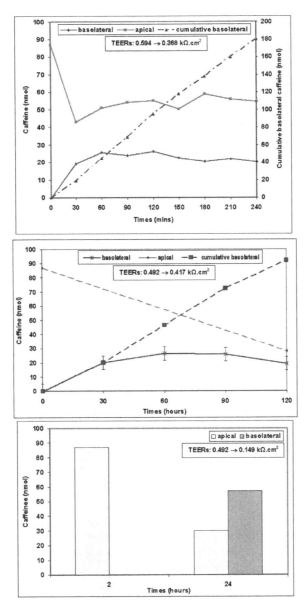

Fig. 3. Bioassay of caffeine using simulated transit method (top panel: model A; using 2 transwell-inserts), static apical solution method (middle panel: model B; using 4 transwell-inserts), and static apical and basolateral solution procedures for 22 h (bottom panel: model C; using 2 transwell-inserts)[13]

---

[13] Model A: apical side is replenished every 30 min, Model B: basolateral side is refreshed every 30 min, Model C: both apical and basolateral are not replenished for 22 h

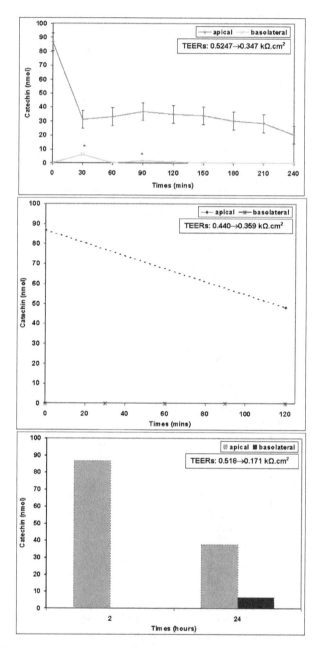

Fig. 4. (+) Catechin transport using simulation of transit chyme (top panel: model A; using 2 transwell inserts), static apical solution methods (middle panel: model B; using 4 transwell inserts), and static apical and basolateral solution after 22 h (bottom panel: model C; using 4 transwell inserts)

β–carotene. There are always reductions of apical levels but not necessarily accompanied by release into the basolateral side (Figure 6). Meanwhile, β-carotene completely disappears in the 22 h static model, both from the apical and basolateral sides although TEER values drops from 0.497 to 0.125 kΩ.cm². β-carotene may diffuse better than lycopene, as indicated by the β-carotene apical disappearances; however, neither is translocated. This may be related to intrinsic solubility, as β-carotene is more soluble than lycopene in the mixed aqueous/organic solvents. In the semi dynamic model after 120 min, apical β-carotene decreases and in the static model after 22 h, β-carotene disappears completely.

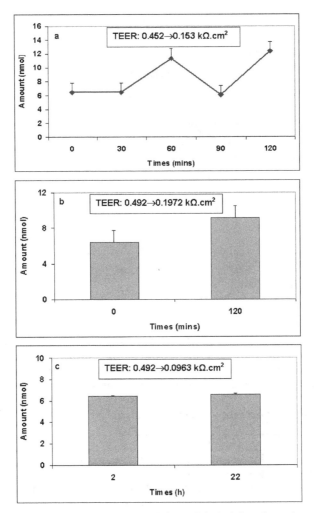

Fig. 5. Apical lycopene bioassay; **a** transit model (model A), **b** basolateral renewals (model B), **c** static model (model C) in buffer-0.5% DMSO

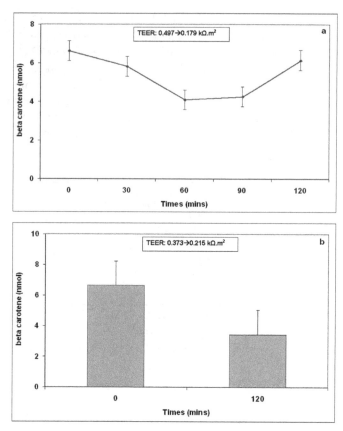

Fig. 6. Apical β-Carotene in HBSS-25 mM HEPES contained 0.5 % DMSO: **a** transit chyme (model A), **b** static apical solution (model B)

4.3 Dosages

Establishing the most suitable dosages for an optimal health benefit of a phytochemical is not an easy task. As an antioxidant, phytochemicals are generally required in small doses due to its ability to become pro-oxidant. Based on its traditional usage, the doses are commonly determined from folklores, thus the key compounds mostly responsible for their health functions and their mechanisms remain to be explored through epidemiological studies. Table 3 lists what doses studied *in vitro* and folklores.

Phytochemicals	Effects	Dosages
Soya saponin (Kang et al., 2010)	• Inhibits metastasis HT-1080 cells • Decrease HT cell growth • Inhibit AFB_1-DNA adduct formation in HepG2 liver cells • Induce apoptosis in SNB 19 glioblastoma cells	• 100-300 µl/mL; 24 h • 150, 300, 600 ppm; 72 h • IC_{50} at 30 µg/mL; 48 h • 25-75 µM; 48 h

Phytochemicals	Effects	Dosages
	• Suppress HTC 15 cell proliferation	• 25-500 ppm
	• Induce macroautophagy	• 100 ppm; 24 h
	• Decrease migratory ability/increase adhesion of B16F10 cells	• 25-75 µM; 12 h
	• Enhance adhesion of MCF7 cells	• 50 µM; 24 h
Soyasapogenol A and B (Kang et al., 2010)	• Suppress HT 29 cell growth	• 6-50 ppm; 72 h
Soyasaponin – soyasapogenol B monoglucuronide mixture (Kang et al., 2010)	• Suppress HT 29 cell growth	• 50 ppm; 72 h
Phytate (Kang et al., 2010)	• Decrease expression of TNF-a and TNF II in Caco-2 cells	• 1, 2.5, and 5 mM; 12 h
	• Inhibit proliferation of HT 29 cells	• 13 mmol.L; 12 h
	• Inhibit growth of MCF-7/Adr cells	• IC$_{50}$ at 1.26 mM; 96 h
	• Inhibit growth of MDA-MB 231cells	• IC$_{50}$ at 1.32 mM; 96 h
	• Inhibit growth of MCF-7 cells	• IC$_{50}$ at 4.18 mM; 96 h
	• Inhibit growth of HepG2 cells	• 0.25-5 mM; 6 d
	• Inhibit growth of LNCaP cells	• 0.5-4 mM; 24 h
	• Inhibit growth of DU145 cells	• 0.25-2 mM; 24 h
Phenolics in colourful potatoes	• Treating gastric ulcer	• 2-3 times a day for no more than 4-6 weeks; drinking diluted water extract of fresh potato (Tan & Rahardja, 2010)
Phytochemicals from luffa [*Luffa cylindrica* Roem.; *Luffa Aegyptica* Mill.; *L. Cattupincina* Ser.; *L. Pentandra* Roxb.]	• To treat intestinal inflammation	• 1-2 times a day; drinking mature seed extract made from 20 g powder in a ½ cup of hot water
	• To improve breast milk production	• Drinking extract of a 6 g of seed and flesh powder
	• To treat asthma	• 2-3 times a day; drinking young luffa juice sweetened with sugar
Phytochemicals from Indian champor weed [*Pluchea indica* (L.)	• For fever and emetic sweat removal	• once a day; consuming 10 g of boiled leaves
	• For body odour removal	• regularly 3 times a day; consuming 10-15 pieces of

Phytochemicals	Effects	Dosages
Less.]	• For relieving gastrointestinal disorders in children	raw or steamed leaves with rice • Consuming 3-5 pieces of crushed leaves mixed with soft rice (porridge) (Dalimartha, 2005; Hariana, 2006).
Phytochemicals from Watercress [*Nasturtium officinale* R. Brown, *N. officinale* W.T. Aiton, *N. nasturtium-aquaticum* (L) H. Karst., *Radicula nasturtium Cav.*,]	• For tuberculosis • For inflamed lung and coughing • For skin irritation • For urinary problems	• 2-3 times a day; consuming soup made from 250 g watercress and pig bone, added with sufficient salt • Consuming soup made from 60 g of watercress and sugar • several times a day; consuming soup of boiled watercress • Consuming soup made from 250 g of watercress and palm sugar (Muchlisah & Hening, 2009)
Phytochemicals from bilimbi [*Averrhoa bilimbi* Linn]	• For hypertension • For acne • For muscle pain • For teeth cavities	• once every three days; drinking extract of 3 bilimbi fruits in 3 glasses of water, concentrated 3 times • 3 times a day; applying a mixture of 6-8 ground bilimbi fruits, a ½ tea spoon of salt, a ¼ glasses of water onto acne • Applying a mixture of 25 pieces of bilimbi leaves, 10 clove, and 15 pepper, ground finely, added with a small amount of vinegar, at suffering body/tissues • Chewing 5 pieces of bilimbi fruits with a little salt and at the suffering teeth (Hariana, 2006).
Phytochemicals from Glossy nightshade, Black nightshade [*Solanum americanum*	• For urethra infection	• twice a day; drinking a ½ glasses of extract of 30 g of black nightshade fruits with *Hedyotis diffusa* grass, and *Phyllantus urinearia* in a 3 glasses of water,

Phytochemicals	Effects	Dosages
Miller, *Solanum nodiflorum* Jacq, *Solanum ningrum* auct non L.]	• For eczema or dermatitis • For xeropthalia • For cervical erosion • For pektay	concentrated twice • twice a day; consuming 60 g of boiled shrub • 3 times a day; chewing around 15 black nightshade fruits • 1-2 times a week for 8 weeks; applying a mixture of ground boiled-black nightshade fruits at the suffering tissues • 3 times twice a week; drinking a ½ glasses of decoction of 30 g ground black nightshade fruits and *Celosia cristata* flowers in a 3 glasses of water, and concentrated (Dalimartha, 2008)
Phytochemicals from Waxy gourd [*Benincasa hispida* (Thunb) Cogn., *B. cerifera savi*, *Cucurbita hispida* Thunb. *Lagenaria dasystemon* Miq]	• Curing hemorrhoid • To treat diabetes	• once a day for 14 days for adult; given infusion liquid of 1 waxy gourd fruit as big as a palm hand, added by 10 pieces of anises/fennels, a ±1cm length of *Alixa stellata*, and a tea spoon of honey; (Kementerian Lingkungan Hidup, 2011) • Consuming 100-150 g boiled or juiced waxy guard (Wijayakusuma, 2008)
Phytochemicals from Lemon basil [*Ocimum americanum, O. citriodorum, O. africanum, O. canum Sims, O. brachiatum Blume*]	• To ease people suffering from early ejaculation, late menstruation, breast milk and gas cleanser in the human body, and for removing fever	• twice a day; drinking a ½ glasses of decoction of 15 g lemon basil grass in a 2 glass of water for 15 minutes (Hariana, 2006)

Table 2. Resume of dosages used in studies regarding phytochemicals health effects and in folklores[14].

---

[14] The information of Indonesian medicinal folklores is obtained through a collaboration project between Korean Food Research Institution and Bogor Agricultural University, Indonesia in 2011.

5. Recommended daily allowance

5.1 Recommended daily allowance

Recommended uses and maximum limits of uses in modern public health management are limited. The ancient uses are based on folklores and old documents. This information should be followed up with proper scientific investigations and documentations. Even for broccoli which is extensively studied, the recommended daily intake has not been officially established. US national cholesterol education program recommends adult subject to consume 2 g of phytosterol/d for optimally lowering LDL-C and coronary heart disease risks by 10% (Kang et al., 2010). The mechanism of this is still vague but it is known that phytosterol/phytostanol does not necessarily present simultaneously with cholesterol to control cholesterol absorption.

5.2 Public health management

There is limited information on detailed diet prescription aiming at treating a particular disease, except those recorded in ancient medications. Dieticians usually arrange diets for patients not aiming for disease treatments but to meet certain nutritional requirements to improve their stamina or immune system to combat their physiological problems. Mechanism for phytochemical health benefits have been studied extensively. Current understanding shows that public health would take benefits from diet management for prevention and maintaining public health instead of treating it. Many research results found scientific base of phytochemicals. For example, liminoids has increasingly proven positive health effects including induction of glutathione S-transferase, inhibiting cancers growth, and lowering cholesterols (Kang et al., 2010), yet officially, this still has not been established for recommended daily allowance. On the other hand, information from ancient medicinal prescriptions as listed in Table 3 is mostly in the form of decoction of the phytochemical sources and the boiled water is drunk. Interesting research area is to establish whether such preparation preserve biological functions of the phytochemicals or, instead, the methods modify molecular form of the phytochemicals that is a much safer and/or more bioactive than its original forms.

5.3 Phytochemicals incorporation in diets

Phytochemicals are commonly consumed as supplements either in capsules, tablets, or powders. The incorporation of such ingredients in food products may or may not face problems of stability, especially at its extraction step and formulation and food processing in which heating is one of predominant aspects for generating food palatability. Most conventional food preparations are of high risks on phytochemical instability. Attempt to improve food technology remains inconclusive. Health effect study indicates that enriched ground beef with soy phytosterol reduces total cholesterol, LDL-C, and TC/HDL cholesterol by 9.3, 14.6, and 9.1%, respectively (Vermeulen, 2009). Such attempts require standardization for establishment of functional food regulations.

5.4 Phytochemical demands per capita

In order to maintain health where phytochemicals are involved, a daily recommended allowance similar to other nutrients is required. Therefore, prior to daily recommended allowance establishment, there is a need for dosage allowance for each bioactive. Similarly, when recommended allowance has been established, food chain supply needs to provide necessary quantity of the phytochemical sources for people. Such data are currently unavailable, and thus, a database and information system for it needs to be established.

6. Conclusion

Phytochemicals bioavailability is strongly dependent on cell wall compositions of the food matrices they originate from, structural chemistry of the phytochemicals, history of processing, as well as individual human gastrointestinal system. Determination of phytochemical bioavailability is increasingly developed using both *in vitro* and *in vivo* approaches, and yet the results are still inconclusive. The main challenge is to develop an *in vitro* model that can represent human *in vivo* condition for practical uses. On the other hand, many aspects of bioavailability is not well understood, prompting further research and database for recommended dosages and consequently per capita phytochemical demands for public health management. Currently, folklores are the main sources of public health management using phytochemicals and database remains to be pursued for better scientific base of folklores practices.

7. References

Berardini, N.; Carle, R. & Schieber, A. (2004). Characterization of gallotannins and benzophenone derivatives from mango (*Mangifera indica* L. cv. 'Tommy Atkins') peels, pulp and kernels by high-performance liquid chromatography electrospray ionization mass spectrometry. *Rapid Communications in Mass Spectrometry*, 18, (2004), pp. 2208 - 2216.

Awad, H.M.; Boersma, M.G.; Boeren, S.; van Bladeren, P.J.; Vervoort, J. & Rietjens, I.M. (2002). The regioselectivity of glutathione adduct formation with flavonoid quinone/quinone methides is pH-dependent. *Chem Res Toxicol*, 15, (2002), pp. 343 - 351.

Bohm, V. & Bitsch, R. (1999). Intestinal absorption of lycopene from different matrices and interactions to other carotenoids, the lipid status, and the antioxidant capacity of human plasma. *Eur J Nutr*, 38, (1999), pp. 118 - 125.

Bugianesi, R.; Salucci, M.; Leonardi, C.; Ferracane, R.; Catasta, G.; Azzini, E. & Maiani, G. (2004). Effect of domestic cooking on human bioavailability of naringenin, chlorogenic acid, lycopene and beta-carotene in cherry tomatoes. *Eur J Nutr [NLM - MEDLINE]*, 43, (2004), pp. 360.

Dalimartha, S. (2005). *Tanaman Obat di Lingkungan Sekitar*. Puspa Swara, Depok

Dalimartha S. (2008). *Atlas Tumbuhan Obat Indonesia*. Jilid 5. Pustaka Bunda, Depok

de Freitas, V. & Mateus, N. (2001). Structural features of procyanidin interactions with salivary proteins. *J Agric Food Chem.*, 49, (2001), pp. 940-945.

Epriliati, I. Nutriomic analysis of fresh and processed fruits through the development of an *in-vitro* model of human digestive system, PhD dissertation, The University of Queensland.

Erlund, I.; Freese, R.; Marniemi, J.; Hakala, P. & Alfthan, G. (2006). Bioavailability of Quercetin from Berries and The Diet. *Nutr Cancer*, 54, 1, (2006), pp. 13–17

Frank, J. (2004). *Dietary Phenolic Compounds and Vitamin E Bioavailability–Model studies in rats and humans*. Doctoral dissertation. ISSN 1401-6249, ISBN 91-576-6453-6. Department of Food Science, Swedish University Agricultural Science

Friedman, M. & Jurgens, H. S. (2000). Effect of pH on the stability of plant phenolic compounds. *J Agric Food Chemistry*, 48, (2000). pp. 2101-2110.

Ginjom, I.R.H. Health aspects of wine antioxidants: composition and *in vitro* bioavailability. PhD dissertation. The University of Queensland.

Glahn, R.P.; Cheng, Z.; Welch, R.M. & Gregorio, G.B. (2002). Comparison of iron biaovailability from 15 rice genotypes: studies using an *in vitro* digestion/caco-2 cell culture model. *J Agric Food Chem.*, 50, (2002), pp. 3586 - 3591.

Glahn, R.P.; Lai, C.; Hsu, J. & Thompson, J.F. (1998). Decreased citrate improves iron availability from infant formula: Application of an *in vitro* digestion/Caco-2 cell culture model. *The Journal of Nutrition*, 128, (1998), pp. 257.

Hariana, A. (2006). *Tanaman Obat dan Khasiatnya*. Seri1. Penebar Swadaya, Jakarta

Johnson, E.J. (1998). Human studies on bioavailability and plasma response of lycopene. *Proc Soc Exp Biol Med*, 218, (1998), pp. 115 - 120.

Johnson, L.R. (2001). *Gastrointestinal Physiology*. 6th ed., Mosby, ISBN 0-323-01239-6 St. Louis

Kang, J.; Badger, T.M.; Ronis, M.J.J.; & Wu, X. (2010). Non-isoflavone Phytochemicals in Soy and Their Health Effects. *J. Agric. Food Chem.* 58, (2010), pp. 8119–8133

Kidd, P. & Head, K. (2005). A review of the bioavailability and clinical efficacy of milk thistle phytosome: A silybin-phosphatidylcholine complex (Silipos®). *Alternative Medicine Rev.*, 10, 3, (2005), pp. 193-203

Konishi, Y.; Kobayashi, S. & Shimizu, M. (2003). Tea polyhenols inhibit the transport of dietary phenolic acids mediated by the monocarboxyclic acid transporters (MCT) in intestinal caco-2 cell monolayers. *J Agric Food Chem.*, 51, (2003), pp. 7296 - 7302.

Kostic, D.; White, W. & Olson, J. (1995). Intestinal absorption, serum clearance, and interactions between lutein and beta-carotene when administered to human adults in separate or combined oral doses. *Am J Clin Nutr*, 62, (1995), pp. 604 - 610.

Kementerian Lingkungan Hidup. (2011). Potensi sumberdaya genetik tanaman: Bligu (*Benincasa hispida (Thunb.) Cogn*). http://bk.menlh.go.id/sdg/ [Accessed June 5, 2011]

Kumar, G. P.; Sudheesh, S.; Ushakumari, B.; Valsa, A. K.; Vijayakumar, S.; Sandhya, C. & Vijayalakshmi, N.R. (1997). A comparative study on the hypolipidemic activity of eleven different pectins. *Journal of Food Science and Technology Mysore*, 34, (1997), pp. 103 - 107.

Larrauri, J.A.; Goni, I.; MartinCarron, N.; Ruperez, P. & SauraCalixto, F. (1996). Measurement of health-promoting properties in fruit dietary fibres: Antioxidant capacity, fermentability and glucose retardation index. *Journal of the Science of Food and Agriculture*, 71, (1996), pp. 515 - 519.

Manach, C.; Williamson, G.; Morand, C.; Scalbert, A. & Remesy, C. (2005). Bioavailability and bioefficacy of polyphenols in humans. I. Review of 97 bioavailability studies. *American Journal of Clinical Nutrition*, 81, (2005), pp. 230S-242.

Manners, G.D.; Jacob, R.A.; Breksa III, A.P.; Schoch, T.K. & Hasegawa, S. (2003). Bioavailability of Citrus Limonoids in Humans. *J. Agric. Food Chem.*, 51, (2003), pp. 4156-4161

Mao, X.; Chai, Y. & Lin, Y-F. (2007). Dual regulation of ATP-sensitive potassium channel by caffeine. *Am J Physiol Cell Physiol*, 292, (2007), pp. C2239 - 58.

Miyazaki, S., Kubo, W., Itoh, K., Konno, Y., Fujiwara, M., Dairaku, M., Togashi, M., Mikami, R. and Attwood, D. 2005. The effect of taste masking agents on in situ gelling pectin formulations for oral sustained delivery of paracetamol and ambroxol. *International Journal of Pharmaceutics*, 297, 38 - 49

Moreno, D.A.; Carvajal, M.; L´opez-Berenguer, C. & Garc´ıa-Viguera, C. (2006). Chemical and biological characterisation of nutraceutical compounds of Broccoli. *J Pharmaceu Biomed Anal*, 41, (2006), pp. 1508–1522

Muchlisah, F. & Hening, S. (2009). *Sayur dan bumbu dapur berkhasiat obat*. Penebar Swadaya, Jakarta

Nagao, A.; Maeda, M.; Lim, B. P.; Kobayashi, H. & Terao, J. (2000). Inhibition of [beta]-carotene-15,15'-dioxygenase activity by dietary flavonoids. *The Journal of Nutritional Biochemistry*, 11, (2004), pp. 348 - 355.

Nagao, A. 2004. Oxidative conversion of carotenoids to retinoids and other products. *The Journal of Nutrition*, 134, (2004), PP. 237S.

Noe, V.; Penuelas, S.; Lamuela-Raventos, R.M.; Permanyer, J.; Ciudad, C.J. & Izquerdo-Pulido, M. (2004). Epicatechin and cocoa polyphenolic extract modulate gene expresión in human Caco-2 cells. *J Nutr.*, 134, (2004), pp. 2509-2516

Nunan, K.J.; Sims, I.M.; Bacic, A.; Robinson, S.P. & Fincher, G.B. (1998). Changes in cell wall composition during ripening of grape berries. *Plant Physiol.*, 118, (1998). pp. 783–792

Passamonti, S.; Terdoslavich, M.; Franca, R.; Vanzo, A.; Tramer, F.; Braidot, E.; Petrussa, E. & Vianello, A. (2009). Bioavailability of flavonoids: A Review of their membrane transport and the function of bilitranslocase in animal and plant organisms. *Current Drug Metabolism*, 10, (2009). pp. 369-394

Pizziol, A.; Tikhonoff, V.; Paleaeri, C.D.; Russo, E.; Mazza, A.; Ginocchio, G.; Onesta, C.; Pavan, L.; Casiglia, E. & Dessina, A.C. (1998). Effects of caffeine on glucose tolerance: a placebo-controlled study. *Eur J Clin Nutr*, 52, (1998), pp. 846 - 9.

Sabboh-Jourdan, H.; Valla, F.; Epriliati, I. & Gidley, M.J. (2011). Organic acid bioavailability from banana and sweet potato using an *in vitro* digestion and Caco-2 cell model. *Eur J Nutr.*, 50, 1, (2011), pp. 31-40, DOI: 10.1007/s00394-010-0112-0

Schneeman, B. O. & Gallaher, D. (1985). Effects of dietry fiber on digestive enzyme activity and bile acids in the small intestine. *Proc Soc Exp Biol Med*, 180, (1985), pp. 409 - 414.

Stracke, B.A.; Ru¨fer, C.E.; Bub, A.; Briviba, K.; Seifert, S.; Kunz, C. & Watzl, B. Bioavailability and nutritional effects of carotenoids from organically and conventionally produced carrots in healthy men. *Br J Nutr.*, 101, (2009), pp. 1664–1672

Stolle-Smits, T.; Beekhuizen, J.G.; Kok, M.T.C.; Pijnenburg, M.; Recourt, K.; Derksen, J. & Voragen, A.G.J. (1999). Changes in cell wall polysaccharides of green bean pods during development. *Plant Physiology*, 121, (October 1999), pp. 363–372,

Tan, H.T. & Rahardja, K. (2010). *Obat-obat sederhana untuk gangguan sehari-hari*. PT Gramedia Pustaka Utama, Jakarta

Vahouny, G.V. & Cassidy, M.M. (1985). Dietary fibres and absorption of nutrients. *Proc Soc Exp Biol Med*, 180, (1985), pp. 432 - 446.

van den Berg, H. (1999). Carotenoid interactions. *Nutrition Reviews*, 57, 1 (1999), pp.

van het Hof, K.H.; West, C.E.; Weststrate, J.A. & Hautvast, J.G.A.J. (2000). Dietary factors that affect the bioavailability of carotenoids. *The Journal of Nutrition*, 130, (2000), pp. 503 - 506.

Vermeulen, M. (2009). Isothiocyanates from cruciferous vegetables: Kinetics, biomarkers and effects. Thesis. Wageningen University, Wageningen, The Netherlands ISBN 978-90-8585-312-1

Wijayakusuma, H. (2008). *Bebas Diabetes ala Hembing*. Puspa Swara, Jakarta

Williams, A.W. (1998). Factors influencing the uptake and absorption of carotenoids. *Proc Soc Exp Biol Med*, 218, (1998), pp.106 - 108.

Williamson, G. (2004). Common features in the pathways of absorption and metabolism of flavonoids. IN MESKIN, M. S., BIDLACK, W. R., DAVIES, A. J., LEWIS, D. S. & RANDOLPH, R. K. (Eds.) *Phytochemicals*. Boca Raton, CRC Press.

Xu, X.; Wang, Y.; Constantinou, A.; Stacewicz-Sapuntzakis, M.; Bowen, P. & van Breemen, R. (1999). Solubilization and stabilization of carotenoids using micelles: Delivery of lycopene to cells in culture. *Lipids*, 34, (1999), pp. 1031 - 1036.

Ye, L.X.; Dinkova-Kostova, A.T.; Wade, K.L.; Zhang, Y.S.; Shapiro, T.A. & Talalay, P. (2002). Quantitative determination of dithiocarbamates in human plasma, serum, erythrocytes and urine: pharmacokinetics of broccoli sprout isothiocyanates in humans. *Clinica Chimica Acta*, 316, 1-2,. (2002), pp. 43-53.

Yun, S.M.; Habicht, J.P.; Miller, D.D. & Glahn, R. P. (2004). An *in vitro* digestion/Caco-2 cell culture system accurately predicts the effects of ascorbic acid and polyphenolic compounds on iron bioavailability in humans. *J Nutr.*, 134, (2004), pp. 2717 - 2721.

10

Polyphenol Antioxidants and Bone Health: A Review

L.G. Rao[1], N. Kang[2] and A.V. Rao[2]
[1]Department of Medicine, St. Michael's Hospital, University of Toronto,
[2]Department of Nutritional Sciences, Faculty of Medicine, University of Toronto,
Canada

1. Introduction

Osteoporosis is a skeletal disease characterized by bone loss and structural deterioration of the bone tissue, leading to an increase in bone fragility and susceptibility to fractures, most frequently in the hip, wrist and spine (Sendur *et al.*, 2009). Bone loss is associated with such factors as age, menopause in women, smoking, alcohol excess, calcium and vitamin D deficiency, low weight and muscle mass, anticonvulsant and corticosteroid use as well as certain co-morbid conditions such as rheumatoid arthritis (Javaid *et al.*, 2008). Worldwide, it has been estimated that fractures caused by osteoporosis account for approximately one in three among women and approximately one in five among men over the age of 50. Although the mechanisms underlying osteoporosis are not fully understood, there is evidence suggesting that oxidative stress caused by reactive oxygen species (ROS) is associated with its pathogenesis (Sahnoun *et al.*, 1997; Basu *et al.*, 2001; Rao *et al.*, 2007).

Oxidative stress is a condition that can be characterized by an imbalance of pro-oxidants and antioxidants with the scale being tipped towards an excess of pro-oxidants, creating abnormally high concentrations of ROS. ROS are a family of highly reactive, oxygen-containing molecules and free radicals, including hydroxyl (OH ⁻) and superoxide radicals (O2 ⁻), hydrogen peroxide (H_2O_2), singlet oxygen, and lipid peroxides (Juránek and Bezek, 2005). Several recent studies reported the impact of oxidative stress on osteoclast differentiation as well as on its function resulting to an increase in bone resorption (Garrett *et al.*, 1990; Bax *et al.*, 1992; Mody *et al.*, 2001; Lean, 2003). Furthermore, recent *in vitro* studies have shown the important detrimental role of ROS on osteoblast activity (Park *et al.*, 2005; Bai *et al.*, 2004; Bai *et al.*, 2005). In addition to *in vitro* and animal models, there is also increasing clinical evidence that oxidative stress might be involved in the pathogenesis of osteoporosis (Melhus *et al.*, 1999; Sontakke & Tare., 2002; Basu *et al.*, 2001; Maggio *et al.*, 2003).

Antioxidants are known to mitigate the damaging effects of oxidative stress on cells. Epidemiological evidence has indicated a link between dietary intake of antioxidants and bone health. Fruits and vegetables are important sources of antioxidant phytochemicals that have been shown to play an important role in bone metabolism. Higher consumption of fruits and vegetables has been correlated with a reduction in the risk for the development of osteoporosis. (Arikan *et al.*, 2011; Prentice *et al.*, 2006; Macdonald *et al.*, 2004; Macdonald *et al.*, 2008; Palacios *et al.*, 2006; Tucker *et al.*, 1999; Lister *et al.*, 2007; New, 2003; Trzeciakiewicz *et al.*, 2009).

Category	Subclass	Structure	Common Flavonoid	Food Examples
Phenolic acids	Hydroxycinnamic acids		Caffeic acid	coffee beans
	Hydroxybenzoic acids		Gallic acid	gallnuts, sumac, witch hazel, tea leaves, oak bark,
Flavonoids	Anthocyanidins		Cyanidin	berries, purple cabbage, beets, grape seed extract, and red wine
	Flavanols		Catechins	white, green and black teas
			Theaflavins	black teas
			Proanthocyanidins	chocolate, fruits and vegetables, red wine, onion, apple skin
	Flavanones		Hesperidin	citrus fruits
			Narigenin	citrus fruits
			Silybin	blessed milk thistle
	Flavonols		Quercetin	red and yellow onions, tea, wine, apples, cranberries, buckwheat, beans
	Flavones		Apigenin	chamomile, celery, parsley
			Tangeritin	tangerine and other citrus peels
			Luteolin	celery, thyme, green peppers,
	Isoflavones		Genistein	soy, alfalfa sprouts, red clover, chickpeas, peanuts, other legumes.

Stilbenes		HO HO—⬡—COOH	Resveratrol	gapes skins, red wine
Lignans		HO HO—⬡—O OH HO	Secoisolaiciresinol	flaxseeds

Table 1. The different categories of polyphenols, their chemical structures and sources

Of particular interest among the antioxidant phytochemicals present in fruits and vegetables are the polyphenols. Polyphenols can be sub classified as non-flavonoids and flavonoids. Ellagic acid and stilbenes are among the major non-flavonoid polyphenols. Included in the flavonoid polyphenols are the anthocyanins, catechins, flavones, flavonols and isoflavones. The different categories of polyphenols, their chemical structures and sources are shown in Table 1.

Numerous studies have shown the health-promoting properties of polyphenols, providing additional mechanisms through which they promote skeletal health by reducing resorption caused by high oxidative stress (Trzeciakiewicz et al., 2009; Tucker, 2009; Hunter et al., 2008). The antioxidant properties of polyphenols have been widely studied and reported in the literature (Liu et al., 2005; Miyamoto et al.,1998; Rassi et al., 2002; Viereck et al., 2002; Ward et al., 2001; Shen et al., 2011; Rao et al., 2007). They strongly support the role of polyphenols in the delayed onset or reduction in the progression of osteoporosis. The protective effects of polyphenols against diseases, including osteoporosis, have generated new expectations for improvements in health. This review will focus mainly on the role of polyphenols in osteoporosis and present results of studies undertaken in our laboratory.

2. Oxidative stress, antioxidants and osteoporosis

Oxidative stress occurs when the production of free radicals through a number of cellular events exceeds the ability of the cell's antioxidant defense to eliminate these oxidants (Baek et al., 2010). These free radicals have the ability to change the integrity of, and thus, damage several biomolecules, such as DNA, proteins and lipids (Baek et al., 2010). There is increasing evidence that oxidative stress is responsible for the pathophysiology of the aging process and may also be involved in the pathogenesis of atherosclerosis, neurodegenerative diseases, cancer, and diabetes. Recently, ROS were shown to be responsible for the development of osteoporosis (Sahnoun et al., 1997; Basu et al., 2001; Rao et al., 2007; Altindag et al., 2008; Becker, 2006; Feng & McDonald, 2011). Several in vitro and animal studies have shown that oxidative stress diminishes the level of bone formation by reducing the differentiation and survival of osteoblasts (Baek et al., 2010). Furthermore, it has been reported that ROS activate osteoclasts and thus, enhance bone resorption (Baek et al., 2010). The presence of ROS in osteoclasts was also demonstrated by Rao et al. in 2003 Recent evidences from a few clinical studies have also revealed that ROS and/or antioxidant systems might play a role in the pathogenesis of bone loss (Rao et al., 2007; Mackinnon et al., 2010; Abdollahi et al., 2005).

A number of studies have shown that antioxidants have a fundamental role in preventing postmenopausal osteoporosis. For instance, estrogens, whose antioxidant activity is essential in protecting women of reproductive age from cardiovascular disease, stimulate osteoblastic activity through specific receptors, thus favouring bone growth (Banfi et al., 2008). Antioxidant deficiency has been shown to have adverse effect on bone mass (Maggio et al. 2003).

Antioxidant enzymes are regarded as the markers of antioxidant defense mechanism against bone resorption. Several studies have investigated the relationship between antioxidant enzymes such as glutathione peroxidase (GP_x) and catalase (CAT) and osteoporosis (MacKinnon *et al.*, 2011; Hahn *et al.*, 2008; Maggio *et al.*, 2003; Sontakke & Tare, 2002).

Recently, many dietary antioxidant nutrients have also been reported to decrease the oxidative stress that takes part in bone-resorptive processes (Rao *et al.*, 2007; Weber, 2001; Peters & Martini, 2010; Macdonald *et al.*, 2004). In addition to the antioxidant enzymes and nutrients, studies have also been directed towards the role of antioxidant phytochemicals such as the carotenoids in osteoporosis which will not be covered here, but has previously been reviewed (Rao & Rao, 2007; Sahni *et al.*, 2009; Tucker, 2009).

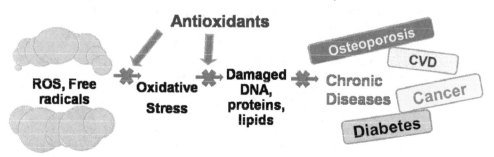

Fig. 1. The role of oxidative stress in osteoporosis and how/where antioxidants play a role in mitigating ROS

3. Natural phytochemical antioxidants

Within the last decade, there has been an increased interest on polyphenols as a result of the *in vitro* evidence demonstrating that they may have numerous benefits to human health, mainly due to their antioxidative and free radical quenching properties (Hendrich, 2006; Lotito & Frei 2006; Heinonen, 2007; Stevenson & Hurst 2007; Aron & Kennedy 2008; Lopez-Lazaro, 2009; Saura-Calixto *et al.* 2007). It is therefore hypothesized that polyphenols may aid in the prevention of aging-associated diseases, particularly cardiovascular diseases, cancers, and osteoporosis.

Polyphenolic compounds are the products of the secondary metabolism of plant and are an essential part of human diet (Goldberg, 2003; Stevenson & Hurst 2007; D'Archivio *et al.*, 2007; Saura-Calixto *et al.* 2007). To date, more than 8,000 polyphenols that have one common structural feature have been identified, a phenol, which is an aromatic ring possessing at least one hydroxyl substituent (Hendrich, 2006; Scalbert & Williamson, 2000; Harborne, 1993). The main classes of polyphenols include phenolic acids, flavonoids, stilbene, and lignans (Spencer *et al.*, 2008; D'Archivio *et al.*, 2007). Figure 1 illustrates the different groups of polyphenols, the chemical structures and food sources. Their total dietary intake can range up to 1 gram/day, which is considerably higher than that of all other classes of phytochemicals (Velioglu *et al.*, 1998). There is much evidence demonstrating that polyphenols improve the status of different oxidative stress biomarkers. However, there is uncertainty regarding both the relevance of these biomarkers as predictors of disease risk and the appropriateness of the different methods used.

Polyphenol Class	Reference	Principal polyphenol	Model	Main findings
Phenolic Acids	Papoutsi et al., (2008)	Ellagic acid (10-100nM)	KS483	↑ nodule formation
	Ayoub et al., (2009)	3-methoxyellagic acid (25ug/ml)	HOS58 & SaOS-2	↑ mineralization of bone cell
Flavonoids	Zhang et al. (2009)	Naringin	bone mesenchymal stem cells (BMSCs)	Dose-specific (1–100 µg/ml) of the naringin solution may enhance the proliferation and osteogenic differentiation of human BMSCs
	Choi (2007)	Apigenin	MC3T3-E1 cells	Apigenin (0.01 mM) increased the growth of MC3T3-E1 cells and caused a significant elevation of alkaline phosphatase (ALP) activity and collagen content in the cells
	Kim et al. (2011)	Luteolin	Bone marrow cells were prepared by removing from the femora and tibiae of ICR mice	luteolin decreased differentiation of both bone marrow mononuclear cells and Raw264.7 cells into osteoclasts, inhibited the bone resorptive activity of differentiated osteoclasts.
	Choi (2011)	Kaempferol	MC3T3-E1 cells	induced the activation of PI3K (phosphoinositide 3-kinase), Akt (protein kinase B), and CREB (cAMP-response element-binding protein). This may prevent or reduce degerneration of osteoblasts
	Wattel et al. (2004)	Quercetin	RAW 264.7 cells, peripheral blood monocytic cells (PBMC)	Quercetin (0.1–10 mM) decreased osteoclastogenesis in a dose dependent manner in both models with significant effects observed at low concentrations, from 1 to 5 mM
Isoflavones	Sugimoto & Yamaguchi (2000)	Daidzein	MC3T3-E1 cells	increase alkaline phosphatase activity
	Rassi et al. (2002)	Daidzein	osteoclasts from young female piglets	inhibits development of osteoclasts from cultures of porcine bone marrow and reduces bone resorption
	Viereck et al. (2002)	Genistein	mature human osteoblasts (hOB)	up-regulated OPG production 2–6-fold in a time- and dose-dependent manner, neutralizing RANKL
Lignans	Hasegawa et al. (2010)	Honokiol	bone marrow cells of 6wk old mice	Inhibits osteoclast differentiation by suppressing the activation of MAPKs (p38 MAPK, ERK and JNK)
Stilbenes	Chang et al. (2006)	Piceatannol	immortalized fetal osteoblasts (hFOB), and osteosarcoma cells (MG-63)	piceatannol increased BMP-2 synthesis, induced osteoblasts maturation and differentiation
	Kupisiewicz et al. (2010)	Modified resveratrol analogues	Myeloma cell lines U266 and OPM-2	Resveratrol analogues showed an up to 5,000-fold increased potency to inhibit osteoclast differentiation and promoted osteoblast maturation compared to resveratrol.

Table 2. Polyphenols- *In vitro* studies

4. Polyphenols and osteoporosis

There has been an increase interest in the field of bone health and nutrients, and within the last decade, it has been well recognized that some polyphenols, whether ingested as supplements or with food, do in fact improve bone health status. Currently, most of the research on polyphenols and their effects has emerged from *in vitro* and *in vivo* studies with only a few clinical studies available. Compounds present in fruits and vegetables influence bone health as shown with *in vitro* osteoblast cell culture. On the other hand, epidemiologic studies tend to have mixed results with regards to the protective effects of polyphenol consumption against osteoporosis. Tables 2, 3, and 4 illustrate some of the recent *in vitro, in vivo* and clinical studies that have been reported in the literature, respectively.

Polyphenol Class	Reference	Substance given	Principal polyphenol	Model	Dose per day	Main findings
Phenolic Acids	Chen (2010)	Blueberries	Phenolic acid mixture	Sprague-Dawley rats		Increase serum osteoblast progenitors, increased osteoblast differentiation, reduced osteoclastogenesis, increase bone mass
	Zych et al. (2010)		Ferulic,caffeic, *p-*coumaric, chlorogenic, clohexanecarbox ylic acid	Wistar Cmd:(WI)W U rats	10 mg/kg p.o.	caffeic acid worsened bone mechanical properties
	Folwarczna et al. (2010)		Curcumin	Wistar Cmd:(WI)W U rats	10 mg/kg, po	no sig. improvement of bone mineralizasation or mechanical properties
	Folwarczna et al. (2009)		Caffeic, *p-*coumaric, chlorogenic acid	Wistar Cmd:(WI)W U rats	10 mg/kg p.o.	caffeic acid ↓ bone mass, p-coumaric acid ↑ bone mass/body mass ratio and bone mineral mass/body mass ratio in long bones
Flavonoids	Devareddy et al. (2008)	Blueberries	Variety of phenolic acids and flavonols	OVX rat	5% w/w	Ovx resulted in loss of whole-body, tibial, femoral, and 4th lumbar BMD by approximately 6%. Blueberry treatment was able to prevent the loss of whole-body BMD and had an intermediary effect on prevention of tibial and femoral BMD
	Arjmandi et al. (2010)	(1) 2% Fructooligosacchari des (FOS); 5% FOS+7.5% DP; 2% FOS+5% DP; 2% FOS+2% DP	Variety	OVX rat		diet of 5% FOS + 7.5% dried plum was most effective in reversing both right femur and fourth lumbar BMD and fourth lumbar

	polyphenol (equivalent to 7.5% DP powder); (5) 2% FOS+7.5% DP juice; (6) 2% FOS+7.5% DP puree; (7) 2% FOS+7.5% DP pulp skins; (8) 2% FOS+7.5% raisin; (9) 2% FOS+7.5% fig; (10) 2% FOS+7.5% date; (11) 2% FOS+7.5% blueberry; (12) 2% FOS+0.25% HMB; and (13) 0.25% HMB.				calcium loss while significantly decreasing trabecular separation. No significant effects of treatment on serum or urine measures of bone turnover.
Shen et al. (2008)	Green tea polyphenols (GTP)	(-)Epigallocatechin gallate	OVX rat	0.1% or 0.5% concentration of GTP in drinking water	GTP supplementation increased urinary epigallocatechin and epicatechin concentrations, femur BMD, decreased urinary 8-hydroxy-2'-deoxyguanosine and urinary calcium levels; no effect on serum estradiol
Shen et al. (2010)	Green tea polyphenols (GTP)	(-)Epigallocatechin gallate	40 female CD rats	0.5% concentration of GTP in drinking water	GTP supplementation increased urinary epigallocatechin and epicatechin concentrations and showed higher values for femur BMC, BMD and serum OC, but lower values for serum TRAP, urinary 8-OHdG and spleen mRNA expression of TNF-α and COX-2 levels.
Shen et al. (2011)	Green tea polyphenols (GTP)	(-)Epigallocatechin gallate	50 OVX	0.5% concentration of GTP in drinking water	GTP supplementation resulted in increased serum osteocalcin concentrations, bone mineral density, and trabecular volume, number, and strength of femur; increased trabecular volume and thickness and bone formation in both the proximal tibia and periosteal tibial shaft
Das et al. (2005)	Black tea extract	Theaflavin	Bilaterally oophorecto	2.5% aqueous	BTE increase serum estradiol level

				mized rats	BTE at a single dose of 1 ml /100 g body weight	
	Chiba et al. (2003)	hesperidin & α-glucosylhesperidin	Hesperidin & α-glucosylhesperidin	OVX mice	0.5 g/100 g hesperidin, 0.7 g/100 g α-glucosylhesperidin	hesperidin or α-glucosylhesperidin restored BMD caused by OVX, α-glucosylhesperidin significantly prevented loss of trabecular bone volume and trabecular thickness in the femoral distal metaphysis
	Park et al. (2008)	apigenin	Apigenin	OVX rats	10 mg/kg	apigenin increased the mineral content and density of the trabecular bone at the neck of the left femur, decreased body weight and dietary consumption
	Kim et al. (2011)	luteolin	Luteolin	OVX mice	5 and 20 mg/kg	luteolin increased bone mineral density and bone mineral content of trabecular and cortical bones in the femur as compared to those of OVX controls
	Do et al. (2008)	Rubus coreanus	Anthocyanin	OVX rats	100 & 200 mg/kg	RCM increased femur trabecular bone area in a dose-dependent manner in ovariectomized rats, increased osteoblast differentiation and osteoclast apoptosis.
	Horcajada-Molteni et al. (2000)	Rutin	Rutin	OVX rats	2.5 g/kg	Rutin prevented decrease in both total and distal metaphyseal femoral mineral density by slowing down resorption and increasing osteoblastic activity caused by OVX,
Isoflavones	Arjmandi et al. (1998)	Soy protein	Genistein	72 OVX rats	1462 mg/kg genistein, 25.1 mg/kg daidzin, 11.3 mg/kg daidzein	no effect on BMC
	Lee et al. (2004)	Soybean	Glycitein	24 OVX rats	6.25 g/kg	soybean isoflavone appear to prevent bone loss in femur and lumber vertebrae via a

						different mechanism of estrogen
	Miyamoto et al (1998)	8-isopentenylnaringenin	8-isopentenylnaringenin	OVX rats	30 mg/day	8-isopentenyl naringenin prevented decrease in BMD and bone turnover markers
Lignans	Xiao et al. (2011)	Sambucus williamsii HANCE (SWH)	Lignans	56 OVX/6J specific-pathogen-free (SPF) female mice	17b-oestradiol (3·2 mg/kg), SWH (60% ethanol crude extract; 1·0 g/kg), SWA (water eluate; 0·570 g/kg), SWB (30% ethanol eluate; 0·128 g/kg) or SWC (50 and 95% ethanol eluates; 0·189 g/kg)	SWC significantly restored bone mineral density and improved bone size and bone content in femur and tibia
	El-Shitany et al. (2010)	Silymarin	Silymarin	OVX rats	50 mg/kg	protected trabecula thickness, decreased serum levels of ALP and increased serum levels of both calcium and phosphorus
	Ward et al. (2001)	Flaxseed	Secoisolariciresinol diglucoside	20 Sprague-Dawley male rats	293 μmol SDG/kg	exposure to a diet with flaxseed during lactation through to early adolescence can reduce bone strength, but lignan does is not the mediator, no sig. change in BMD and BMC those fed flaxseed
Stilbenes	Pearson et al. (2008)	Resveratrol	Resveratrol	Male C57BL/6NI A mice	100 mg/kg or 400 mg/kg	Both diets improved distal trabecular tissue mineral density (TMD) and bone volume to total volume ratio over the entire femur compared to control
	Liu et al. (2005)	*trans-Resveratrol*	Resveratrol	OVX rat	0.7 mg/kg	epiphysis BMD and bone calcium content was significantly greater with resveratrol treatment than that in the OVX group, no differences in femoral midpoint BMD

Table 3. Polyphenols- *In vivo* Studies

Polyphenol Class	Reference	Substance given	Principal polyphenol	Model	Dose per day	Main findings
Flavonoids	Hardcastle et al. (2011)	None	Catechin	perimenopausal Scottish women		flavanones were negatively associated with bone-resorption markers, association between energy-adjusted total flavonoid intakes and BMD at the femoreal neck and lumbar spine, annual percent change in BMD was associated with intakes of procyanidins and catechins
Isoflavones	Chen et al. (2004)	Soy isoflavone	Daizein	203 postmenopausal women	placebo: 0 mg isoflavones + 500 mg calcium, mid-dose:40 mg isoflavones+ 500 mg calcium, high-dose:80 mg isoflavones + 500 mg calcium	no effect on BMD in all groups, effect of soy isoflavones on BMC at the total hip and trochanter was less strong in women in early menopause or in those with higher body weight, nonsignificantin BMC in those with a high level of dietary calcium intake
	Arjmandi et al. (2005)	Soy protein	Daizein	87 postmenopausal women	25 g protein and 60 mg isoflavones	Whole body and lumbar BMD and BMC significantly decreased, and BSAP and osteocalcin increasedin control and soy groups
	Kenny et al. (2009)	Soy protein + isoflavone tablets	Isoflavones	131 postmenopausal women >65 years old	18 g soy protein and 105 mg isoflavone tablets	no differences in BMD
Lignans	Cornish et al. (2009)	Flaxseed	Secoisolaricir esinol diglucoside	50 men, 50 postmenopausal women		no effect on BMD
	Dodin et al. (2005)	Flaxseed	Secoisolaricir esinol diglucoside	199 menopausal women		no sig. change in BMD

Table 4. Polyphenols - Clinical Studies

There have been several results suggesting that the combination of polyphenolic compounds found naturally in fruits and vegetables may reduce the risk of osteoporosis via increasing bone mineral density (Wu *et al.*, 2002; Morton *et al.*, 2001; Melhus *et al.*, 1999; Leveille *et al.*, 1997; Singh, 1992). In 1992, Singh was able to show that polyphenols afford protection against oxidative stress-induced bone damage during strenuous exercise. Similarly, Melhus was able to show its counteractive effect of polyphenols among smokers (Melhus *et al.*, 1999).

5. Research results on the role of polyphenols in osteoporosis from the author's laboratory

Previous *in vitro* results from our laboratory have shown that a supplement rich in a variety of polyphenols commercially known as greens+^{TM}, is more effective in stimulating

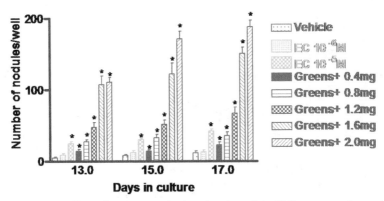

Fig. 2. Dose dependent effect of greens+^{TM} (g+) and epicatechin (EC) compared to vehicle. (p<0.05)

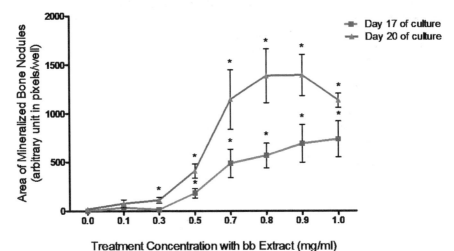

Fig. 3. Time and dose-dependent effects of bone builder^{TM} on mineralized bone nodule area in SaOS-2 cells (p< 0.05).

osteoblasts to form more bone nhodules in a dose-dependant manner than epicatechin, the main polyphenol found in green tea (Fig. 2). Our laboratory also studied the effects of a second supplement, bone builder™, which is rich in minerals, vitamins and nutrients. Similarly to the greens+™, the water-soluble bone-builder extract had a significant dose-dependent stimulatory effect on bone nodules formation (Fig. 3). Figure 4 shows that when the two supplements, greens+™ and bone builder™, were tested as combination, the effects were six times more effective than either one alone. This led us to believe that synergistic effects of greens+™ and bone builder™ may have a beneficial effect on osteoporosis. We then conducted a clinical evaluation of this nutritional supplement greens+ bone builder™ Results have shown that there was an increase in total antioxidant capacity after 8 weeks of treatment compared to placebo (Fig 4). as well as a decrease in both lipid and protein oxidation over a 4 and 8-weeks of intervention with greens+ bone builder™ compared to placebo (Fig. 6 & 7). This suggests that the nutritional supplement may have a beneficial effect on bone health by mitigating the effects of oxidative stress.

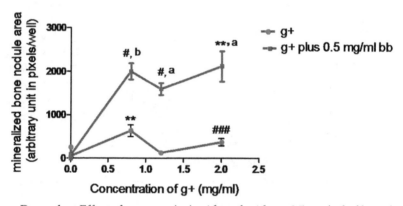

Fig. 4. Dose Dependent Effect of greens + (g+) with and without 0.5 mg/ml of bone builder (bb) on the area of mineralized bone nodules in osteoblasts SaOS-2 Cells. * p<0.0005, **p<0.005; ***p<0.05; # p<0.0001; ## p<0.001; ### p<0.01; significance differences were found when treatment with g+ plus 0.5 mg/ml bb was compared to treatment with g+ alone as follows: a\b< 0.0001; bp< 0.005

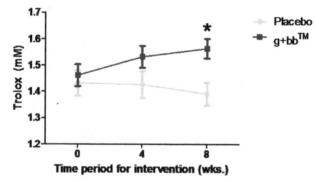

Fig. 5. The effect of nutritional intervention with g+bb™ compared to placebo on serum total antioxidant capacity (p<0.05).

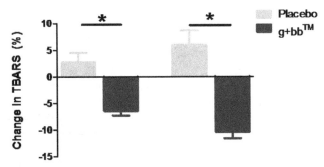

Fig. 6. Change in TBARS over 4 and 8-weeks of nutritional intervention with g+bb™ compared to placebo (p<0.001).

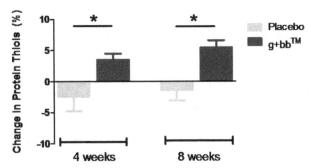

Fig. 7. Change in protein oxidation over 4 and 8-weeks of nutritional intervention with g+bb™ compared to placebo (p<0.05).

6. Conclusions

Although epidemiologic studies are practical for the evaluation of human health effects on the physiologic concentrations of polyphenols, reliable data on polyphenol contents of foods are limited. This review has shown that polyphenols or polyphenol-rich diets can provide significant protection or treatment for the development and progression of osteoporosis. Keeping in mind that many nutrients are co-dependent, and they may interact among themselves and others. The complexity of these interactions may possibly be the reason why many studies show controversial or inconsistent results regarding the effects of a single nutrient or groups of nutrients in bone health. Based on current knowledge, polyphenols offer a platform for the prevention of many human chronic diseases involved with oxidative stress, including osteoporosis.

To value the actual significance of food phenolics, it is necessary to investigate not only their bioavailability, but also their mechanisms of action and their possible synergism with other constituents either in the diet or within the human body, as well as the polyphenolic content and composition of foods. We have attained this goal by studying the nutritional supplement greens+™, which is rich in polyphenols and their interactions with minerals, vitamins and nutrients that were present in the nutritional supplement bone builder™.

7. References

Abdollahi, M., Larijani, B., Rahimi, R. & Salari, P. (2005). Role of oxidative stress in osteoporosis. *Therapy*, 2(5), 787-796.

Arikan, D. C., Coskun, A., Ozer, A., Kilinc, M., Atalay, F., & Arikan, T. (2011). Plasma selenium, zinc, copper and lipid levels in postmenopausal turkish women and their relation with osteoporosis. *Biological Trace Element Research*, 144(1-3), 407-417.

Altindag, O., Erel, O., Soran, N., Celik, H., & Selek, S. (2008). Total oxidative/anti-oxidative status and relation to bone mineral density in osteoporosis. *Rheumatol Int*, 28(4), 317-321.

Arjmandi, B. H., Birnbaum, R., Goyal, N. V., Getlinger, M. J., Juma, S., Alekel, L., et al. (1998). Bone-sparing effect of soy protein in ovarian hormone-deficient rats is related to its isoflavone content. *The American Journal of Clinical Nutrition*, 68(6 Suppl), 1364S-1368S.

Arjmandi, B. H., Getlinger, M. J., Goyal, N. V., Alekel, L., Hasler, C. M., Juma, S., et al. (1998). Role of soy protein with normal or reduced isoflavone content in reversing bone loss induced by ovarian hormone deficiency in rats. *The American Journal of Clinical Nutrition*, 68(6 Suppl), 1358S-1363S.

Arjmandi, B. H., Johnson, C. D., Campbell, S. C., Hooshmand, S., Chai, S. C., & Akhter, M. P. (2010). Combining fructooligosaccharide and dried plum has the greatest effect on restoring bone mineral density among select functional foods and bioactive compounds. *Journal of Medicinal Food*, 13(2), 312-319.

Arjmandi, B. H., Lucas, E. A., Khalil, D. A., Devareddy, L., Smith, B. J., McDonald, J., et al. (2005). One year soy protein supplementation has positive effects on bone formation markers but not bone density in postmenopausal women. *Nutrition Journal*, 4, 8.

Aron, P. M., & Kennedy, J. A. (2008). Flavan-3-ols: Nature, occurrence and biological activity. *Molecular Nutrition & Food Research*, 52(1), 79-104.

Ayoub, N. A., Hussein, S. A., Hashim, A. N., Hegazi, N. M., Linscheid, M., Harms, M., et al. (2009). Bone mineralization enhancing activity of a methoxyellagic acid glucoside from a feijoa sellowiana leaf extract. *Die Pharmazie*, 64(2), 137-141.

Baek, K. H., Oh, K. W., Lee, W. Y., Lee, S. S., Kim, M. K., Kwon, H. S., et al. (2010). Association of oxidative stress with postmenopausal osteoporosis and the effects of hydrogen peroxide on osteoclast formation in human bone marrow cell cultures. *Calcified Tissue International*, 87(3), 226-235.

Banfi, G., Iorio, E. L., & Corsi, M. M. (2008). Oxidative stress, free radicals and bone remodeling. *Clinical Chemistry and Laboratory Medicine : CCLM / FESCC*, 46(11), 1550-1555.

Basu, S., Michaelsson, K., Olofsson, H., Johansson, S., & Melhus, H. (2001). Association between oxidative stress and bone mineral density. *Biochem Biophys Res Commun*, 288(1), 275-279.

Bax, B. E., Alam, A. S. M. T., Banerji, B., Bax, C. M. R., Bevis, P. J. R., Stevens, C. R., et al. (1992). Stimulation of osteoclastic bone resorption by hydrogen peroxide. *Biochemical and Biophysical Research Communications*, 183(3), 1153-1158.

Becker, C. (2006). Pathophysiology and clinical manifestations of osteoporosis. *Clinical Cornerstone*, 8(1), 19-27.

Chang, J. K., Hsu, Y. L., Teng, I. C., & Kuo, P. L. (2006). Piceatannol stimulates osteoblast differentiation that may be mediated by increased bone morphogenetic protein-2 production. *European Journal of Pharmacology, 551*(1-3), 1-9.

Chen, J. R., Lazarenko, O. P., Wu, X., Kang, J., Blackburn, M. L., Shankar, K., et al. (2010). Dietary-induced serum phenolic acids promote bone growth via p38 MAPK/beta-catenin canonical wnt signaling. *Journal of Bone and Mineral Research : The Official Journal of the American Society for Bone and Mineral Research, 25*(11), 2399-2411.

Chen, Y. M., Ho, S. C., Lam, S. S., Ho, S. S., & Woo, J. L. (2004). Beneficial effect of soy isoflavones on bone mineral content was modified by years since menopause, body weight, and calcium intake: A double-blind, randomized, controlled trial. *Menopause (New York, N.Y.), 11*(3), 246-254.

Chiba, H., Uehara, M., Wu, J., Wang, X., Masuyama, R., Suzuki, K., et al. (2003). Hesperidin, a citrus flavonoid, inhibits bone loss and decreases serum and hepatic lipids in ovariectomized mice. *The Journal of Nutrition, 133*(6), 1892-1897.

Choi, E. M. (2007). Apigenin increases osteoblastic differentiation and inhibits tumor necrosis factor-alpha-induced production of interleukin-6 and nitric oxide in osteoblastic MC3T3-E1 cells. *Die Pharmazie, 62*(3), 216-220.

Choi, E. M. (2011). Kaempferol protects MC3T3-E1 cells through antioxidant effect and regulation of mitochondrial function. *Food and Chemical Toxicology : An International Journal Published for the British Industrial Biological Research Association, 49*(8), 1800-1805.

Cornish, S. M., Chilibeck, P. D., Paus-Jennsen, L., Biem, H. J., Khozani, T., Senanayake, V., et al. (2009). A randomized controlled trial of the effects of flaxseed lignan complex on metabolic syndrome composite score and bone mineral in older adults. *Applied Physiology, Nutrition, and Metabolism = Physiologie Appliquee, Nutrition Et Metabolisme, 34*(2), 89-98.

D'Archivio, M., Filesi, C., Di Benedetto, R., Gargiulo, R., Giovannini, C., & Masella, R. (2007). Polyphenols, dietary sources and bioavailability. *Annali Dell'Istituto Superiore Di Sanita, 43*(4), 348-361.

Das, A. S., Das, D., Mukherjee, M., Mukherjee, S., & Mitra, C. (2005). Phytoestrogenic effects of black tea extract (camellia sinensis) in an oophorectomized rat (rattus norvegicus) model of osteoporosis. *Life Sciences, 77*(24), 3049-3057.

Devareddy, L., Hooshmand, S., Collins, J. K., Lucas, E. A., Chai, S. C., & Arjmandi, B. H. (2008). Blueberry prevents bone loss in ovariectomized rat model of postmenopausal osteoporosis. *The Journal of Nutritional Biochemistry, 19*(10), 694-699.

Do, S. H., Lee, J. W., Jeong, W. I., Chung, J. Y., Park, S. J., Hong, I. H., et al. (2008). Bone-protecting effect of rubus coreanus by dual regulation of osteoblasts and osteoclasts. *Menopause (New York, N.Y.), 15*(4 Pt 1), 676-683.

Dodin, S., Lemay, A., Jacques, H., Legare, F., Forest, J. C., & Masse, B. (2005). The effects of flaxseed dietary supplement on lipid profile, bone mineral density, and symptoms in menopausal women: A randomized, double-blind, wheat germ placebo-controlled clinical trial. *The Journal of Clinical Endocrinology and Metabolism, 90*(3), 1390-1397.

El-Shitany, N. A., Hegazy, S., & El-Desoky, K. (2010). Evidences for antiosteoporotic and selective estrogen receptor modulator activity of silymarin compared with ethinylestradiol in ovariectomized rats. *Phytomedicine : International Journal of Phytotherapy and Phytopharmacology, 17*(2), 116-125.

Feng, X., & McDonald, J. M. (2011). Disorders of bone remodeling. *Annual Review of Pathology, 6*, 121-145.

Folwarczna, J., Zych, M., & Trzeciak, H. I. (2010). Effects of curcumin on the skeletal system in rats. *Pharmacological Reports : PR, 62*(5), 900-909.

Folwarczna, J., Zych, M., Burczyk, J., Trzeciak, H., & Trzeciak, H. I. (2009). Effects of natural phenolic acids on the skeletal system of ovariectomized rats. *Planta Medica, 75*(15), 1567-1572.

Garrett, I. R., Boyce, B. F., Oreffo, R. O., Bonewald, L., Poser, J., & Mundy, G. R. (1990). Oxygen-derived free radicals stimulate osteoclastic bone resorption in rodent bone in vitro and in vivo. *J Clin Invest, 85*(3), 632-639.

Goldberg, G. (2003). *Plants: Diet and health: The report of the british nutrition foundation task force.* Oxford, UK.: Blackwell Science for the British Nutrition Foundation.

Hahn, M., Conterato, G. M. M., Frizzo, C. P., Augusti, P. R., da Silva, J. C. N., Unfer, T. C., et al. (2008). Effects of bone disease and calcium supplementation on antioxidant enzymes in postmenopausal women. *Clinical Biochemistry, 41*(1-2), 69-74.

Harborne, J. B. (1993). *The flavonoids: Advances in research since 1986.* London: Chapman and Hall.

Hardcastle, A. C., Aucott, L., Reid, D. M., & Macdonald, H. M. (2011). Associations between dietary flavonoid intakes and bone health in a scottish population. *Journal of Bone and Mineral Research : The Official Journal of the American Society for Bone and Mineral Research, 26*(5), 941-947.

Hasegawa, S., Yonezawa, T., Ahn, J. Y., Cha, B. Y., Teruya, T., Takami, M., et al. (2010). Honokiol inhibits osteoclast differentiation and function in vitro. *Biological & Pharmaceutical Bulletin, 33*(3), 487-492.

Heinonen, M. (2007). Antioxidant activity and antimicrobial effect of berry phenolics--a finnish perspective. *Molecular Nutrition & Food Research, 51*(6), 684-691.

Hendrich, A. B. (2006). Flavonoid-membrane interactions: Possible consequences for biological effects of some polyphenolic compounds. *Acta Pharmacologica Sinica, 27*(1), 27-40.

Horcajada-Molteni, M. N., Crespy, V., Coxam, V., Davicco, M. J., Remesy, C., & Barlet, J. P. (2000). Rutin inhibits ovariectomy-induced osteopenia in rats. *Journal of Bone and Mineral Research : The Official Journal of the American Society for Bone and Mineral Research, 15*(11), 2251-2258.

Hunter, D. C., Skinner, M. A., & Lister, C. E. (2008). Impact of phytochemicals on maintaining bone and joint health. *Nutrition (Burbank, Los Angeles County, Calif.), 24*(4), 390-392.

Javaid, M. K., & Holt, R. I. (2008). Understanding osteoporosis. *Journal of Psychopharmacology (Oxford, England), 22*(2 Suppl), 38-45.

Juranek, I., & Bezek, S. (2005). Controversy of free radical hypothesis: Reactive oxygen species--cause or consequence of tissue injury? *General Physiology and Biophysics, 24*(3), 263-278.

Kenny, A. M., Mangano, K. M., Abourizk, R. H., Bruno, R. S., Anamani, D. E., Kleppinger, A., et al. (2009). Soy proteins and isoflavones affect bone mineral density in older women: A randomized controlled trial. *The American Journal of Clinical Nutrition, 90*(1), 234-242.

Kim, T. H., Jung, J. W., Ha, B. G., Hong, J. M., Park, E. K., Kim, H. J., et al. (2011). The effects of luteolin on osteoclast differentiation, function in vitro and ovariectomy-induced bone loss. *The Journal of Nutritional Biochemistry, 22*(1), 8-15.

Kupisiewicz, K., Boissy, P., Abdallah, B. M., Hansen, F. D., Erben, R. G., Savouret, J. F., et al. (2010). Potential of resveratrol analogues as antagonists of osteoclasts and promoters of osteoblasts. *Calcified Tissue International, 87*(5), 437-449.

Lean, J. M., Davies, J. T., Fuller, K., Jagger, C. J., Kirstein, B., Partington, G. A., et al. (2003). A crucial role for thiol antioxidants in estrogen-deficiency bone loss. *J Clin Invest, 112*(6), 915-923.

Lee, Y. B., Lee, H. J., Kim, K. S., Lee, J. Y., Nam, S. Y., Cheon, S. H., et al. (2004). Evaluation of the preventive effect of isoflavone extract on bone loss in ovariectomized rats. *Bioscience, Biotechnology, and Biochemistry, 68*(5), 1040-1045.

Leveille, S. G., LaCroix, A. Z., Koepsell, T. D., Beresford, S. A., Van Belle, G., & Buchner, D. M. (1997). Dietary vitamin C and bone mineral density in postmenopausal women in washington state, USA. *Journal of Epidemiology and Community Health, 51*(5), 479-485.

Lister, C., Skinner, M., & Hunter, D. (2007). Fruits, vegetables and their phytochemicals for bone and joint health. *Curr Top Nutraceut Res, 5,* 67–82.

Liu, Z. P., Li, W. X., Yu, B., Huang, J., Sun, J., Huo, J. S., et al. (2005). Effects of trans-resveratrol from polygonum cuspidatum on bone loss using the ovariectomized rat model. *Journal of Medicinal Food, 8*(1), 14-19.

Lopez-Lazaro, M. (2009). Distribution and biological activities of the flavonoid luteolin. *Mini Reviews in Medicinal Chemistry, 9*(1), 31-59.

Lotito, S. B., & Frei, B. (2006). Consumption of flavonoid-rich foods and increased plasma antioxidant capacity in humans: Cause, consequence, or epiphenomenon? *Free Radical Biology & Medicine, 41*(12), 1727-1746.

Maggio, D., Barabani, M., Pierandrei, M., Polidori, M. C., Catani, M., Mecocci, P., et al. (2003). Marked decrease in plasma antioxidants in aged osteoporotic women: Results of a cross-sectional study. *J Clin Endocrinol Metab, 88*(4), 1523-1527.

Macdonald, H. M., Black, A. J., Aucott, L., Duthie, G., Duthie, S., Sandison, R., et al. (2008). Effect of potassium citrate supplementation or increased fruit and vegetable intake on bone metabolism in healthy postmenopausal women: A randomized controlled trial. *The American Journal of Clinical Nutrition, 88*(2), 465-474.

Macdonald, H. M., New, S. A., Golden, M. H., Campbell, M. K., & Reid, D. M. (2004). Nutritional associations with bone loss during the menopausal transition: Evidence of a beneficial effect of calcium, alcohol, and fruit and vegetable nutrients and of a detrimental effect of fatty acids. *The American Journal of Clinical Nutrition, 79*(1), 155-165.

Mackinnon, E. S., Rao, A. V., & Rao, L. G. (2011). Dietary restriction of lycopene for a period of one month resulted in significantly increased biomarkers of oxidative stress and bone resorption in postmenopausal women. *The Journal of Nutrition, Health & Aging, 15*(2), 133-138.

Melhus, H., Michaelsson, K., Holmberg, L., Wolk, A., & Ljunghall, S. (1999). Smoking, antioxidant vitamins, and the risk of hip fracture. *J Bone Miner Res, 14*(1), 129-135.

Miyamoto, M., Matsushita, Y., Kiyokawa, A., Fukuda, C., Iijima, Y., Sugano, M., et al. (1998). Prenylflavonoids: A new class of non-steroidal phytoestrogen (part 2). estrogenic effects of 8-isopentenylnaringenin on bone metabolism. *Planta Medica, 64*(6), 516-519.

Mody, N., Parhami, F., Sarafian, T. A., & Demer, L. L. (2001). Oxidative stress modulates osteoblastic differentiation of vascular and bone cells. *Free Radical Biology & Medicine, 31*(4), 509-519.

Morton, D. J., Barrett-Connor, E. L., & Schneider, D. L. (2001). Vitamin C supplement use and bone mineral density in postmenopausal women. *J Bone Miner Res, 16*(1), 135-140.

New, S. A. (2003). Intake of fruit and vegetables: Implications for bone health. *The Proceedings of the Nutrition Society, 62*(4), 889-899.

Palacios, C. (2006). The role of nutrients in bone health, from A to Z. *Critical Reviews in Food Science and Nutrition, 46*(8), 621-628.

Papoutsi, Z., Kassi, E., Chinou, I., Halabalaki, M., Skaltsounis, L. A., & Moutsatsou, P. (2008). Walnut extract (juglans regia L.) and its component ellagic acid exhibit anti-inflammatory activity in human aorta endothelial cells and osteoblastic activity in the cell line KS483. *The British Journal of Nutrition, 99*(4), 715-722.

Park, J. A., Ha, S. K., Kang, T. H., Oh, M. S., Cho, M. H., Lee, S. Y., et al. (2008). Protective effect of apigenin on ovariectomy-induced bone loss in rats. *Life Sciences, 82*(25-26), 1217-1223.

Pearson, K. J., Baur, J. A., Lewis, K. N., Peshkin, L., Price, N. L., Labinskyy, N., et al. (2008). Resveratrol delays age-related deterioration and mimics transcriptional aspects of dietary restriction without extending life span. *Cell Metabolism, 8*(2), 157-168.

Peters, B. S., & Martini, L. A. (2010). Nutritional aspects of the prevention and treatment of osteoporosis. *Arq Bras Endocrinol Metab, 54*(2), 179-185.

Prentice, A., Schoenmakers, I., Laskey, MA., de Bono, S., Ginty, F. & Goldberg, GR. (2006). Nutrition and bone growth and development. *Proc Nutr Soc 65*, 348–360.

Rao, A. V., & Rao, L. G. (2007). Carotenoids and human health. *Pharmacological Research, 55*(3), 207-216.

Rao, L. G., Krishnadev, N., Banasikowska, K., & Rao, A. V. (2003). Lycopene I--effect on osteoclasts: Lycopene inhibits basal and parathyroid hormone-stimulated osteoclast formation and mineral resorption mediated by reactive oxygen species in rat bone marrow cultures. *J Med Food, 6*(2), 69-78.

Rao, L. G., Mackinnon, E. S., Josse, R. G., Murray, T. M., Strauss, A., & Rao, A. V. (2007). Lycopene consumption decreases oxidative stress and bone resorption markers in postmenopausal women. *Osteoporos Int, 18*(1), 109-115.

Rassi, C. M., Lieberherr, M., Chaumaz, G., Pointillart, A., & Cournot, G. (2002). Down-regulation of osteoclast differentiation by daidzein via caspase 3. *Journal of Bone and Mineral Research : The Official Journal of the American Society for Bone and Mineral Research, 17*(4), 630-638.

Sahni, S., Hannan, M. T., Blumberg, J., Cupples, L. A., Kiel, D. P., & Tucker, K. L. (2009). Inverse association of carotenoid intakes with 4-y change in bone mineral density in elderly men and women: The framingham osteoporosis study. *The American Journal of Clinical Nutrition, 89*(1), 416-424.

Sahnoun, Z., Jamoussi, K., & Zeghal, KM. (1997). Free radicals and antioxidants: human

Saura-Calixto, F., Serrano, J., & Goñi, I. (2007). Intake and bioaccessibility of total polyphenols in a whole diet. *Food Chemistry, 101*, 492–501.

Scalbert, A., & Williamson, G. (2000). Dietary intake and bioavailability of polyphenols. *The Journal of Nutrition, 130*(8S Suppl), 2073S-85S.

Sendur, O. F., Turan, Y., Tastaban, E., & Serter, M. (2009). Antioxidant status in patients with osteoporosis: A controlled study. *Joint Bone Spine, 76*(5), 514-518.

Shen, C. L., Cao, J. J., Dagda, R. Y., Tenner, T. E.,Jr, Chyu, M. C., & Yeh, J. K. (2011). Supplementation with green tea polyphenols improves bone microstructure and quality in aged, orchidectomized rats. *Calcified Tissue International, 88*(6), 455-463.

Shen, C. L., Wang, P., Guerrieri, J., Yeh, J. K., & Wang, J. S. (2008). Protective effect of green tea polyphenols on bone loss in middle-aged female rats. *Osteoporosis International : A Journal Established as Result of Cooperation between the European Foundation for Osteoporosis and the National Osteoporosis Foundation of the USA, 19*(7), 979-990.

Shen, C. L., Yeh, J. K., Cao, J. J., Chyu, M. C., & Wang, J. S. (2011). Green tea and bone health: Evidence from laboratory studies. *Pharmacological Research : The Official Journal of the Italian Pharmacological Society, 64*(2), 155-161.

Shen, C. L., Yeh, J. K., Cao, J. J., Tatum, O. L., Dagda, R. Y., & Wang, J. S. (2010). Green tea polyphenols mitigate bone loss of female rats in a chronic inflammation-induced bone loss model. *The Journal of Nutritional Biochemistry, 21*(10), 968-974.

Singh, V. N. (1992). A current perspective on nutrition and exercise. *The Journal of Nutrition, 122*(3 Suppl), 760-765.

Sontakke, A. N., & Tare, R. S. (2002). A duality in the roles of reactive oxygen species with respect to bone metabolism. *Clin Chim Acta, 318*(1-2), 145-148.

Spencer, J. P., Abd El Mohsen, M. M., Minihane, A. M., & Mathers, J. C. (2008). Biomarkers of the intake of dietary polyphenols: Strengths, limitations and application in nutrition research. *The British Journal of Nutrition, 99*(1), 12-22.

Stevenson, D. E., & Hurst, R. D. (2007). Polyphenolic phytochemicals – just antioxidants or much more? *Cellular & Molecular Life Sciences, 64*, 2900-16.

Sugimoto, E., & Yamaguchi, M. (2000). Stimulatory effect of daidzein in osteoblastic MC3T3-E1 cells. *Biochemical Pharmacology, 59*(5), 471-475.

Trzeciakiewicz, A. (2009). When nutrition interacts with osteoblast function: molecular mechanisms of polyphenols. *Nutrition Research Reviews, 22*, 68-81.

Tucker, K.L. (2009). Osteoporosis Prevention and Nutrition. *Current Osteoporosis Reports, 7*(4), 111.

Tucker, K. L., Hannan, M. T., Chen, H., Cupples, L. A., Wilson, P. W., & Kiel, D. P. (1999). Potassium, magnesium, and fruit and vegetable intakes are associated with greater bone mineral density in elderly men and women. *The American Journal of Clinical Nutrition, 69*(4), 727-736.

Velioglu, Y. S., Mazza, G., Gao, L., & Oomah, B. D. (1998). Antioxidant activity and total phenolics in selected fruits, vegetables, and grain products. *Journal of Agricultural Food & Chemistry, 46*, 4113–4117.

Viereck, V., Grundker, C., Blaschke, S., Siggelkow, H., Emons, G., & Hofbauer, L. C. (2002). Phytoestrogen genistein stimulates the production of osteoprotegerin by human trabecular osteoblasts. *Journal of Cellular Biochemistry, 84*(4), 725-735.

Ward, W. E., Yuan, Y. V., Cheung, A. M., & Thompson, L. U. (2001). Exposure to flaxseed and its purified lignan reduces bone strength in young but not older male rats. *Journal of Toxicology and Environmental Health.Part A, 63*(1), 53-65.

Wattel, A., Kamel, S., Prouillet, C., Petit, J. P., Lorget, F., Offord, E., et al. (2004). Flavonoid quercetin decreases osteoclastic differentiation induced by RANKL via a mechanism involving NF kappa B and AP-1. *Journal of Cellular Biochemistry, 92*(2), 285-295.

Weber, P. (2001). Vitamin K and bone health. *Nutrition, 17*(10), 880-887.

Wu, C. H., Yang, Y. C., Yao, W. J., Lu, F. H., Wu, J. S., & Chang, C. J. (2002). Epidemiological evidence of increased bone mineral density in habitual tea drinkers. *Archives of Internal Medicine, 162*(9), 1001-1006.

Xiao, H. H., Dai, Y., Wan, H. Y., Wong, M. S., & Yao, X. S. (2011). Bone-protective effects of bioactive fractions and ingredients in sambucus williamsii HANCE. *The British Journal of Nutrition*, 1-8.

Zhang, P., Dai, K. R., Yan, S. G., Yan, W. Q., Zhang, C., Chen, D. Q., et al. (2009). Effects of naringin on the proliferation and osteogenic differentiation of human bone mesenchymal stem cell. *European Journal of Pharmacology, 607*(1-3), 1-5.

Zych, M., Folwarczna, J., Pytlik, M., Sliwinski, L., Golden, M. A., Burczyk, J., et al. (2010). Administration of caffeic acid worsened bone mechanical properties in female rats. *Planta Medica, 76*(5), 407-411.

11

Phytochemical Studies of Fractions and Compounds Present in Vernonanthura Patens with Antifungal Bioactivity and Potential as Antineoplastic

Patricia Isabel Manzano Santana[1], Mario Silva Osorio[2],
Olov Sterner[3] and Esther Lilia Peralta Garcìa[1]
[1]*Laboratorio Bioproductos,*
Centro de Investigaciones Biotecnológicas del Ecuador, CIBE-ESPOL,
[2]*Laboratorio de Productos Naturales de la Facultad de Ciencias*
Naturales y Oceanográficas de la Universidad de Concepción,
[3]*Centre for Analysis and Synthesis, Lund University,*
[1]*Ecuador*
[2]*Chile*
[3]*Sweden*

1. Introduction

Phytochemical research is closely related to the needs of finding new and effective pharmaceuticals. Searching for plant substances that are capable forbeing used to develop new therapeutic drugs against catastrophic recognized illnesses such as cancer, diabetes and AIDS is one of the main topics that researchers around the world have been focusing.

The wonderful plant diversity of South America and more specifically from the Amazon region has around 30-50% of the worlds biodiversity therafor it is an important source for this type of study. Beside the significant undiscovered resources from these regions, ancestral knowledge of indigenous peoples is another relevant and complementary source for biodiscovery programs. Traditional healers guard centuries of accumulated knowledge about natural medicinal resources of this region. These ancient "physicians" hold the key to discovering new drugs that could benefit millions of people around the world. The Amazon forest has contributed dozens of substances to western medicine. Among the best known are the "curare"; a key component of modern anesthetics and quinine, the first contribution of "natural medicine" to treat malaria[1].

Study of new plant species and the structural elucidation of its bioactive molecules are the most important aims of phytochemical research which is in constant technological development.

---

[1] Fundación Icaro. La medicina tradicional de los pueblos indígenas amazónicos: Descubriendo la Amazonía europea. Disponible en el sitio: http://www.fundacion-icaros.org/index.php/component/content/article/8-descubriendo-la-amazonia-europea

Initial phytochemical screening and further isolation, purification and identification of molecules structure have made a major breakthrough with the development of new methods of chromatography and spectroscopy. The establishment of new and more effective bioassays is also one of the essential aspects that support biodiscovery programs today.

This chapter contains the main results on the phytochemical study of *Vernonanthura patens* leaves which according to ancestral knowledge, have been used to treat different diseases in humans.

2. Botanical classification, general characteristics and ethnobotanical knowledge on *Vernonanthura patens*

Vernonanthura patens is a wild plant broadly distributed throughout America. It grows from 0 to 2200 meters above sea level in the Ecuadorian coastal region. Folk medicine uses its leaves cooked to combat malaria, postpartum treatment and for healing infected wounds of animals by washing with a plant mixture which includes *V. patens* leaves (Blair, 2005).

It is also used against headaches, to clean and heal wounds (Kvist *et al.*, 2006); treatment of leishmaniasis (Gachet *et al.*, 2010); preparation of antivenom (Tene *et al.*, 2007) and as a poultice of leaves to combat athlete's foot (Valadeau *et al.*, 2009). Its usefulness for treating certain types of cancer has also been referred by indigenous healers. There is however there are few chemical studies about this species

2.1 *Vernonanthura patens* (Kunth) H. Rob. botanical classification and general characteristics

Species *V. patens* belongs to the *Asteraceae* family, quoting 60 synonyms and one basionym (*Vernonia patens* Kunth) (ARS-GRIN, 2009). Referred to *Vernonia patens* HBK in the list of lignocellulose species investigated in Ecuador, it is a source of raw material for pulping and papermaking (Acuña, 2000). It is also commercially important in the beekeeping industry, and is ranked as one of the most important honeybee plants from Tundo, Olmedo and Loja (Camacho, 2001) for its excellent production and availability of nectar and pollen (Ramirez *et al.*, 2001).

In the Ecuadorian province of Zamora it is one of four ecologically important species belonging to the typical families of disturbed forests that are been regenerated (Camacho, 2001; REMACH, 2004). It is now registered as representative tree species of secondary forests in Ecuadorian coastal zone (Aguirre, 2001).

The species has the following synonyms (Blair, 2005):

Cacalia patens (Kunth), Kuntze
C. aschenborniana (Schauer) Kuntze
C. baccharoides (Kunth) Kuntze
C. haenkeana (DC.) Kuntze
C. lanceolaris (DC.) Kuntze
C. suaveolens (H.B.K.) Kuntze
Vernonanthura patens (Kunth) H. Rob
Vernonia ascherbotniana Schauer
V. lanceolaris D.C.

Phytochemical Studies of Fractions and Compounds Present in Vernonanthura Patens with Antifungal
Bioactivity and Potential as Antineoplastic

217

V. micradenia DC.
V. monsonensis Hieron
V. pacchensis Benth
V. salamana Gleason
V. suaveolens Kunt
V. treberbaneri Hieron

2.1.1 Taxonomy

Taxon	*Vernonanthura patens* (Kunth) H. Rob
Genus	*Vernonanthura*
Family	*Asteraceae* (alt. Compositae)
Number	415138
Synonyms	*Vernonia patens* Kunth (basionym)
Place of publication	Phytologia 73:72, 1992
Verified name	02-Jun-2008 by systematic botanists of ARS. Last update: 02-Jun-2008 (ARS-GRIN, 2009)

2.1.2 Vernacular names

Table 1 presents a list of vernacular names that are assigned to *V. patens* according to the countries it is grown.

Country/Location		Vernacular name	References
Colombia	Tulua, Valle del Cauca-	Yasmiande, varejón	Blair, 2005
	Valle del Cauca	Pebetero	Terreros *et al*, proyecto ECOFONDO-ACDI 2004-2009
Costa Rica		Cusuco	Chavarría *et al*., 1998
		Tuete, tuete blanco	Rodríguez, 2005
Ecuador	Prov. Loja and El Oro	Laritaco	Tobías, 1996
	Prov. Guayas	Chilco Blanco	León, 2006
	Quinindé, Bilsa, Viche, Esmeraldas, Muisne and Salina Prov. Esmeralda	Chilca	REMACH, 2004
El Salvador Chalatenango		Sukunang	PROMABOS a, 2006
Guatemala		Xuqunán Xuquinái	PROMABOS, 2006
Panamá		Salvia blanca, Sanalego	Diéguez et al, 2006

Table 1. List of vernacular names assigned to *V. patens*

2.1.3 Geographical distribution

V. patens is native from America and can be found in Belize, Costa Rica, Brazil, Venezuela, Panama, Bolivia, Mexico and Ecuador according to the data reported by Missouri Botanical Garden[2].

---

[2] Tropicos.org. Missouri Botanical Garden. 23 Jun 2011.http://www.tropicos.org/Name/2740044.

2.1.4 Habitat

V.patens grows wild in the inter-Andean forest located in the south of Ecuador; its maximum height is 3-6 meters and its altitudinal distribution is between 0 and 2000 meters above sea level (Tobías, 1996; León, 2006). This species has been identified in the vegetal community of dry forests at the south-west of Ecuador[3].

This species is sometimes grown or kept in farms after its spontaneous appearance. Generally it can be found near the forest trail and on the edge of the rivers. Flowering and fruiting occurs between May and October.

2.1.5 Botanical information

V. patens (Figure 1), is a small branched shrub, growins up to six meters high with furrowed stems and ferruginous trichomes. Alternate leaves are petiolate, narrowly lanceolate, petiole tomentose with ferruginous trichomes, 4-11mm long; the leaves are entirely or weakly serrate, rounded base with a sharp or acuminate apex leaves are 7-15 cm long and 1.3 - 1.2 cm wide, the adaxial surface is bright and the abaxial is pubescent or puberulent, subcoriaceous, penninerved. Inflorescence is paniculate, terminal, extended branched with the endings scorpioid, provided with leaves and bracts, capitates sessile and very shortly pedicellate, with numerous bell-shaped flowers, 8 mm long, 4-5 sets bracts imbricated, tomentose and of dark brown color, corolla glabrous, about 5 mm long, weakly pubescent achenes, pappus hairs-layered irregular shaped edges that are about 7 mm long. A detailed description of the botanical characteristics of this species has been published by Blair (2005).

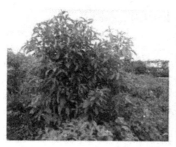 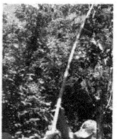

Fig. 1. *Vernonanthura patens* (laritaco). It grows wild in different Ecuadorian areas belonging to the provinces of Loja, El Oro, Guayas, Manabí and Los Ríos.

2.2 Ethnomedical information

In Ecuador the inhabitants of the south-west of Loja and the Marcabelí region of El Oro province recognize both its healing power and analgesic action. They use the leaves of *V. patens* to wash wounds and to relieve headaches. It is also employed as anti-inflammatory to soothe coughs and against certain types of cancers. In addition, a veterinary practice is described as it can heal infected wounds by washing with a mixture of plants that includes leaves from this species (Blair, 2005). Other interesting uses have been also reported.

---

[3] http://www.darwinnet.org/index.php?option=com_content&view=article&id=153%3Aarticulos-cientificos-y-reportes-&catid=25%3Acontenido&Itemid=1

Gacheta *et al.*, (2010) informed its usefulness for leishmanianis treatment; Tene *et al* (2007) indicating its use in the preparation of antivenon and the use of "laritaco" leaves in poultices to combat athlete's foot is referred by Valadeau *et al.*, (2009).

Different uses of *V. patens* have been registered in other South American countries. In the Bolivian community of Tacama, the juice of the plant stem is applied against conjunctivitis (Tacana, 1999) and in Colombia the watery brews of the aerial parts mixed with "panela"[4], white wine and rosemary are used against malaria. It is also used to relieve pain due to labor and to purge (Blair, 2005).

2.3 Biological and chemical activity

There are very few biological and chemical studies of the specie *V. patens*. The only results published so far refer to the antimalarial activity against *Plasmodium falciparum*, Itg2 strain (Blair, 2005) ,anti-*Leishmania* activity (Valadeau *et al.*, 2009) of the leaves of this species and no antiprotozoal activity against different strains of Leishmania (Fournet, 1994). On the chemical composition of the species, reports lack of sesquiterpene lactones and sesquiterpenes present in the aerial parts (Mabry, 1975; Jakupovic, 1986). There are some references on genus *Vernonanthura* that show the presence of diterpenes compounds (Portillo *et al.*, 2005; Valadeau *et al.*, 2009), flavonoids (Borkosky *et al.*, 2009; Mendonça *et al.*, 2009), triterpenes (Tolstikova *et al.*, 2006, Gallo *et al.*, 2009), saponins (Borkosky *et al.*, 2009) and sesquiterpene lactones. In addition, different biological activities have been described assuming that certain chemical groups could be responsible for the therapeutic properties attributed to species of this genus (Pollora *et al.*, 2003, 2004; Portillo *et al.*, 2005; Bardon *et al.*, 2007).

These were the main factors that led to the Laboratorio Bioproductos Centro de Investigaciones Biotecnológicas del Ecuador to undertake a chemical-pharmacological study of *Vernonanthura patens* leaves from plants growing in Ecuadorian areas. Such investigations are part of the Biodiscovery Program developed by this center.

3. Phytochemical screening

As an initial step of thephytochemical screening research allows to determine qualitatively the main groups of chemical constituents present in a plant. This screening can guide the subsequent extraction and / or fractionation of extracts for the isolation of groups of interest. The phytochemical screening routine is performed by extraction with suitable solvents of increasing polarity and the application of color reactions (Miranda & Cuellar, 2001).

These reactions are characterized by their selectivity to types or groups of compounds, their simplicity, short time consuming and capacity to detect small amount of compounds using a minimum requirement of laboratory equipment. The results are recorded by the presence (+) or absence (-) of the color reactions.

---

[4] "Panela" is a unrefined sugarcane product obtained from the boiling and evaporation of sugarcane juice. It contains sucrose and fructose and is a typical product of Latin America, but can be finding in certain Asian countries.

The general outline of steps followed for performing the phytochemical screening of *V. patens'* leaves is presented in Figure 2, while the analysis of the extracts obtained at different polarities is schematically shown in Figure 3. This methodology has been referred previously (Miranda & Cuellar, 2000; Manzano *et al.*, 2009).

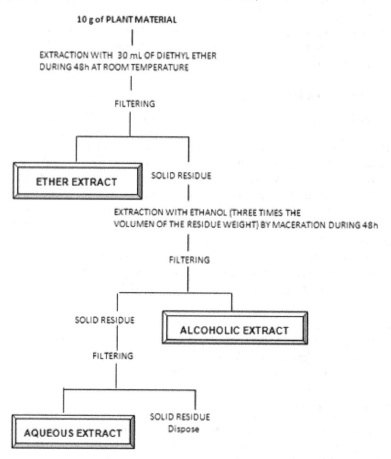

Fig. 2. General procedure used for performing the phytochemical screening of *V. patens* leaves.

The plant material of adult leaves of *Vernonanthura patens* (laritaco) were used from plants at the vegetative state which were growing in the citadels "July 25", "Imbabura" and "June 24" and all belonget to the Canton Marcabelí, province El Oro, Ecuador. Leaves were collected at early morning at different dates during the months of December to February in 2009 and 2010.

Botanical identification was performed and voucher specimens of the herbs were prepared and deposited at the National Herbarium of Ecuador (QCNE) and a duplicated sample (CIBE37) was kept as herbal witness in the laboratory of the CIBE-ESPOL Bioproducts. Prior

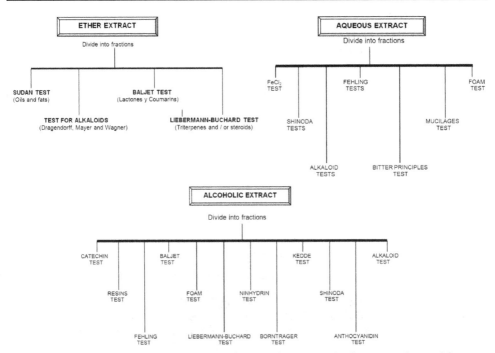

Fig. 3. Chemical reactions carried out in each type of V. *patens'* leaf extracts obtained from using solvents of different polarity.

consent was obtained and authorized by the corresponding agencies of the government. The fieldwork and data collection were conducted in accordance with the institutional, national and international principles and guidelines for using and conserving plant biodiversity.

For conducting the phytochemical screening, extraction and fractionation, leaves samples were dried using an automatic dryer (45 °C, 8 hours) and then pulverized in a blender and screened. The fraction that remained in the sieve of 2 mm in diameter was collected and kept in polyethylene bags of low density at 24 °C.

The result of phytochemical screening is presented in Table 2. This reveals moderate to low concentration of essentials oils, alkaloids, reducing compounds, phenols, tannins, flavonoids, quinones, saponins, triterpenes and steroids. Some of these chemical compounds have been associated to antibacterial, antifungal, antiprotozoal and citotoxicity properties and thus have a potential therapeutic use (Nweze *et al.*, 2004; Reuben *et al.*, 2008; Vital *et al.*, 2010).

4. Plant extracts, fractions and compounds

The dry plant material (67 g of leaves of *V. patens*) was subjected to successive extractions with HPLC grade methanol by maceration in a closed container and in the absence of light. The extraction time was eight days and was conducted until total depletion of plant material; agitator and a rotary evaporator were used for solvent recovery.

Chemical groups	Essays	Extracts		
		Ether	Alcoholic	Aqueous
Essential oils, fatty compounds	Sudan	+		
Alkaloids	Dragendorff Mayer		+	+
Aminoacids	Ninhidrine		-	-
Antocianidine	Antocianidine		-	-
Cardiotonic	Kedde		-	-
Reducing compounds	Fehling		-	+
Phenols and tannins	Ferric chloride		+	+
Flavonoids	Shinoda		-	+
Lactones	Baljet		-	-
Mucilages	Mucilages		-	-
Bitter principles	Bitter principles		-	-
Quinones	Börntrager		+	-
Resins	Resins		-	-
Saponins	Foam		+	+
Triterpenes and steroids	Lieberman-Buchard	+	+	-

Table 2. Chemical groups detected in *V. patens* leaves through the phytochemical screening.

The extract was evaporated to dryness, yielding 7g (10.44%) of methanol extract. The methanol residue was subjected to fractionation by successive column chromatography (CC) packed with activated silica from 60 to 200 mesh; elution was performed with solvents of increasing polarity using mixtures of hexane and ethyl acetate (10, 9:1 , 8:2, 3:7, 10) (Table 3). The extracts were analyzed by thin layer chromatography (TLC) on 60 F254 silica gel cromatofolios (Merck) with fluorescent indicator and a solvent system hexane / ethyl acetate (9:1). Plates were observed under UV light at 254 and 366 nm wavelengths.

Solvent	Proportion (%)
Hexane	100
Hexane/ethyl acetate	90:10
Hexane/ethyl acetate	80:20
Hexane/ethyl acetate	30:70
Ethyl acetate	100
Ethyl acetate/methanol	70:30

Table 3. Solvents and proportions used in the chromatographic column fractionation of *V. patens*.

Six fractions were obtained (Figure 6): Fr 1 hexane (79mg), Fr 2 Hex / EtOAc 90:10 (1370mg), Fr 3 Hex / EtOAc 80:20 (0.60 mg), Fr 4 Hex / EtOAc 30:70 (0.41mg), Fr 5 EtOAc (0.21 mg), fraction 6 EtOAc / MeOH 70:30 (1760m g) and three pure compounds of the EtOAc fraction 10 and 20% (Figure 7): 57 mg of the compound [1] , 20 mg of the compound [2] and 90 mg of the compound [3].

The isolated fractions with different solvents from methanol extract of leaves of *V. patens* by column chromatography, have not been referred to this species, resulting in a high mass in the hexane fraction (79mg) compared with other extracted fractions. Nevertheless, methanol, ethyl acetate and hexane extracts from other plant species had showed a relevant antimicrobial activity (Ramya *et al.*, 2008).

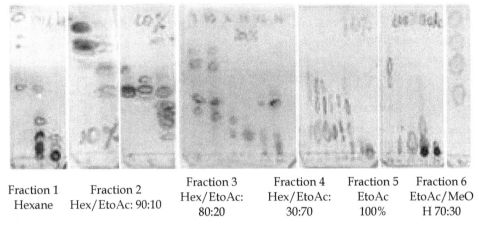

| Fraction 1 | Fraction 2 | Fraction 3 | Fraction 4 | Fraction 5 | Fraction 6 |
| Hexane | Hex/EtoAc: 90:10 | Hex/EtoAc: 80:20 | Hex/EtoAc: 30:70 | EtoAc 100% | EtoAc/MeOH 70:30 |

Fig. 6. Isolated fractions from methanol extract of *V. patens*

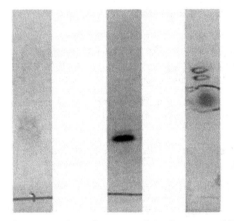

Compound 1   Compound 2   Compound 3

Fig. 7. Chromatographic plate (TLC) showing the three pure compounds isolated from *V. patens*. Pure compounds were isolated from Fr 2 Hex / EtOAc 90:10 (1370mg).

5. Bioassays

Assays for screening the bioactivity of natural products has had an impressive history of development and is one of the keys for discovering new natural bioactive compounds.

In this study, a qualitative preliminary evaluation of the antifungal capacity of fractions and pure compounds isolated were conducted in order to select the most active. Those selected were re-evaluated to quantify their ability to inhibit fungal growth.

The diffusion method (Avello *et al.,* 2009) in potato dextrose agar (PDA) was used to determine the antifungal activity of fractions and pure compounds isolated from *V. patens* leaves at 100 and 200 µg mL⁻¹. Dilutions were made with dimethylsulfoxide (DMSO) 10%.

Strains of *Fusarium oxysporum* and *Penicillium notatum,* isolated from infected *Pinus radiata* and *Citrus sinense* fruits and maintained in the Collection of Fungi at University of Concepcion were used.

Holes of 5 mm Ø were made in the agar with a sterile cork borer and filled with 20 μL of each concentration of fractions and pure compounds. DMSO 10% was used as negative control in each plate. A disc (5 mm Ø) of already grown fungus was placed in the center of Petri dishes and incubated at 22 °C. Evaluations were during two weeks.

Experimental design was completely randomized and each assay was performed in triplicate. Descriptive statistics of the experimental data was made in order to represent and point out its most important features.

Most relevant antifungal activity was observed in fraction 1 (100% hexane) and pure compounds 1 and 3 at the both concentrations tested.

The hexane fraction inhibited the growth of both fungal species tested. Highest inhibition exerted against *Penicillium notatum* (80.2%) and *Fusarium oxysporum* (81.5%) occurred when using 200 μg mL^{-1} of this fraction. Statistical differences (P≤0,05) with negative controls indicated that DMSO did not influence the results of biological evaluation.

Pure compounds showed selective inhibition properties and a certain concentration dependence in its antifungal activity. Compound 1 showed a rate of inhibition of 50 and 90% (100 and 200 μg mL^1 respectively) against *Penicillium notatum* while compound 3 was capable to inhibit 80 and 100% of the *Fusarium oxysporum* growth for each assayed concentrations.

Screening for antifungal activity of fractions and pure compounds of *V. patens* has been conducted for the first time. The potential of these results is relevant.

6. Structural identification and quantitative analysis of the fractions and isolated compounds

6.1 Chemical characterization of the fraction with antifungal activity

The isolated fraction with antifungal activity were analyzed for structural identification by gas chromatography-mass spectrometry (GC-MS) using an Agilent 7890A gas chromatograph with an Agilent 5975 detector (Avondale, PA.USA) equipped with a column HP-5MS of 5m long (0.25 mm in diameter and 0.25 cm inside diameter). Helium was used as the carrier gas; the analytical conditions were: initial temperature: 100 ° C (increasing 8 ° C per minute to a final temperature of 250 ° C); inlet temperature and mass detector: 250 ºC and 300 °C respectively. The mass detector was used in scan mode ("scan") with a range of 100 to 400 amu.

According to this technique and the analytical conditions described, this chromatogram was obtained and is as shown in Figure 8.

Using the library computer and taking into consideration those compounds that exceeded the 90% of confidence, structures of 33 components could be assigned (Table 4).

The compounds identified are mostly hydrocarbons, a logical result given the solvent used. There was a relative abundance of possible bicyclical sesquiterpenos (peaks 1-5) and of the acyclic triterpeno squalene (peak 30). For the sesquiterpenos exist antecedents of antimicrobial activity (Gregori *et al* ., 2005) and for the escualeno reports of activity antioxidant, antitumor

Phytochemical Studies of Fractions and Compounds Present in Vernonanthura Patens with Antifungal
Bioactivity and Potential as Antineoplastic

225

and antimicrobial activities, in addition to its beneficial effect for preventing cardiovascular diseases by reducing cholesterol and triglycerides (Garcia *et al.*, 2010).

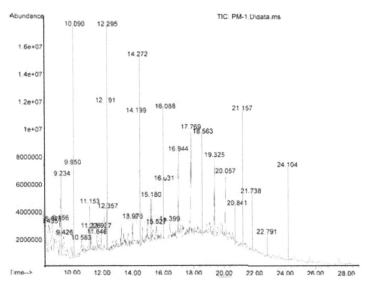

Fig. 8. Analytical gas chromatogram of the hexane fraction of *Vernonanthura patens*.

For this reason, it is possible to hypothesis that antifungal activity of *V. patens* against *F. oxysporum* and *P. notatum* which has been determined could be directed related to the squalene presence despite not being the main component of the fraction tested. The remaining compounds, individually or collectively, could also be involved in the bioactivity demonstrated. The results described here have not been reported previously for *V. patens*.

6.2 Structural identification of isolated compounds

The structures of the three compounds isolated from the hexane soluble fraction by column chromatography were identified by their spectroscopic patterns as compared with references. These pure compounds were identified as Lupeol (compound 1), Acetyl Lupeol (compound 2) and Epi Lupeol (compound 3) (Figure 9).

Spectroscopy was performed in the Laboratory of Organic Chemistry at the University of Lund. ^{1}H NMR (500 MHz) and ^{13}C NMR (125 MHz) were recorded at room temperature with a Bruker DRX500 spectrometer with an inverse multinuclear 5 mm probe head equipped with a shielded gradient coil. The spectra were recorded in $CDCl_3$, and the solvent signals (7.26 and 77.0 ppm, respectively) were used as reference. The chemical shifts (δ) are given in ppm, and the coupling constants (J) in Hz. COSY, HMQC and HMBC experiments were recorded with gradient enhancements using sine shaped gradient pulses. For the 2D heteronuclear correlation spectroscopy the refocusing delays were optimized for $^1J_{CH}$=145 Hz and $^nJ_{CH}$=10 Hz. The raw data were transformed and the spectra were evaluated with the standard Bruker XWIN-NMR software (rev. 010101).

The results that are shown in this chapter are unpublished and have not been previously registered for the species *V. patens*. Even though, the elucidated structures of the pure compounds have been found in other vegetal species, and recognize their diverse biological activity which includes antineoplastic action against certain types of cancer (Gallo & Sarachine, 2009).

Peak	Time retention	Name
1	8.435	α-caryophyllene (sesquiterpene)
2	8.678	Napthalene, 1, 2, 3, 4, 4a, 5, 6, 8a-octahydro-7-methyl-4-methylene-1-(1-methylethyl) - (1 α., 4a. α, 8a. α). (bicyclic sesquiterpene)
3	9.156	Naphthalene, 1, 2, 4a, 5, 6, 8a-hexahydro-4, 7-dimethyl-1-(1-methylethyl) (bicyclic sesquiterpene)
4	9.234	Naphthalene, 1, 2, 3, 5, 6, 8a-hexahydro-4, 7-dimethyl-1-(1-methylethyl) (bicyclic sesquiterpene)
5	9.426	Naphthalene, 1, 2, 4a, 5, 6, 8a-hexahydro-4, 7-dimethyl-1-(1-methylethyl) - [1S-(1. α, 4a. β., 8a. α)] (bicyclic sesquiterpene)
6	9.950	2 - tetradecene (E) -
7	10.090	Hexadecane
8	10.583	2, 6, 10, - trimethyl-pentadecane,
9	11.153	2,6,11-trimetil-dodecano,
10	11.226	2,6,11-trimethyl-dodecane,
11	11.646	Tritetracontano
12	11.937	Heptadecane, 3-methyl-
13	12.191	3 - octadecane, (E) -
14	12.295	Heptadecane
15	12.357	4-methyl-heptadecane,
16	13.976	Octadecane
17	14.199	(E) -3 - eicosane,
18	14.272	Eicosane
19	15.180	Heneicosano
20	15.527	Octadeciloxy –2-Ethanol
21	16.031	Docosenoic
22	16.088	2 - Bromo dodecane
23	16.399	1 - bromo-octadecane
24	16.944	1-iodo-Hexadecane
25	17.769	Tetracosanoic
26	18.563	11-decyl-tetracosanoic
27	19.325	1-chloro-Heptadecosano,
28	20.057	5,14-dibutyl-octadecane
29	20.841	Nonadecane
30	21.157	Squalene
31	21.738	Eicosane
32	22.791	9-octyl-Heptadecane
33	24.104	Hentriacontane

Table 4. Identified compounds in hexane fraction of *V. patens* with antifungal activity.

Phytochemical Studies of Fractions and Compounds Present in Vernonanthura Patens with Antifungal
Bioactivity and Potential as Antineoplastic

227

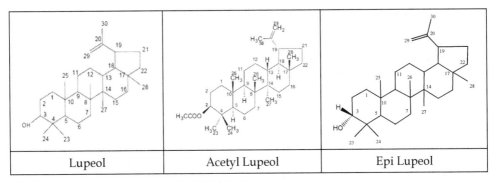

| Lupeol | Acetyl Lupeol | Epi Lupeol |

Fig. 9. Structure of compounds identified in *V. patens*.

7. Concluding remarks

Phytochemical screening of *V. patens* has showed the presence of essentials oils, alkaloids, reducing compounds, phenols, tannins, flavonoids, quinones, saponins, triterpenes and steroids, of which some have been previously associated to important biological activities.

Fractions and pure compounds of this species were screened for the first time for antifungal activity. Hexane fraction and two pure compounds further identified as Lupeol and Epilupeol, were active against two important fungal pathogens at high rate (80-100%). Hexane fraction reduced the growth of *Fusarium oxysporum* in 80% and Epilupeol completely inhibited the *Fusarium oxysporum* growth.

Thirty-three chemical compounds in the hexane fraction from *V. patens* leaves were determined, Of which must are hydrocarbons. Antifungal activity of this fraction can be related to presence of squalene and/or combined activity of others identified compounds. Further research must be done for determining specific bioactivity of identified compounds.

Chemical structures of three isolated compounds were elucidated, corresponding to Lupeol, Acetyl Lupeol and Epi Lupeol. These compounds are recognized for their significant and diverse biological activities, including antimicrobial and antineoplastic actions.

Results of this study show that *V. patens* can be considered as important potential candidate for further chemical and biological researches and justify its inclusion in the biodiscovery program of CIBE.

8. Acknowledgements

This study was supported by grants from SENESCYT and ESPOL (Ecuador)

9. References

Acuña O. (2000). Valoración de las características físico químicas de especies ligno-celulósicas y subproductos agroindustriales en la obtención de pulpa y elaboración

de papel. *Primer encuentro Nacional de productores y artesanos de fibras naturales.*
    Memorias técnicas, Ibarra-Ecuador. Avaliable from
    http://biblioteca.espe.edu.ec/upload/Memorias_Tecnicas.pdf.
Aguirre N. (2001). ECOPAR: *Sistemas forestales en la costa del Ecuador*: una propuesta para la
    zona de amortiguamiento de la reserva Mache – Chindul. University of
    Amsterdam. Programa FACE de Forestación del Ecuador S.A. Quito, Ecuador.
    Available from
    http://www.rncalliance.org/WebRoot/rncalliance/Shops/rncalliance/4C15/9487
    /9F8B/02A1/3D0A/C0A8/D218/9663/Aguirre_et_al_2001_SFCosta2001.pdf
Avello M., Valdivia R., Sanzana R., Mondaca, M., Mennickent S., Aeschlimann V., Bittner
    M., Becerra J. (2009). Extractos antioxidantes y antimicrobianos de *Aristotelia
    chilensis* y *Ugni molinae* y sus aplicaciones como preservantes en productos
    cosméticos . Boletín Latinoamericano y del Caribe de Plantas Medicinales y
    Aromáticas, Vol. 8 (6), pp. 479-486.
Bardón A., Borkoskya S., Ybarra M., Montanaroa S. & Cartagena E. (2007). Bioactive plants
    from Argentina and Bolivia. *Fitoterapia* Vol. 78(3), pp. 227-231.
Borkosky S., Ponce S., Gabriela Juárez G., González M. & Bardón A. (2009). Molusquicida
    Sesquiterpene Lactones from Species of the Tribe Vernonieae (Compositae).
    Chemistry & Biodiversity, Vol. 6(4), pp. 513–519. Avaliable from
    http://onlinelibrary.wiley.com/doi/10.1002/cbdv.200800156/citedby
Blair S. (2005). *Plantas antimaláricas de Tumaco*: Costa Pacífica Colombiana; Vol. 1(347) pp. 84-
    87. Universidad de Antioquia. Avaliable from
    http://books.google.com.ec/books?id=8a7CKa3yXr0C&pg=PA84&lpg=PA84&dq
    =botanica++vernonanthura+patens&source
Camacho A. (2001). *Potencialidad melífera y polinífera de dos zonas de vida de la provincia de Loja.*
    Editores: Pablo Lozano y Zhofre Aguirre. Fundación Ecuatoriana para la
    Investigación y el Desarrollo de la Botánica, Avaliable from
    http://joethejuggler.com/Funbotanica/Boletin9.html
Chavarría F., Masís A., Pérez D., Espinoza R. & Guadamuz A. (1998). Species Page of
    Vernonia patens (Asteraceae). *Species* Home Pages, Área de Conservación
    Guanacaste, Costa Rica. Avaliable from
    http://www.acguanacaste.ac.cr
Diéguez M., Luque D., Domínguez I., Somoza A., Ortega G., Tejada I., Veces A., Gallardo
    M., Araúz Y. & Núñez E. (2006). Convenio de Cooperación ANAM – ACP.
    Monitoreo de la Cuenca Hidrográfica del Canal de Panamá. *Componente de Calidad
    de Agua Región Oriental de la Cuenca del Canal*, pp. 51. Avaliable from
    http://www.pancanal.com/cich/documentos/indice-integridad-biologica.pdf
ECOPAR (2001). *Sistemas forestales en la costa del Ecuador: una propuesta para la zona de
    amortiguamiento de la reserva Mache – Chindul.* University of Amsterdam. Programa
    FACE de Forestación del Ecuador S.A. Quito.
Fournet, A., Barrios, A.A. *Leishmamanicidal and trypanocidal activities of Bolivian medicinal
    plants.* Journal of Ethnopharmacology. 1994. 41:19-37
Gacheta M., Salazar J., Kaiserc M., Brunc R., Navarrete H., Muñoz R., Bauer R. & Schühlya
    W. (2010). *Assessment of anti-protozoal activity of plants traditionally used in Ecuador in
    the treatment of leishmaniasis.* Journal of Ethnopharmacology, pp. 128, 184–197.
Gallo M. & Sarachine M. (2009). *Biological Activities of Lupeol.* International Journal of
    Biomedical and pharmaceutical Sciences. Global Sciences Books. pp. 46-62.
    Avaliable from

Phytochemical Studies of Fractions and Compounds Present in Vernonanthura Patens with Antifungal
Bioactivity and Potential as Antineoplastic

229

http://www.globalsciencebooks.info/JournalsSup/images/0906/IJBPS_3(SI1)46-660.pdf

García Luján, Martínez A., Ortega J. & Castro F. (2010). *Componentes químicos y su relación con las actividades biológicas de algunos extractos vegetales.* Química Viva, Vol. : 9(2) pp. 86-96.

Gregori Valdés Susana. *Estructura y actividad de los antifúngicos.* Revista Cubana de Farmacia 2005. 39(2).

Jakupovic, J., Schmedia-Hirschmann, G. *Hirsutinolides, glaucolides and sesquiterpene lactones in species of Vernonia.* Biochem. Phytochemistry. 1986. 25:145-158.

Kvist L. P., Aguirre Z. & Sánchez O. (2006). *Bosques montanos bajos occidentales en Ecuador y sus plantas útiles.* Botánica Económica de los Andes Centrales Universidad Mayor de San Andrés, La Paz pp. 205-223. Avaliable from http://www.beisa.dk/Publications/BEISA%20Book%20pdfer/Capitulo%2013.pdf

León M. R. & Guiracocha F. G. (2006). Tesis Ing. Agro. *Diversidad vegetal asociada a cacaotales de dos zonas agroecológicas en la región litoral del Ecuador.* 144 pp., ESPOL, Ecuador.

Mabry, T.J., Abdel-Baset, Z. *Systematic implications of flavonoids and sesquiterpene lactones in species of Vernonia.* Biochem. Sist. Ecol. 1975. 2:185.

Manzano, P., Miranda, M., Orellana-Manzano A., García, G., Gutiérrez, Y. & Orellana, T. (2009) *Efecto antiinflamatorio y composición química del aceite de ramas de Bursera graveolens Triana & Planch. (palo santo) de Ecuador.* Revista cubana de plantas medicinales. Vol. 14(3), pp: 45-53. Available in http://scielo.sld.cu/scielo.php?pid=S1028-47962009000300007&script=sci_arttext

Mendonça C., Gonçalves-Esteves V., Esteves R., & Nunes A. (2009). *Palynotaxonomy of vernonanthura H. Rob. (Vernonieae, Asteraceae) Species from southeast Brazil.* Revista Brasil. Bot. Vol. 32(4): pp. 647-662.

Miranda M. & Cuéllar A. (2001). *Farmacognosia y productos naturales,* Editorial Félix Varela, Ciudad de La Habana, pp. 207-222.

Miranda M. & Cuellar A. (2000). *Manual de Prácticas de Laboratorio. Farmacognosia y Productos Naturales. Instituto de Farmacia y Alimentos.* Editorial Félix Varel, Ciudad de La Habana, p. 44-49.

Nweze, E.T. Okafor, J.I. & Njoku, O. (2004). *Antimicrobial Activities of Methanolic extract of Trumeguineesis (Schumm and Thorn) and Morinda lucinda Benth used in Nigerian Herb. Medicinal Practice.* J. Bio. Res. Biotechnol. Vol. 2 (1): pp. 34-46.

Pollora G. C., Bardón A., Catalan C., Gedris E. & Herz W. (2003) *Elephantopus-type sesquiterpene lactones from a Vernonanthura species, Vernonanthura nebularum Biochemical Systematics and Ecology,* Voumen 31(4) : pp. 397-405. Avaliable from http://cat.inist.fr/?aModele=afficheN&cpsidt=14685237

Pollora G. C ., Bardón A., Catalán C., Griffin C. l. & Herz W. (2004). Elephantopus-type Sesquiterpene Lactones from a Second *Vernonanthura* species, *Vernonanthura lipeoensis, Biochemical Systematics and ecology.* Elsevier, Amsterdam. Vol. 32: pp. 619-625. Avaliable from http://cat.inist.fr/?aModele=afficheN&cpsidt=15798184

Portillo A., Vila R., Freixaa B., Ferrob E., Parellac T., Casanovad J. & Cañiguerala S. (2005). *Antifungal sesquiterpene from the root of Vernonanthura tweedieana.* Journal of Ethnopharmacology Vol. 97(1): pp. 49-52.

Promabos (2006). *Proyecto de manejo de abejas y del bosque.* Flora of la palma (Chalatenango, El Salvador), Avaliable from http://www.bio.uu.nl/promabos/flora/alt_index.html

Promabos. (2006). *Proyecto de Manejo de Abejas y Bosques. Árboles melíferos para reforestar.* Xuqunán o Xuquinái, Avaliable from http://www.bio.uu.nl/promabos/arbolesmeliferos/pdf_files/Xuqun%E1n.pdf

Ramírez J., Camacho A., Merino B. & Ureña J. (2001). *Recursos florales y origen botánico de las mieles de las abejas (Apis mellifera, L.) en las provincias de Loja y Zamora Chinchipe.* Área agropecuaria y de recursos renovables. Universidad Nacional de Loja. Revista informática, Avaliable from http://issuu.com/miltonric/docs/recursosflorales#comments.

Ramya S., Kalayansundaram M., Kalaivani T. & Jayakumararaj, R. (2008). *Phytochemical Screening and Antibacterial Activity of Leaf Extracts of Pterocarpusmarsupium Roxb. (Fabaceae).* Ethnobotanical Leaflets Vol. 12: pp. 1029-34.

REMACH, (2004). *Plan de Manejo y Gestión participativa de la reserva ecológica Manche-Chindul,* Avaliable from http://www.darwinnet.org/docs/PlanManejoMacheChindul.pdf.

Reuben, K.D., Abdulrahman F.I., Akan J.C., Usman H., Sodipo O.A. & Egwu G.O. (2008). *Phytochemical Screening and In Vitro Antimicrobial Investigation of the Methanolic Extract of Croton Zambesicus Muell ARG. Stem Bark.* European Journal of Scientific Research, Vol. 23(1) : pp. 134-140

Rodriguez A. (2005). *Vernonia patens Kunth.* INBIO. Instituto Nacional de Biodiversidad. Avaliable from http://darnis.inbio.ac.cr/FMPro?-DB=UBIpub.fp3&-lay=WebAll&-Format=/ubi/detail.html&-Op=bw&id=6713&-Find

Tacana. (1999). *Conozcan nuestros árboles, nuestras hierbas.* Editores UMSA - CIPTA – IRD. La Paz, pp. 27. Avaliable from http://horizon.documentation.ird.fr/exl-doc/pleins_textes/divers10-04/010018852.pdf

Tene V., Malangón O., Vita P., Vidari G., Armijos Ch. & Zaragoza T. (2007). *An ethnobotanical survey of medicinal plants used in Loja and Zamora-Chinchipe, Ecuador.* Journal of Ethnopharmacology Vol. 111: pp. 63–81.

Terreros G. & Adriana M. (2009). *Recuperación del conocimiento ancestral en manejo de plantas con fines medicinales en comunidades étnicas el norte del Cauca y en la vereda la colonia (Yotoco).* Proyecto Regional ECOFONDO-ACDI, Valle-Norte del Cauca, 2004-2009. Avaliable from http://proyecto.ecofondo.org.co/index2.php?option=com_docman&task=doc_vie w&gid=46&Itemid=36.

Tobías. (1996). *EC076. Cañón del río Catamayo.* Darwinnet, Avaliable from http://www.darwinnet.org/docs/Ibas_RT/EC076.pdf.

Tolstikova T. G., SorokingI. V., Tolstikov G. A. Tolstikov A. G. & Flekhter O. B. (2006). *Biological Activity and Pharmacological Prospects of Lupane Terpenoids: I. Natural Lupane Derivatives.* Russian Journal of Bioorganic Chemistry Vol. 32(1): pp. 37–49. Avaliable from http://www.springerlink.com/content/e754t15r23114117/

Valadeau C., Pabon A., Deharo E., Albán–Castillo J., Estévez Y., Lores F., Rojas R., Gamboa D., Sauvain M., Castillo D. & Bourdy G. (2009). Medicinal plants from the Yanesha (Peru): *Evaluation of the leishmanicidal and antimalarial activity of selected extracts. Journal of Ethnopharmacology* pp. 123, 413–422.

Vital, P.G., Velasco Jr, R.N., Demigillo, J.M. & Rivera, W.L. (2010). *Antimicrobial activity, cytotoxicity and phytochemical screening of Ficus septica Burm and Sterculia foetida L. leaf extracts.* Journal of Medicinal Plants Research, Vol. 4(1): pp. 58-63.

12

The Pentacyclic Triterpenes α, β-amyrins: A Review of Sources and Biological Activities

Liliana Hernández Vázquez[1], Javier Palazon[2] and Arturo Navarro-Ocaña[3,*]
[1]Universidad Autónoma Metropolitana, Unidad Xochimilco, Depto. Sistemas Biológicos,
[2]Laboratorio de Fisiología Vegetal, Facultat of Farmacia, Universitat de Barcelona,
[3]Departamento de Alimentos y Biotecnología, Facultad de Química "E" – UNAM,
[1,3]México
[2]Spain

1. Introduction

Pentacyclic triterpenes are ubiquitously distributed throughout the plant kingdom, in a free form as aglycones or in combined forms, and have long been known to have a number of biological effects. The compounds α-amyrin and β-amyrin are commonly found in medicinal plants and oleo-resin obtained by bark incision of several species of *Bursera or Protium* of the Burseraceae family. Both *in vitro* and in *vivo* studies have shown that β-amyrin also has important biological functions.

In light of the considerable interest recently generated in the chemistry and pharmacological properties of amyrins and their analogs, we have undertaken this review in an effort to summarize the available literature on these promising bioactive natural products. The review will detail the recent studies on the chemistry and bioactivity of α, β-amyrins, which is presented in the following sections: the isolation and distribution of α-amyrin and β-amyrin, giving a brief introduction to amyrins as natural products and the methods used in their isolation; the biological activities of amyrins, examining the biological properties associated with these compounds with a focus on their potential chemotherapeutic applications.

2.1 Chemical structure, detection, analysis and sources

2.1.1 Structure

The chemical structure of α-amyrin (3β-hydroxy-urs-12-en-3-ol) is shown in Fig. 1. The chemical formula of α-amyrin is $C_{30}H_{50}O$, its melting point is 184-186 °C (Sirat, et al., 2010), and it presents an MS ion Peak at m/z 426 (M$^+$) (Dias et al., 2011). The infra-red spectrum of α-amyrin is IR u_{max} (KBr) cm^{-1}: 3450, 2895 and 2895. The chemical structure of β-amyrin (3β-hydroxy-olean-12-en-3-ol) is also depicted in (Fig. 1) and its formula is $C_{30}H_{50}O$. The infra-red spectrum of β-amyrin shows the presence of a hydroxyl function and the olefinic moiety at a spectrum of 3360 and 1650 cm^{-1} and MS studies of β-amyrin confirm a parent ion peak at m/z 426 (M$^+$) (Dias et al., 2011), other work of HR-EI-MS m/z: 426.2975 (calcd. for $C_{30}H_{50}O$, 426.3861) (Jabeen et al., 2011). The melting point of β-amyrin is 189-191 °C (Lin et al., 2011).

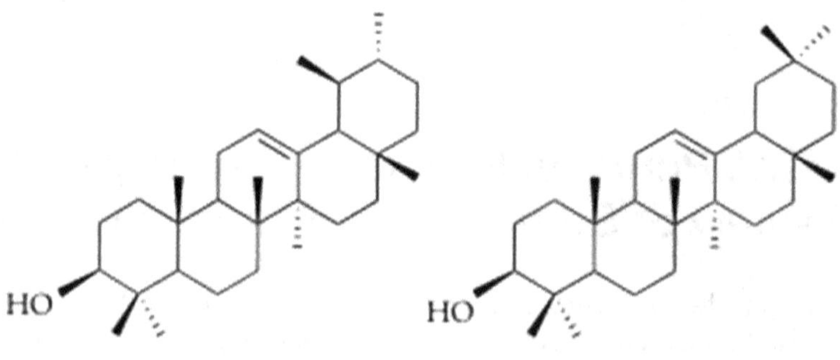

α-amyrin   β-amyrin

Fig. 1. Estructure of amyrins

NMR methods have indisputably become the single most important spectroscopic techniques for the identification and structure elucidation of amyrins. Several ID and 2D NMR methods are now commonly used for the characterization of pentaclyclic triterpenes. These methods incluye ^{1}H and ^{13}C-NMR, APT, DEPT, COSY, HMQC, HMBC and TOCSY. The ^{1}H and ^{13}C-NMR assignments of α- β-amyrin are presented in Table 1, (Dias et al., 2011).

2.1.2 Detection

Amyrins are found in various plants and plant materials such as leaves, bark, wood, and resins. This material has to be pre-treated prior to isolation of the target compounds. First, the plant material is usually dried, then ground into a power and sieved. Second, extractions are carried out with dichloromethane, chloroformo, n-hexane, and methanol. The samples can be subjected to alkaline hydrolysis, derivatization and separation by thin layer chromatography, and the resulting material can be directly subjected to analysis. Gas chromatography (CG) and high performance thin layer chromatography (HPTLC) techniques are the most commonly employed methods to quantitate α-, β-amyrin in plants.

TLC provided an easy and rapid way to study plant extract profiles and partially identify compounds. The first step for the identification of α-amyrin, β-amyrin and 3-epi-lupeol was to compare R$_F$ values of reference standards with those of sample extracts. TLC on silica gel revealed that α-amyrin on tracks 6 and 15, β-amyrin on track 14 and the α-, β-amyrin mixture on track 16, as well as two standards, all had the same R$_F$ (Fig. 2). The α-amyrin band was observed as brown, while the β-amyrin band appeared violet, as did the band for the α-, β-amyrin mixture. TLC analysis revealed the presence of α-amyrin, β-amyrin and 3-epi-lupeol by a comparison of the position and color of the triterpene spots with those of authentic compounds (Fig. 2). The bands of α- and β-amyrin or their mixture were observed in all commercial resin tracks 1-5 and medicinal plant tracks 8-13, while 3-epi-lupeol track 7 was detected only in the commercial Mexican Copal resins tracks 1-4. Attempts were made to separate the α-, β-amyrin mixture, which had appeared homogenous on TLC, but without success. These results showed that TLC can be used as a simple method for a preliminary analysis of these triterpenes in extracts of commercial resins and plants, but cannot be employed for the analysis of the α-, β-amyrin mixture. (Hernández-Vázquez et al., 2010)

Position	α-amyrin		β-amyrin	
	δ^1H	$\delta^{13}C$	δ^1H	$\delta^{13}C$
1		38.7		38.7
2		28.7		27.2
3	3.16 (dd, J = 5.1; 11.2)	79.6	3.15 (dd, J = 4.4; 10.8)	79.3
4		38.7		38.5
5	0.67 (d, J = 11.6)	55.1	0.68 (d, J = 11.0)	55.1
6		18.4		18.6
7		32.2		32.4
8		40.7		39.8
9		47.7		47.6
10		36.6		36.9
11		23.3		23.6
12	5.06 (t, J = 3.2)	124.4	5.12 (t, J = 3.2)	121.7
13		139.5		145.2
14		42.0		41.7
15	1.94 (td, J = 4.5; 13.5 Hβ)	27.2	1.89 (td, J = 4.0; 14.0 Hβ)	26.2
16	1.76 (td, J = 5.0; 13.5 Hβ)	26.6	1.70 (td, J = 4.3; 13.5 Hβ)	26.1
17		33.7		32.6
18		59.0		47.2
19		39.6	1.93 (dd, J = 4.0; 13.7 Hβ)	46.8
20		39.6		31.0
21		31.2		34.7
22	1.85 (dt, J = 3.0; 7.0)	41.5	1.80m	37.1
23	0.93s	28.1	0.77s	28.0
24	0.74s	15.6	0.90s	15.4
25	0.73s	15.6	0.73s	15.4
26	0.89s	16.8	0.93s	16.8
27	1.01s	23.2	1.19s	25.9
28	0.94s	28.1	1.07s	28.4
29	0.85 (d, J = 6.0)	17.4	0.87s	33.8
30	0.73 (d, J = 7.0)	21.4	0.80s	23.7

Table 1. The ^1H and ^{13}C-NMR Spectral Data of α- and β-amyrin

α-Amyrin, β-amyrin and other triterpenes were analysed by TLC and HPLC, the chromatographic techniques including silica gel and reversed-phase (C18RP) TLC and C18 RP-HPLC using UV and mass spectrometric (MS) detection with APCI (Martelanc et al., 2009). HPTLC combined with densitometry has been used to analyse the triterpenoids α-, β-amyrin and the oleanolic acid content of acetone and ethyl acetate extracts of the leaves of *Jovibara sobolifera* (Sims) (Szewczyk et al., 2009). The detection and/or quantitation of α-, β-amyrin either in plants or plant products using GC methods requires pre-derivatization of the samples, for example, acetylation or trimethylsilylation. Sometimes a sample clean-up employing silica gel columns or liquid-liquid partition is also necessary.

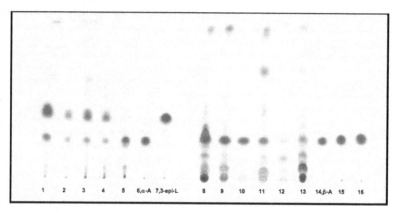

Fig. 2. TLC plate. Tracks: 1=MCT; 2=MCS; 3=MCN; 4=MCP; 5=MER; 6 and 15=α-amyrin; 7=3-*epi*-lupeol; 8=Dandelion; 9=Olive; 10=Cancerina; 11=Nance wastes; 12=Bearberry; 13=Pot marigold; 14=β-amyrin; 15=α-amyrin and 16=mixture α-, β-amyrin.

2.1.3 Analysis

Gas chromatography (CG) is applied to determine the concentration of α-, β-amyrin and α-, β-amyrin mixtures. The chemical composition of the essential oil of Lemon Catnip (*Nepeta cataria* L. var. citriodora Balbis) was determined by CG-MS, and α-amyrin was detected in the hydrodistilled volatile of Lemon Catnip (Wesolowska et al., 2011). α-amyrin has also been determined in the kernel fats of the shea tree (*Vitellaria paradoxa*; Sapotaceae) of sub-Saharan countries (Akihisa et al., 2010). CG of the apolar extract from *Clusia Minor* L. leaves led to the identification of 25 compounds, lupeol and α-amyrin being the most abundant triterpenoids (Mangas-Marin et al., 2008). CG-MS fingerprints for cerumen from the stingless bee *Tetragonula carbonaria* in South East Queensland, Australia, showed trace quantities of TMS ethers of β-amyrins (Massaro et al., 2010). Studies on the constituents of yellow Cuban propolis by CG-MS revealed the presence of large amounts of triterpenic alcohols including β-amyrin, (Márquez-Hernández et al., 2010). Solid-phase extraction and GC-MS were developed to separate and enrich only sterols from unsaponifiables of vegetable, hazelnut and olive oils, detecting sterols, lupeol and δ-, β-amyrin (Azadmard-Damirchi et al., 2010). Epicuticular and intracuticular waxes from both adaxial and abaxial surfaces of *Kalanchoe daigremontiana* leaves (Hamet et Perr. De la bathie) were analyzed by CG. All wax mixtures were found to contain triterpenoids and fatty acids, the triterpenoid fraction containing small amounts of β-amyrin (van Maarseveen & Jetter., 2009). Fatty acid, phytosterol, and polyamine conjugate profiles of corn edible oils were analyzed by GC-MS and HPLC, and a few minor sterols and β-amyrin were identified and quantified using GC-FID (Moreau et al., 2009). Fatty acids, phytosterols and tocopherols of Milk thistle (*Silybum marianum*) seeds were determined in four varieties grown in Ardebil-Iran. In this study using TLC-GC, dimethylsterols were predominant followed by cycloartenol and β-amyrin, (Fathi-Achachlouei, Azadmard-Damirchi., 2009). CG proved an effective method for quantitative measurement of the β-sitosterol content of white mulberry (*Morus alba*) leaves and bark without derivatization. Sterols, lupeol and α–, β-amyrin were identified in leaves and bark by GC-FID analysis (Böszörményi et al., 2009). GC and CG-MS were used to analyse hexane extracts from seven oleoresins of *Protium* species. High concentrations of α- and β-amyrin were identified in *P. strumosum* (64%) and *P. tenuifolium* (66.7%) (Silva et al., 2009). Finally, the analytical performances of three atmospheric-pressure sources, electrospray (ESI), atmospheric-pressure chemical ionization (APCI) and atmospheric-pressure photoionization (APPI), were evaluated for the analysis of pentacyclic triterpenes in liquid chromatography-mass spectrometry (LC-MS) (Zarrouk et al., 2010). The developed LC-MS method was used to characterize pentacyclic triterpenes in tree plant extracts. The main component of birch bark was betulin and the extracts of Okume resin exhibited high amounts of α- and β-amyrin (Rhourri-Frih et al., 2008). Other technique used to quantitate and determine amyrins is Reversed-Phase High Performance Liquid Chromatography (RP-HPLC). HPLC was used for analysis of some isomeric plant triterpenoids (α-amyrin and β-amyrin δ-amyrin, lupeol, lupenon, lupeol acetate, cycloartenol acetate, ursolic acid oleanolic acid and two sterols) (Martelanc et al., 2009), other studies was for analysis of medicinal plants and Mexican Copal resins (Hernández-Vázquez et al., 2010) and resin obtained from species of the genus *Protium* (Burseraceae) (Dias et al., 2011).

2.1.4 Sources of α-, β-amyrins

α-amyrin is a triterpene of natural origin isolated from various sources, most notably plant resins. Considerable amounts (up to g/kg) of this triterpene are available in the resins of *Bursera* and *Protium* species of the *Burseraceae* family. Other known sources of α-amyrin include Mexican copal (5 g/kg) (Hernández-Vázquez, et al., 2010), *Cassia obtusifolia* (140 mg/kg) (Sob et al., 2010) and the resin of *Commiphora holtziana* (syn. *Commiphora erythraea*) (200 mg/kg) (Manguro, et al., 2009). The most important sources of β-amyrin include lotus (*Nelumbo nucifera* Gaertn) bee pollen (3 g/kg) (Xu. et al., 2011), bark of "cuachalalate" (*Amphipterygium adstringens*) (2.4 g/kg) (Rosas-Acevedo et al., 2011), semi-preparative isolation from resin of *Protium* (α-amyrin 1g /kg and β-amyrin 1.7 g/Kg) (Dias et al., 2011), *Eucalyptus globulus* biomass residues from the pulping industry (326 mg/kg) (Domingues et al., 2010), *Ficus carica* latex (1.2 g/kg) (Oliveira et al., 2010), root bark of *Ficus cordata* (20 mg/kg), steam bark *Ficus cordata* (200 mg/kg) (Kuete et al., 2008) and leaves and bark of *Byrsonima crassa* Niedenzu (IK) (1.3 g/kg) (Higuchi et al., 2008). Mixtures of α and β–amyrin were obtained from steam bark residues of *Byrsonima crassifolia* (Nance) (9 g/kg) (Hernández-Vázquez et al., 2010), leaves of *Byrsonima fagifolia* Niedenzu (2.3 g/Kg) (Higuchi et al., 2008) and leaves of *Pouteria gardnerii* (Mart & Miq) Bahemi gave α-, β-amyrin and other triterpenes (Silva et al., 2009).

Plants reported since 2008 to possess α-amyrin, β-amyrin and a α, β-amyrin mixture in minor amounts (detected and isolated) are listed here. α-Amyrin has been isolated from the resin of *Boswellia carterii* Birdw (Wang et al., 2011), detected in stemwood and bark from *Populus x euramericana* (Xu et al., 2010), isolated (65 mg/kg) from the n-hexane extract of the leaves of *Melastoma malabathricum* L (Sirat et al., 2010), identified in the methanol extract of the stem bark of *Poncirus trifoliate* (Feng et al., 2010), isolated (1 mg/kg) from the methanol extract of the stem bark of the African tree *Antiaris Africana* Engler (Vouffo et al., 2010), detected in seed oil of Saskatoon berries (*Amelanchier alnifolia* Nutt.) (Bakowska-Barczak et al., 2009), isolated (23 mg/kg) from the methanol extract of stem bark and leaves of *Ficus pandurata* Hance (Ramadan et al., 2009), dried rhizomes of *Nelumbo nucifera* (Chaudhuri et al., 2009), and detected in bread wheat (Nurmi et al., 2008).

Plant	α-amyrin	β-amyrin	α/β-amyrin	Ref
Mexican copal	5g/Kg			Hernandez-Vazquez et al., 2010
Cassia obtusifolia	0.14g/kg			Sob et al., 2010
Commiphora holtziana (syn. *Commiphora erythraea*)				Manguro, et al., 2009.
Nelumbo nucifera Gaertn		3g/kg		(Xu. et al., 2011)
Amphipterygium adstringens		2.4g/kg		Rosas-Acevedo et al., 2011
Protium sp	3.1g/kg	1.7g/Kg		Dias et al., 2011
Eucalyptus globulus		0.3g/kg		Domingues et al., 2010
Ficus carica		1.2g/Kg		Olivera et al 2010
Ficus cordata		0.2g/Kg		Kuete et al., 2008
Byrsonima crassa Niedenzu (IK)		1.3g/kg		(Higuchi et al., 2008.
Byrsonima crassifolia (Nance)			9g/kg	Hernández-Vázquez et al., 2010
Byrsonima fagifolia			2.3g/Kg	Higuchi et al., 2008
Pouteria gardnerii (Mart & Miq)			X	Silva et al., 2009

Table 2. List of selected materials containing α-, β-amyrin and α/β-amyrins

β-Amyrin has been isolated and detected in various materials: an ethanolic fraction of oleo-gum-resin from *Ferula gummosa* (Jalali et al., 2011), the plant *Carpobrotus edulis*, (Martins et al., 2011), the leaves of *Clerodendrum inerme* (L.) (22.5 mg/kg) (Parveen et al., 2010), the chloroform and ethyl acetate fractions of the methanolic extract of *Carpobrutus edulis* (Martins et al., 2010), chloroform extract of aerial parts of the plants or calli of *Euphorbia tirucalli* L. (Uchida et al., 2010), seed oil of *Capparis spinosa* (Tlili et al., 2011), chloroform extract of the leaves of *Ficus benjamina* (var. camosa) (Moraceae) (Simo et al., 2009), leaves (2 mg/kg) of *Pyrenacantha staudii*, (Falodun et al., 2009), ethanol extract of leaves of *Olea europea* L. (Wang et al., 2009), ethyl acetate extract of apple peels of the Red Delicious variety (*Malus domestica* Borkh) (He et al., 2008), air-dried leaves of *Tectona philippinensis*, an endemic and endangered Philippine medicinal plant (Ragasa et al., 2008), a mixed benzene and chloroform extract of leaves of *Rhus alata* (Parveena et al., 2008), and an extract of stem bark of *Piptadenia Africana*, a western Cameroonian plant (Mbouangouere et al., 2008).

An α- and β-amyrin mixture has been detected in the following plants: *n*-hexane and chloroform extracts of the epicuticular wax layer of *Mandevilla guanabarica* and *Mandevilla moricandiana*, (Cordeiro et al., 2011), an ethanolic extract of roots of *Salacia amplifolia*, (Wang et al., 2011), and chloroform extracts of Blue Honeysuckle (*Lonicera caerulea* L.) (Palíkova et al., 2008).

A multitude of extraction and isolation schemes have been used for the procurement of α-amyrin, β-amyrin and an α/β amyrin mixture. Typically, dry material (resins, leafs and stem barks) is extracted with hexane or another non-polar solvent, (Fig. 3), and the resulting extract is directly subjected to column or thin layer chromatography. An alternative procedure is sequential fractionation by silica gel columns using various solvents. The amyrins are not readily visible on TLC plates UV (λ = 254 and 365 nm) but are easily detected following exposure to iodine vapors, anisaldehyde-H_2SO_4 or vanillin-H_2SO_4 spray reagents.

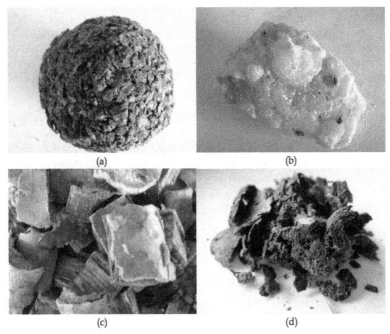

(a)   (b)

(c)   (d)

Fig. 3. Sources of amyrins; a) Copal Piedra, b) White Copal, c) Bursera bark, d) Propolis

2.2 An overview of pharmacological activities of α, β-amyrins

α, β-amyrins have been shown to exhibit various pharmacological actitivies *in vitro* and *in vivo* conditions against various health-related conditions, including conditions such as inflammation, microbial, fungal, and viral infections and cancer cells.

2.2.1 Anti-microbial and anti-fungal

The antimicrobial properties of *n*-hexane and methanol extracts of *Bombax malabaricum* flowers were examined against different bacterial, fungal and yeast strains. The methanol extract was highly active against *Staphylococcus aureus*, *Bacillus subtilis*, *Stretoccocus faecalis*, *Neisseria gonorrehea*, *Pseudomonas aeruginosa* and *Candida albicans*, whereas the *n*-hexane extract displayed moderate-to-weak activities against the same test microorganisms. An *n*-hexane extract afforded sterols including α-amyrin (El-Hagrassi et al., 2011). A bioassay-guided fractionation of *n*-hexane extracts of *Bursera simaruba* (L) Sarg. leaves resulted in the isolation and identification of five sterols and β-amyrin. Additionally, *n*-hexane extracts have displayed anti-inflammatory activity on adjuvant-carrageenan-induced inflammation in rats (Carretero et al., 2008). α-Amyrin and other compounds have been proposed as possible biomarkers for the fungal resistance of grape-vine leaves (*Vitis vinifera*) (Batovska et al., 2008).

β-Amyrin has been found to exhibit antifungal and antimicrobial activity against some microbes. The antifungal activity of *Melia azedarach* L. leaves was investigated against *Ascochyta rabiei* (Pass.) Lab., the cause of destructive blight disease of chickpea (*Cicer arietinum* L.). Bioassay-guided fractionation revealed that the chloroform fraction of the methanolic extract of *M. azedarach* leaves was highly effective against *A. rabiei*. Six compounds, namely β-sitosterol (1), β-amyrin (2), ursolic acid (3), benzoic acid (4), 3,5-dimethoxybenzoic acid (5) and maesol (6), were isolated from this fraction. All compounds showed antifungal activity, β-amyrin being the most effective, with an MIC value of 0.0156 mg mL^{-1} (Jabeen et al., 2011).

In a recent study on the leaves of *Siraitia grosvenorii*, β-amyrin and other bioactive compounds were obtained, and their activities against the growth of oral bacterial species *Streptococcus mutans*, *Actinobacillus actinomycetemcomitans*, and *Fusobacterium nucleatum* and the yeast *C. albicans* were evaluated *in vitro*. β-amyrin only exhibited a slight inhibition of *Streptococcus mutans* and *Fusobacterium nucleatum* (Zheng et al., 2011). Bioassay-guided fractionation of the methanol extract of the stem bark of *Klainedoxa gabonensis* Pierre ex Engl. (Irvingiaceae) afforded 12 compounds: four flavonoids and eight (including β-amyrin) triterpenes. Antimicrobial activities in the triterpenoids ranged from low to non-existent (Wansi et al., 2010). In this study, the *in vitro* antibacterial activity of the methanolic extract and isolated compounds from the bark of *Byrsonima Crassifolia* against twelve bacteria and the yeast *C. albicans* was investigated. Eight known compounds, β-amyrin, betulin, betulinic and oleanolic acid, quercetin, epicatechin, gallic acid and β-sitosterol, were isolated and evaluated for their antimicrobial activity. Bacterial growth was inhibited by β-amyrin, olenolic and gallic acid at concentrations ranging from 64 to 1088 μg.mL^{-1} (Rivero-Cruz et al., 2008).

2.2.2 Anti-inflammatory activity

Hexane extracts of *Bursera simaruba* (L.) Sarg. leaves display an anti-inflammatory effect on adjuvant-carrageenan-induced inflammation in rats. In order to isolate and identify the active compounds of the hexane extract, we performed a preliminary phytochemical study and a bioassay-directed fractionation using the carrageenan-induced paw oedema test in mice. From the nine fractions (A–I) obtained, A and E showed the strongest anti-inflammatory activity, comparable to that of the reference drug phenylbutazone. Sterols and α-amyrin have been isolated and characterized from these fractions, the evidence suggesting that these bioactive compounds may play a key role in the anti-inflammatory effects of *B. Simaruba* extracts (Carretero et al., 2008).

Ligustrum (privet) plants are used by Chinese physicians to prevent and cure hepatitis and chronic bronchitis. Three common *Ligustrum* plant spp., namely *Ligustrum lucidum* Ait. (LL), *L. pricei* Hayata (LP) and *L. sinensis* Lour. (LS) were collected to assess their analgesic/anti-inflammatory effects on chemical-induced nociception and carrageenan-induced inflammation in rodents. The methanol extracts from *Ligustrum* plant leaves effectively inhibited nociceptive responses induced by 1% acetic acid and 1% formalin. LP and LL reduced the edema induced by 1% carrageenan. The most potent *Ligustrum* plant was LP, which also reduced abdominal Evans blue extravasations caused by lipopolysaccharide, lipoteichoic acid, autocrines and sodium nitroprusside. The triterpenoid content of the three

Ligustrum spp. was measured by HPLC, the highest content of β-amyrin, betulinic acid and lupeol being found in LP. This work suggested that these three triterpenoids are responsible for the anti-inflammatory potency of LP (Wu et al., 2011).

A recent report describes that the roots of *Calotropis gigantea* (Linn.) R.Br, traditionally used in India to treat asthma, possess anti-lipoxygenase activity, it was found that intraperitoneal administration of indomethacin did not block edema formation, but edema was inhibited by montelukast and methanolic extracts of *C. gigantea* roots. This result indicates that the extract from *C. gigantea* was responsible for the inhibition of the lipoxygenase pathway in the arachidonate metabolism. Therefore, it can be concluded that *C. gigantea* may have a similar mechanism of action as dexamethasone as well as antioxidant and anti-lipoxygenase effects, possibly due to the presence of α-amyrin and β-amyrin (Bulani et al., 2011).

Aqueous and organic extracts of *Acacia visco* Lor. Ap Griseb (Fabaceae) were tested for anti-inflammatory activity in experimental rat models. The extracts revealed an anti-inflammatory effect against carrageenan-induced oedema, phospholipaseA-induced oedema, and cotton pellet-induced granuloma without any acute toxic effects. Among the class of compounds characterized from *A. visco* leaves, the triterpenoids lupeol, α-amyrin and β-amyrin may be mainly responsible for these anti-anflammatory properties (Padernera et al., 2010). α-, β-Amyrin ameliorates L-arginine-induced acute pancreatitis in rats. It has been demonstrated that the crude resin of *Protium heptaphyllum* (March.) has an α- and β-amyrin ratio of 63:37. The mixture of both compounds and methylprednisolone treatments significantly (P < 0.05) attenuated the L-arginine-induced increases in pancreatic wet weight/body weight ratio, and decreased the serum levels of amylase and lipase, and TNF-α and IL-6, in comparison with the vehicle control. Also, pancreatic levels of MPO activity, TBARS, and nitrate/nitrite were significantly lower. The conclusion of this study is that α, β-amyrin has the potential to combat acute pancreatitis by acting as an anti-inflammatory and antioxidant agent (Melo et al., 2010).

Another study has shown the systemic preventive or therapeutic anti-inflammatory action of the triterpenes α- and β-amyrin in TNBS-induced colitis in mice. It was found that α–, β-amyrin is as efficacious as dexamethasone in reversing the macroscopic and microscopic outcomes of TNBS-induced colitis, including the restoration of cytokine balance. Furthermore, the results also indicate that inhibition of NF-κB and CREB activation is certainly the main mechanism through which these triterpenes exert their anti-inflammatory action (Vitor et al., 2009). Another report demonstrated for the first time that α–, β-amyrin isolated from *Protium heptaphyllum* modulates acute periodontal inflammation in rats by reducing neutrophil infiltration, oxidative stress and the production of proinflammatory cytokine TNF-a, and suggests that these triterpenes might be useful as a therapeutic agent for the treatment of gingivitis and to retard the progression of periodontitis (Holanda-Pinto et al., 2008).

2.2.3 Other pharmacological activities

α- and β-Amyrin have been tested for a variety of other biological activities. An anti-ulcer effect of *Cytocarpa procera* and *Amphipterygium adstringens* was assayed on experimental gastric injury in rats and phytochemical analysis allowed the identification of β-amyrin and β-sitosterol in *A. adstringens* (Rosas-Acevedo et al., 2011). The triterpenoids β-amyrin, cohulupone and garcinielliptone were isolated from the pericarp, heartwood and seed of *Garcinia subelliptica*, respectively, and the three compounds showed an inhibitory effect on xanthine oxidase. Treatment of NTUB1, a human bladder cancer cell, with β-amyrin or β-amyrin in cotreatment with cisplatin for 24 h resulted in a reduced viability of cells. This work suggested that β-amyrin exhibited weak cytotoxic activities against NTUB1 cells (Lin et al., 2011). The antiproliferative effects of *n*-hexane, chloroform and aqueous methanol extracts prepared from the whole plant of *Centaurea arenaria* M.B. ex Willd. were investigated against cervix adenocarcinoma (HeLa), breast adenocarcinoma (MCF7) and skin epidermoid carcinoma (A431) cells, using the MTT assay. Only the flavonoids and lignans showed moderate activity against these cell lines and β-amyrin was inactive (Csapi et al., 2010). From the ethyl acetate fraction of the stem bark of *Camellia japonica*, three new triterpenoids, 3-β-O-acetyl-16b-hydroxy-12-oxoolean, 3β-O-acetyl-16β-hydroxy-11-oxoolean-12-ene, and 3-β-O-acetyl-16β-hydroxyolean-12-ene, along with seven known compounds, 3-α-hydroxy-1-oxofriedelan, friedelin, 3-β-friedelanol, canophyllol, 3-oxofriedelan-1(2)-ene, β-amyrin, camellenodiol, and camelledionol, were isolated. Their structures were established on the basis of spectroscopic analysis and chemical evidence. The isolated compounds were tested *in vitro* for their cytotoxic activities against the A549, LLC, HL-60 and MCF-7 cancer cell lines. Among them, β-amyrin exhibited weak cytotoxicity against A549 and HL-60 cancer cell lines with IC (50) values of 46.2 and 38.6 μM, respectively (Thao et al., 2010). Another report showed that the methanol extract obtained from soxhlet extraction of leaves of *Ardisia elliptica* Thunberg (Myrsinaceae) contained α- and β-amyrin, determined by GS-MS. The leaf extract inhibited platelet aggregation with an IC_{50} value of 167 μg/mL, using bioassay guided fractionation. β-Amyrin was isolated and purified showing an IC_{50} value of 4.5 μg/mL, while that of aspirin was found to be 11 μg/mL, indicating that β-amyrin is more potent that aspirin in inhibiting collagen-induced platelet aggregation (Ching et al., 2010). Two triterpenes, β-amyrin and 12-oleanene 3β, 21β-diol, were isolated as a mixture from the chloroform soluble fraction of an ethanolic extract of *Duranta repens* (Verbanaceae) stem. The mixture was highly effective against the larvae of *Culex quinquefasciatus* Say (Diptera: Culicidae) as a mosquitocide. *C. quinquefasciatus* is a potential vector of *Wuchereria bancrofti* (Filarioidae), the causative agent of human lymphatic filariasis (Nikkon et al., 2010). One study has examined the potential trypanocidal activity of different plant species growing in the Brazilian Cerrado, after *in vitro* screening of 20 extracts obtained from 10 plants. The phytochemical analysis of the most active extracts (hexane extracts) allowed the identification of β-amyrin, α-amyrin, lupeol and other triterpenes and sterols. The results showed that pure amyrins are inactive whereas the *n*-hexane leaf extract of *Tibouchina stenocarpa* cogn. Melastomataceae was active. The trypanocidal activity of the extract may be due to the presence of other compounds (Cunha et al., 2009).

3. Conclusion

α- and β-Amyrin are bioactive compounds commonly found in leaves, barks and resins. Such plant material is an interesting source of these triterpenoids, as it allows for easy extraction. Extensive research over the last four years has identified α- and β-amyrin in several plants and the pure compounds have shown anti-microbial, anti-inflammatory and other interesting biological activities. Amyrins are also involved in the biosynthetic pathways of other biologically active compounds such as avenacine, centellosides, glycyrrhizin or ginsenosides. The development of biotransformation systems to convert amyrins into these or other compounds would open new ways for using α- and β-amyrins as a source of bioactive plant secondary metabolites more scarcely distributed in the plant kingdom. In this context, the bioconversion of α-amyrin into centellosides in *Centella asiatica* cell cultures has been recently reported (Hernandez-Vazquez et al., 2010).

4. Acknowledgement

We thank the PAPIIT-UNAM, IN223611 and CONACYT, CB2009 IN 129061, for financial support.

5. References

Akihisa, T., Kojima, N., Katoh, N., Ichimura, Y., Suzuki, H., Fukatsu, M., Maranz, S. & Masters, E. (2010). Triterpene alcohol and fatty composition of sea nuts from seven African countries, *Journal of the Oleo Science*, 59 2(7): 351-360. ISSN: 1347-3352

Azadmard-Damirchi, S., Nemati, M., Hesari, H., Ansarin, M. & Fathi-Achalouei, B. (2010) Rapid separating and enrichment of 4.4´-dimethylsterols of vegetable oils by solid-phase extraction, *Journal of American Oil Chemical Society*, 87: 1155-1159. ISSN: 003-021X

Bakowska-Barczak, A. M., Schieber, A. & Kalodziejczyk, P. (2009). Charaterization of Saskatoon berry (*Amelanchier alnifolia* Nutt.) seed oil, *Journal of Agricultural and Food Chemistry*, 57: 5401-5406. ISSN:1520-5118

Batovska, D. I., Todorova, I. T., Nedelcheva, D. V., Parushev, S. P., Atanassov, A. J., Hvarleva, T. D., Djakova, G. J., bankova, V. S. (2008). Preliminary study on biomarkers for the fangal resitence in *Vitis vinifera* leaves, *Journal of Plant Physiology*, 165: 791-795. ISSN: 0176-1617

Börzörményi, A., Szarka, S., Héthelyi É., Gyurján, I., László, M., Simándi, B., Szoke. É. & Lemberkovics, É. (2009) Triterpenes in traditional an d supercritical fluids extracts of *Morus alba* and stem bark, *Acta Chromatographica*, 4: 659-669. ISSN 1231-2522

Bulani, V., Biyani, K., Kale, R., Joshi, U., Charhate, K., Kumar, D. & Pagore, R. (2011). Inhibitory effect of *Calotropis gigantea* extract on ovalbumin-induced airway inflammation and Arachidonic acid induced inflammation in a murine model of asthma, *International Journal of Current Biological and Medical Science* 1(2): 19-25. ISSN 2231-6256

Carretero, M. E., López-Pérez, J. L., Abad, M. J., Bermejo, P., Tillet, S., Israel. A. & Noguera-P, B. (2008). Preliminary study of the anti-inflammatory activity of hexane extract and fraction from *Bursera simaruba* (Linneo) Sarg. (Burseraceae) leaves, *Journal of Ethnopharmacology*, 116: 11-15. ISSN: 0378-8741

Chaudhuri, P. C. & Deepika, S. (2009). A new lipid and other constituents from the rhizomes of *Nelumbo nucifera*, *Journal of Asian Natural Products Research*, 11(7): 583-587. ISSN: 1477-2213

Ching, J., Chua, T., Chin, L., Lau, A., Pang, Y., Jaya, J. M., Tan, C. & Koh, H. (2010). β-Amyrin from *Ardisia elliptica* Thunb. Is more potent than aspirin in inhibiting collegen-induced platelet aggregation, *Indian Journal of Experimental Biology*, 48: 275-279. ISSN 0975-1009

Cordeiro, S. Z., Simas, N. K., Arruda, R. C. O. & Sato, A. (2011). Composition of epicuticular wax layer of two species of *Mandevilla* (Apocynoideae, Apocynaceae) from Rio de Janeiro, Brazil, *Biochemical Systematics and Ecology*, 39: 198-202. ISSN 0305-1978

Csapi, B., Zsuzsanna, H., Zupkó, I., Berényi, A., Forgo, P., Szabó, P & Hohmann, J. (2010). Bioactivity-guided isolation of antiproliferative compounds from *Centaurea arenaria*, *Phytotherapia Research*, 24: 1664-1669. ISSN 1099-1573

Cunha, W.R., Dos Santos, F. M., Peixoto, J. A., Veneziani, C. S., Crotti, A. E. M., Siva, M. L. A., Filho, A. A. S., Albuquerque, S., Turatti, I. C. C & Bastos, J. K. (2009). Screeing of plantas extracts from the Brazilian Cerrado for their *in vitro* trypanocidal activity, *Pharmaceutical Biology*, 47(8): 744-749. ISSN 1744-5116

Dias, M. M., Hamerski, L. & Pinto, A. (2011). Separacao semipreparative de α e β-amyrina por cromatografia líquida de alta eficiencia, *Qumica Nova*, 34(4): 704-706. ISSN 1678-7064

Domingues, R. M. A., Sousa, G. D. A., Freire, C. S. R., Silvestre, A. J. D. & Pascoal-Neto, C. (2010). *Eucalyptus globulus* biomass residues from pulping industry as a source of high value triterpenic compounds, *Industrial Crops and Product*, 31: 65-70. ISSN: 0926-6690

El-Hagrassi, A. M., Ali, M. M., Osman, A. F. & Shaaban, M. (2011). Phytochemical investigation and biological studies of *Bombax malabaricum* flowers, *Natural Products Research*, 25(2): 141-151. ISSN: 1029-2349

Falodun, A., Chaudhry, A. M. A. & Choudhary, I. M. (2009). Phytotoxic and chemical investigations of a Nigerian medicinal plant, *Research Journal of Phytochemistry*, 3(1): 13-17. ISSN: 1819-3471

Fathi-Achachlouei, B. & Azadmard-Damirchi, S. (2009) Milk thistle seed oil constituents from different varieties grown in Iran, *Journal of American Oil Chemical Society*, 86: 643-649. ISSN: 003-021X

Feng, T., Wang, R., Cai, X., Zheng, T. & Luo, X. (2010). Anti-human immunodeficiency virus-1 constituents of the Bark of *Poncirus trifoliata*, *Chemical Pharmaceutical Bulletin*, 58(7): 971-975. ISSN: 0009-2363

He, X. & Lui, R. L. (2008). Phytochemicals of apple peels: isolation, structure, elucidation, and their antiproliferative and antioxidant activities, *Journal of Agricultural and Food Chemistry*, 56: 9905-9910. ISSN: ISSN 1520-5118

Hernandez-Vázquez, L., Mangas, S., Palazón, J. & Navarro-Ocaña, A. (2010) Valuable medicinal plants and resins: Comercial phytochemicals whith bioactive properties, *Industrial Crops and Products*, 31: 476-480. ISSN: 0926-6690

Hernandez-Vázquez, L., Bonfil, M., Moyano, E., Cusido, R. M., Navarro-Ocaña, A. & Palazón, J. (2010), Conversion of α-amyrininto centellosides by plant cell cultures of *Centella asiatica*, *Biotechnology Letters*, 32(2): 94-104. ISSN: 0141-5492

Higuchi, C. T., Pavan, F. R., Leite, Sannomiya, M., Vilegas, W., Leite, S. R. A., Sacramento, L. V. & Sato, D. N. (2008). Triterpenes and antitubercular activity of *Byrsonima crassa*, *Quimica Nova*, 31(7): 1719-1721. ISSN: 1678-7064

Higuchi, C. T., Sannomiya, F. R., Pavan, F. R., M., Leite, S.R. A., Sato, D. N., Sacramento, L. V. S. Vilegas, W. & Leite, C. Q. F. (2008). *Byrsonima fagifolia* Niedenzu Apolar

Compounds with antitubercular activity, *Evidence-Based Complementary and Alternative Medicine*, 2011: 1-5. ISSN: 1741-4288

Holanda Pinto, S. A., Pinto, L. M. S., Cunha, G. M. A., Chaves, M. H., Santos, F. A. & Rao, V. S. (2008). Anti-inflammatory effect of α, β-Amyrin, a pentacyclic triterpene from *Protium heptaphyllum* in rat model of acute periodontitis, *Inflammopharmacology*, 16: 48-52. ISSN: 0925-4692

Jabeen, K., Javaid, A., Ahmad, E. & Athar, M. (2011). Antifungal compounds from *Melia azederach* leaves for management of *Ascochyta rabiei*, the cause of chickpea blight, *Natural Products Research*, 25(3): 264-276. ISSN: 1029-2349

Jalali, H. T., Ebrahimian, Z. J., Evtuguin, D. V. & Neto, C. P. (2011). Chemical composition of oleo-gum-resin from *Ferula gummosa*, *Industrial Crops and Products*, 33: 549-553. ISSN: 0926-6690

Kuete, V., Ngameni, B., Simo, C. C. F., Tankeu, R. K., Ngadjui, B. T., Meyer, J. J. M., Lall, N. & Kuiate, J. R. (2008). Antimicrobial activity of the crude extracts and compounds from *Ficus chlamydocarpa* and *Ficus cordata*, *Journal of ethnopharmacology*, 120: 17-24. ISSN: 0378-8741

Lin, K., Huang, A., Tu, H., Lee, L., Wu, C., Hour, T., Yang., S., Pu., Y & Lin, C. (2011). Xanthine oxidase inhibitory triterpenoid and phloroglucinol from guttiferaceous plants inhibit growth and induced apoptosis in human NTB1 cells through a ROS-dependent mechanism, *Journal of Agricultural and Food Chemistry*, 59: 407-414. ISSN: 1520-5118

Mangas-Marín, R., Montes de Oca-Porto, R., Bello-Alarcón, A., Nival Vázquez-Lavín, A. (2008) Caracterización por cromatografía de Gases/Espectrofotometría de Masas del Extracto Apolar de las hojas de *Clusia minor* L, *Latin American Journal of Pharmacy (formerly Acta Farmaceutica Bonaerense)*, 27(5): 747-51. ISSN 0326-2383

Manguro, L. O. A., Opiyo, S. A., Herdtweck, E. & Lemmen, P. (2009) Triterpenes of *Commiphora holtziana* oleo-gum resin, *Canadian Journal of Chemistry*, 87: 1173-1179. ISSN: 1480-3291

Marquez-Hernandez, I., Cuesta-Rubio, O., Campo-Fernández, M., Rosado-Perez, A., Montes de Oca-Porto, R., Piccinelli, A.L. & Rastrelli, L. (2010) Studies on the constituents of yellow Cuban propolis: GC-MS Determination of Triterpenoids and Flavonoids, *Journal of Agricultural and Food Chemistry*, 58: 4725-4730. ISSN: 1520-5118

Martelanc, M., Vovk, I. & Simonovska, B. (2009) Separation and identification of some common isomeric plant triterpenoids by thin-layer and high-performance liquid chromatography, *Journal of Chromatography A.*, 1216: 6662-6670. ISSN: 0021-9673

Martins, A., Vasas, A., Schelz, Z. S., Viveiros, M., Molnár, J., Hohmann, J. & Amaral, L. (2010).Constituents of *Carpobrotus edulis* Inhibit P-glycoprotein of MDR1-transfected mouse lymphoma cells, *Anticancer Research*, 30: 829-835. ISSN: 1791-7530

Martins, A., Vasas, A., Viveiros, M., Molnár, J., Hohmann, J. & Amaral, L. (2011). Antibacterial properties of compounds isolated from *Carpobrotus edulis*, *International Journal of Antimicrobial Agents*, 37: 438-444. ISSN 0924-8579

Massaro, F. C., Brooks ,P. R., Wallace, H. M. & Russell, F. D. (2011). Cerumen of Australian singles bees (*Tretragonula carbonariua*): gas chromatography-mass spectrometry fingerprint and potential anti-inflammatory properties, *Naturwissenschaften*, 98 (4) 329-337. ISSN: 1432-1904

Mbouangouere, R. N., Tane, P., Choudhary, M- P., Djemgou, P. C., Ngadjui, B. T. & Ngamga, D. (2008). Pipthadenol A-C and α-glucosidase inhibitor from *Piptadenia africana*, *Research Journal of Phytochemistry*, 2(1): 27-34. ISSN: 1819-3471

Melo, C. M., Carvalho, K. M. M. B., Neves, J. C. S., Morais, T. C., Rao, V. S., Santos, F. A., Brito, G. A. B. & Chaves, M. H. (2010). α,β-amyrin, a natural triterpenoid ameliorates L-arginne-induced acute pancreatitis in rats, *World Journal of Gastroenterology*, 16 (34): 4272-4280. ISSN: 1007-9327

Moreau, R.A., Lampi, A. M. & Hicks, K.B. (2009) Fatty Acid, Phytosterol and Polyamine Conjugates Profiles of Edible Oils Extracted from Corn Germn, Corn Fiber, and Corn Kernels. *Journal of American Oil Chemical Society*, 86(12): 1209-1214. ISSN: 003-021X

Nikkon, F., Salam, K. A., Yeasmin, T., Mosaddik, A., Khondkar P. & Haque, M. E. (2010). Mosquitocidal triterpenes from the stem of *Duranta repens*, *Pharmaceutical Biology*, 48(3): 264-268. ISSN: 1744-5116

Nurmi, T., Nyström, L., Edelmann, M., Lampi, A. & Pironen, V. (2008). Phtosterols in wheat genotypes in the HEALTHGRAIN diversity screen, *Journal of Agricultural and Food Chemistry*, 56: 9710-9715. ISSN: 1520-5118

Oliveira, A. P., Silva, L. R., Andrade, P. B., Valentão, P., Silva, B. M., Goncalves, R, F., Pereira, J. A. & Pinho, P. G., (2010) Further Insight into the látex metabolite profile of *Ficus carica*, *Journal of Agricultural and Food Chemistry*, 58: 10855-10863. ISSN: 1520-5118

Palíková, I., Heinrich, J., Bednár, P., Marhol, P., Kren, V., Cvak, L., Valentová, C., Ruzicka, F., Holá, V., Kolár, M., Simánek, V. & Ulrichová, J. (2008). Constituents and antimicrobial properties of blue honeysucke: A novel source for phenolic antioxidants, *Journal of Agricultural and Food Chemistry*, 56: 11883-11889. ISSN: 1520-5118

Parveen, M., Ghalib, R. M., Mehdi, S. H., Mattu, R. U. H. & Ali, M. (2009). A novel antimicrobial triterpenic acid from the leaves of *Ficus benjamina* (var. *comosa*), *Journal of Saudi Chemical Society*, 13: 287-290. ISSN: 1319-6103

Parveen, M., Khanam, Z., Ali, M. & Rahman, S.Z. (2010). A novel lupene-type triterpenic glucoside from the leaves of *Clerodendrum inerme*, *Natural Product Research*, 24(2): 167-176. ISSN: 1029-2349

Parveena, M., Basudan, O. A., Mushfiq, M. & Ghalib, R. M. (2008). A new benzofuranic acid from the leaves of *Rhus alata*, *Natural Product Research*, 22(5): 371-382. ISSN: 1478-6419

Pedernera, A. M., Guardia, T., Calderón, C. E. G., Rotelli, A. E., de la Rocha, N. E., Saad, J. R., López Verrilli, M. A., Aseff, S. G. & Pelzer, L.E. (2010). Anti-inflammatory effect of *Acacia visco* extracts in animal models, *Inflammopharmacology*, 18: 253-260. ISSN: 0925-4692

Ragasa, C. Y-, Lapina, M. C., Lee, J. J., Mandia, E. H. & Rideout, J. A. (2008). Secondary metabolites from *Tectona philippinensis*, *Natural Product Research*, 22(9): 820-824. ISSN: 1478-6419

Ramadan, M., Ahmad, A. S., Nafady, A. M. & Mansour, A. I. (2009). Chemical composition of the stem bark and leaves of *Ficus pandurata* Hance, *Natural Product Research*, 23(13): 1218-1230. ISSN: 1029-2349

Rhourri-Frih, B., Chaimbault, P., Claude,B., Lamy, C., André, P. & Lafosse, M. (2008). Analysis of pentacyclic triterpenes by LC-M. A comparative study between APCL and APPI, *Journal of Mass Spectrometry*, 44: 71-80. ISSN: 1387-3806

Rivero-Cruz, F., Sánchez-Nieto, S., Benítez, G., Casimiro, X., Ibarra-Alvarado, C., Rojas-Molina, A. & Rivero-Cruz, B. (2009). Antibacterial compounds isolated from *Byrsonima crassifolia*, *Revista Latinoamericana de Química*, 37(2): 155-163. ISSN: 0370-5943

Rosas-Acevedo, H., Terrazas, T., González-Trujano M. E., Guzmán, Y. & Soto-Hernández, M. (2011) Anti-ulcer activity of *Cyrtocarpa procera* analogous to that of *Amphipterygium adstringens*, both assayed on the experimental gastric injury in rats, *Journal of Ethnopharmacology*, 134: 67-73. ISSN: 0378-8741

Silva, A. M., Simeoni, L. A. & Silveira, D. (2009) Genus Pouteria: Chemistry and biological activity, *Brazilian Journal of Pharmacognosy*, 19(2A): 501-509. ISSN: 0102-695X

Silva, J. R. A, Zoghbi, M. G. B., Pinto. A., Godoy, R. L. O. and Amaral, A.C. F. (2009) Analysis of the hexane extracts from seven oleoresins of *Protium* species, *Journal of Essential Oil Research*, 21(4): 305-308. ISSN: 1041-2905

Simo, C. C. F., Kouam, S. F., Poumale, H. P., Simo, I. K., Ngadjui, B. T., Green, I. R. & Krohn, K. (2008) Benjaminamide: A new ceramide and other compounds from the twigs of *Ficus benjamina* (Moraceae), *Biochemical Systematics and Ecology*, 36: 238-243. ISSN: 0305-1978

Sirat, H. M., Susanti, D., Ahmad, F., Takayama, H. & Kitajima, M. (2010). Amides, triterpene and flavonoids from the leaves of *Melastoma malabathricum* L., *Journal of Natural Medicine*, 64: 492-495. ISSN 1861-0293

Sob, S. V. T., K. Wabbo, H. K., Tchinda, A. T., Tane, P., Ngadju, B. T. & Ye, Y. (2010) Anthraquinones, sterols, triterpeniods and xanthones from *Cassia obtusifolia*, *Biochemical Systematics and Ecology*, 38:342-345. ISSN: 0305-1978

Szewczyk, K., Komsta, L. & Skalska-Kaminska, A. (2009) Densitometric HPTLC method for analysis of triterpenoids in the leaves of *Jovibarba sobolifera* (Sims.) Opiz (Hen and Chickens houseleek), *Journal of Planar Chromatography*, 22(85): 367-369. ISSN: 0993-4173

Thao, N. T. P., Hung, T. M., Lee, M. K., Kim, J. C., Min, B. S. & Bae, K. (2010). Triterpenoids from *Camellia japonica* and Their Cytotoxic Activity, *Chemical Pharmaceutical Bulletin*, 58(1): 121- 124. ISSN: 0009-2363

Tlili, N., El Guizani, T., Nasri, N., Khaldi, A. & Triki, S. (2011). Protein, lipid, aliphatic and triterpenic alcohol content of caper seeds "*Capparis spinosa*", *Journal American Oil Chemical Society* 88: 265-270. ISSN: 0003-021X

Uchida, H., Ohyama, K., Suzuki, M., Yamashita, H., Muranaka, T. & Ohyama, K. (2010). Triterpenoid levels are reduced during Euphorbia *tirucalli* L. callus formation, *Plant Biotechnology*, 27: 105-109. ISSN: 1342-4580

Van Maarseveen, C. & Jetter, R. (2009). Composition of the epicuticular and intracuticular wax layers on *Kalanchoe daigremontiana* (Hamet et Perr. de la Bathie) leaves, *Phytochemistry*, 70: 899-906. ISSN: 0031-9422

Vitor, C. E., Figueiredo, C. P., Hara, D. B., Bento, A. F., Mazzuco, T. L & Calixto, J. B. (2009) Therapeutic action and underlying mechanisms of a combination of two pentacyclic triterpenes, α- and β-amyrin, in a mouse model of colitis, *British Journal of Pharmacology*, 157: 1034-1044. ISSN: 1476-5381

Vouffo, B., Dongo, E., Facey, P., Thorn, A., Sheldrick, G., Maier, A., Fiebig, H. & Laatsch, H. (2010). Antiarol cinnamate and africanoside, a cinnamoyl triterpene and a hydroperoxy-cardenolide from the stem bark of *Antiaris africana*, *Planta Medica*, 76: 1717-1723. ISSN: 0032-0943

Wang, F., Li, Z., Cui, H., Hua, H., Jing, Y. & Liang, M. (2011). Two new triterpenoids from the resin of *Boswellia carterii*, *Journal of Asian Natural Products Research*, 13(3): 193-197. ISSN: 1477-2213

Wang, X., Li, C., Shi, Y. & Di, D. (2009). Two new secoiridoid glycosides from the leaves of *Olea europaea* L., *Journal of Asian Natural Products Research*, 11(11): 940-944. ISSN: 1477-2213

Wang, Y., Chen, W., Wu, Z., Xi, Z., Chen, W., Zhao, G., Li, X. & Sun, L. (2011). Chemical consituents from *Salacia amplifolia*, *Biochemical Systematics and Ecology*, 39: 205-208. ISSN: 0305-1978

Wansi, J. P., Chiozem, D. D., Tcho, A. T., Toze, F. A. A., Devkota, K. P., Ndjakou, B. L., Wandji, J. & Sewald, N. (2010). Antimicrobial and antioxidante effects of phenolic constituents from *Klainedoxa gabonensis*, *Pharmaceutical Biology*, 48(10): 1124-1129. ISSN: 1744-5116

Wesolowska, A., Jadczak, D. & Grzeszczuk, M. (2011). GC-MS Analysis of lemon catnip (*Nepeta cataria* L. var. *citriodora* Balbis) essential oil, *Acta Chromatographica*, 23(1): 169-180. ISSN: 0231-2522

Wu, C., Hseu, Y., Lien, J., Lin, L., Lin, Y. & Ching, H. (2011). Triterpenoid contents and anti-Inflammatory properties of the methanol extracts of *Ligustrum* species leaves, *Molecules*, 16: 1-15. ISSN: 1420-3049

Xu, C., Qin, M., Fu, Y., Liu, N., Hemming, J., Holmbom, B. & Willförd, S. (2010). Lipophilic extractives in *Populos x euramericana* "Guariento" stemwood and bark, *Journal of Wood Chemistry and Technology*, 30: 105-117. ISSN: 1532-2319

Xu, X., Dong, J., Mu, X. & Sun, L. (2011). Supercritical CO_2 extraction of oil, carotenoids, squalene and sterols from lotus (*Nelumbo nucifera Gaertn*) bee pollen, *Food and Bioproducts Processing*, 89(1): 47-52. ISSN: 0960-3085

Zarrouk, W., Carrasco-Pancorbo, A., Segura-Carretero, A., Fernandez-Gutierrez, A. & Zarrouk, M. (2010) Exploratory characterization of the unsaponifiable fraction of Tunisdian Virgin Olive Oils by a global approach with HPLC-APCL MS/MS analysis, *Journal of Agricultural and Food Chemistry*, 58: 6418-6426. ISSN: 1520-5118

Zheng, Y., Huang, W., Yoo, J., Ebersole, J. L. & Huang, C. B. (2011). Antibacterial compounds from *Siraitia grasvenorii* leaves, *Natural Products Research*, 25(9): 890-897. ISSN: 1029-2349

13

The Inhibitory Effect of Natural Stilbenes and Their Analogues on Catalytic Activity of Cytochromes P450 Family 1 in Comparison with Other Phenols – Structure and Activity Relationship

Renata Mikstacka[1], Zbigniew Dutkiewicz[1],
Stanisław Sobiak[1] and Wanda Baer-Dubowska[2]
[1]*Departament of Chemical Technology of Drugs, Poznań University of Medical Sciences*
[2]*Department of Pharmaceutical Biochemistry, Poznań University of Medical Sciences*
Poland

1. Introduction

In the last decade, increasing interest in the role of nutrition in disease prevention has been observed. The World Health Organization (WHO) reported that one-third of all cancer deaths could be prevented, and that diet plays a key role in prevention (Bode & Dong, 2009). The term *chemoprevention* introduced and developed by Sporn (2005) and Wattenberg (1985) refers in general to multi-targeted pharmacological and nutritional intervention with the use of naturally occurring or chemically synthesized compounds. For this purpose, dietary phytochemicals believed to be safe for human use seem to be very promising. The importance of natural chemopreventive agents relies on their non-toxicity when given in small amounts for longer periods of time. Moreover, using a combination of phytochemicals provides synergistic or additive preventive effects.

Cancer cell growth arises through a complex multistep process by which cancer cells acquire characteristics of unlimited proliferation potential, lack of response to growth signals, and resistance to cell death. Thus, preventive/therapeutic action of phytochemicals may be directed towards numerous molecular targets that are proteins involved in procarcinogen metabolism, cell transformation and proliferation, and signaling pathways leading to apoptosis of damaged or transformed cells (William et al., 2009). Targeting enzymes of the P450 superfamily may provide one of the strategies for enhancing the efficacy of chemopreventive and therapeutic agents (Swanson et al., 2010).

Mechanistic studies of natural compounds are of great value regarding their characteristics of bioactivity, efficacy, selectivity and potential adverse side effects. Targeted inhibition of metabolic activation of carcinogens and induction of detoxifying enzymes has been considered a fundamental strategy for blocking the early stage of carcinogenesis. For example, inhibition of CYP1 enzymes was one test in the battery of assays employed in screening of potential cancer chemopreventive agents (Gerhauser et al., 2003). Variable dietary exposure to phytochemicals may contribute to some of the inter-individual variation in the pharmacokinetics and pharmacological responses that are observed for drugs such as phenacetin, caffeine, and theophylline, which are substrates for CYP1A2 (Rendic & Di Carlo, 1997). Further research is needed to determine the extent to which the effect of dietary exposure may be modified by genetic polymorphism of xenobiotic metabolizing enzymes.

Phenolics are a diverse group of aromatic compounds broadly distributed in plants. Among this group, stilbenoids are compounds displaying multiple activities of interest with regard to cancer prevention and therapy, and their anticancer properties have been proven in various animal models (Szekeres et al., 2010). In this review, we summarize the results of studies on inhibitory activity of *trans*-resveratrol (3,4',5-trimethoxy-*trans*-stilbene), the best recognized *trans*-stilbene (Figure 1), and its natural and synthetic analogues toward expression and activity of CYPs responsible for procarcinogen activation. We discuss the role of cytochrome family 1 inhibitors in cancer chemoprevention and chemotherapy. Additionally, we compare their effect with other natural phenols occurring in plant foods in relatively high amount and exerting significant bioactivity. Finally, we analyze the use of computational methods for biomolecular docking in structure and activity relationship studies of CYP1 inhibitors.

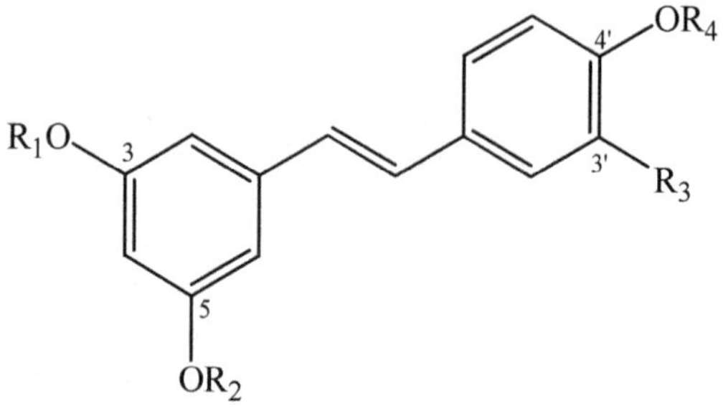

		R_1	R_2	R_3	R_4
1.	*trans*-Resveratrol	H	H	H	H
2.	Piceatannol	H	H	OH	H
3.	Rhapontigenin	H	H	OH	CH_3
4.	Desoxyrhapontigenin	H	H	H	CH_3
5.	Pinostilbene	H	CH_3	H	H
6.	Pterostilbene	CH_3	CH_3	H	H

Fig. 1. Structure of *trans*-resveratrol and its natural analogues

2. Potential strategies targeting CYPs for cancer therapy and prevention

One of the strategies of cancer chemoprevention is directed at drug-metabolizing enzymes such as cytochromes P450 (CYPs), a superfamily which metabolizes a wide spectrum of endogenous and exogenous substrates. Cytochrome P450 family 1 comprises three important isoforms: CYP1A1, CYP1A2 and CYP1B1 that catalyze the activation of procarcinogens such as polycyclic aromatic hydrocarbons, and aromatic and heterocyclic

The Inhibitory Effect of Natural Stilbenes and Their Analogues on Catalytic Activity of Cytochromes P450
Family 1 in Comparison with Other Phenols – Structure and Activity Relationship

249

amines. Additionally, CYP1B1 metabolizes 17β-estradiol (E2) to 4-hydroxyestradiol (4-OH-E2), which is further oxidized by peroxidase to estradiol-3,4-quinone to form a quinone-DNA adducts responsible for estrogen-related carcinogenesis (Liehr et al., 1996). This pathway of metabolism is extensively studied with respect to polymorphism of CYP1 enzymes and its association with carcinogenic metabolite formation (Kisselev et al., 2005).

All members of the human CYP1 family are expressed in extrahepatic tissues. However, CYP1A2 is the only constitutive form of liver enzyme, and as such takes part in metabolism of xenobiotics, including numerous drugs (caffeine, theophylline, methadone, verapamil, propranolol, warfarin, tamoxifen). On the other hand, it is worth mentioning that microbial CYPs are considered as drug targets and may be used as biocatalysts in drug biosynthesis (Lamb et al, 2007).

In humans, CYP1B1 is overexpressed in tumor cells, and this has important implications for tumor development and progression (Castro et al., 2008). It was found that CYP1B1 knockout mice were highly resistant to 7,12-dimethylbenz[a]anthracene induced tumor formation (Gonzalez, 2002). Thus, regulators of the expression and catalytic activity of family 1 cytochromes appear to play an important role in cancer chemoprevention by blocking the initial stages of tumorigenesis. With respect to cancer chemotherapy, CYP1A1 and CYP1B1 have the ability to metabolize cytostatics, diminishing their toxic effect on cancer cells (McFadyen & Murray, 2001). Considering this, the inhibition of CYP1B1, an enzyme up-regulated in many cancers, would be a strategy to prevent the loss of cytostatics effectiveness. On the other hand, the development of anticancer prodrugs specifically activated by CYP1B1 to cytotoxic compounds might be a promising novel strategy in cancer chemotherapy (Bruno & Njar, 2007).

3. Mechanism of the expression of CYP1 genes – AHR as a target for effective chemopreventive approach

Members of the CYP1 family are under the transcriptional control of the aryl hydrocarbon receptor (AHR) localized in cytosol that is activated by polyhalogenated aromatic hydrocarbons, among them 2,3,7,8-tetrachlorodibenzo-p-dioxin (TCDD). AHR agonists are well known environmental pollutants. As a result of activation AHR translocates into the nucleus and forms a dimer with ARNT (aryl hydrocarbon nuclear translocator). The AHR/ARNT complex is characterized by a high affinity to specific DNA recognition sites termed DREs (dioxin response elements) or AHREs (aryl hydrocarbon response element) which upregulate a battery of target genes, including those involved in metabolism of chemical carcinogens such as CYP1A1, CYP1A2 and CYP1B1 (Fig. 2). In this way, agonists induce the expression of xenobiotic metabolizing enzymes (XMEs) that activate procarcinogens to genotoxic forms. Thus, the treatment with AHR antagonists by preventing this undesirable effect might be a chemopreventive strategy.

There are phytochemicals that possess the ability to block agonist interaction with the ligand-binding site of the AHR and agonist induction of the AHR-signaling pathways. In that respect, resveratrol is the best recognized stilbene derivative. Moreover, it is one of the best-characterized chemopreventive phytochemicals (Goswami and Das, 2009). It occurs mainly in small fruits like berries and grapes, peanuts and red wine. Its chemopreventive properties found in studies on animals *in vivo* were described for the first time by Jang and

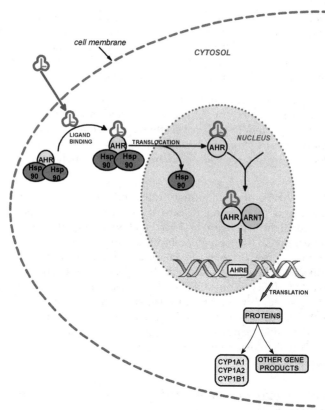

Fig. 2. AHR signaling pathway; L – ligand; Hsp90 – heat shock protein 90; ARNT – aryl hydrocarbon nuclear receptor; AHRE – aryl hydrocarbon response element. AHR/ARNT complexes bind to the DNA recognition sequence AHRE located in regulatory regions of phase I (CYP1A1, CYP1A2, CYP1B1) and phase II drug metabolizing enzymes.

coworkers (Jang et al., 1997). Chen and collaborators have reported that resveratrol strongly inhibited TCDD-induced AHR binding activity in human mammary epithelial (MCF-1-A) cells (Chen et al., 2004). The inhibition of CYP1A1 expression by resveratrol was observed in rat primary hepatocytes (Andrieux et al., 2004). In human HepG2 hepatoma cells, resveratrol inhibited the increase in CYP1A1 mRNA caused by TCDD in a concentration-dependent manner. The induction of transcription of an aryl hydrocarbon-responsive reporter vector containing the CYP1A1 promoter by TCDD was likewise inhibited by resveratrol. Resveratrol also inhibited the constitutive level of CYP1A1 mRNA and reporter vector transcription in human hepatoma HepG2 cells (Ciolino et al., 1998). Resveratrol was also effective in inhibiting CYP1A1 transcription induced by the aryl hydrocarbon dimethylbenz[a]anthracene in human mammary carcinoma MCF-7 cells and B[a]P-treated HepG2 cells (Ciolino et al., 1999). These data demonstrate that resveratrol inhibits aryl hydrocarbon-induced CYP1A activity *in vitro* by directly inhibiting CYP1A1/1A2 enzyme activity, and by inhibiting the signal transduction pathway that up-regulates the expression of carcinogen activating enzymes. The antagonistic action of resveratrol was supported by *in*

The Inhibitory Effect of Natural Stilbenes and Their Analogues on Catalytic Activity of Cytochromes P450
Family 1 in Comparison with Other Phenols – Structure and Activity Relationship

251

vivo experiments on phytochemicals with four different structures, where only resveratrol given topically on mouse epidermis inhibited aryl hydrocarbon hydroxylase (AHH) activity in a dose dependent manner (Table 1) (Szaefer et al., 2004). Moreover, resveratrol has been shown to prevent genotoxicity of B[a]P by inhibiting B[a]P-induced CYP1A1 expression and BPDE-DNA adduct formation in the lungs of mice (Revel et al., 2003).

Treatment	Dose	Activity [pmol/min/mg protein]
Acetone	0.2 ml	65.3 ± 4.6
5,6-Benzoflavone	8 µM	336 ± 17.2
Protocatechuic acid	8 µM	75.3 ± 2.1
	16 µM	83.4 ± 6.4
Chlorogenic acid	8 µM	71.7 ± 3.2
	16 µM	83.9 ± 2.8
trans-Resveratrol	8 µM	18.9 ± 2.6
	16 µM	0.08 ± 0.01

Table 1. Effect of phenolic compounds on mouse epidermal AHH activity

Summarising, resveratrol inhibits AHR-dependent transcription by preventing AHR/ARNT binding to the AHRE. The activity of preventing the conversion of ligand-bound cytosolic AHR into its nuclear DNA-binding form and/or the interaction between the AHR and the transcription initiation complex at the CYP1A1 gene promoter may be an important part of the chemopreventive activity of resveratrol. However, the action of resveratrol is not specific because this natural stilbene as a phytoestrogen is also a potent ER (estrogen receptor) agonist. Recently, experiments on human breast cancer cells revealed that the estrogenic properties of resveratrol and its influence on the ER expression are independent of its ability to inhibit the expression of genes controlled by AHR (MacPherson & Matthews, 2010). New stilbene derivatives of resveratrol that were synthesized appeared to be selective for AHR and devoid of affinity for ER. Among the *trans*-stilbenes synthesized, all displayed a significantly higher affinity than resveratrol for AHR. Substitution of 3- and/or 5-hydroxy groups with chlorine atoms coupled with replacement of 4'-hydroxy with chlorine or a methoxy group yielded selective TCDD antagonists with high affinity for the AHR that was much higher than resveratrol. Interestingly, one of the studied compounds, 3-hydroxy-5-chloro-4'-trifluoromethyl-*trans*-stilbene, was a selective AHR agonist exerting extremely high-affinity to AHR with a K_i of 0.2 nM. None of the compounds studied showed any detectable affinity for the ER that should eliminate estrogen-related risks, such as the increased risk of ER-related cancers (de Medina et al. 2005).

In the Table 2 we summarized the studies on the effects of resveratrol and its derivatives on AHR related expression of CYP1 enzymes. However, the results of *in vivo* experiments on animals are highly dependent on the dose of a studied compound, as well as the duration and manner of its administration. Further, the effect of a studied substance may also be tissue-dependent. The expression of CYP1A1 and CYP1A2-related monooxygenases in hepatic subcellular preparations from resveratrol treated male mice did not differ from the control; while in pulmonary subcellular preparations significantly lower expression of CYP1A1/2 –dependent enzymes was observed (Canistro et al., 2009).

Effect	Compound	Experimental Model	References
AHR translocation ↑ AHRE transactivation ↓	resveratrol	47DRE reporter cell line	Casper et al., 1999
AHR DNA binding ↓, expression and activity of CYP 1A1/1B1 ↓	resveratrol	TCDD-treated MCF-10A cells	Chen et al, 2004
Expression and activity of CYP1A1/1A2 ↓	resveratrol	B[a]P-treated HepG2 cells and DMBA-treated MCF-7 cells	Ciolino et al., 1999
CYP1A1 expression ↓ Induction of transcription of AHR reporter vector containing the CYP1A1 promoter by TCDD ↓ constitutive level of CYP1A1 mRNA and reporter vector transcription ↓	resveratrol	TCDD treated human HepG2 cells	Ciolino et al., 1998
CYP1A1 expression ↓ BPDE-DNA adduct formation ↓	resveratrol	lung tissue from BP-treated mice	Revel et al., 2003
CYP1A1 expression by resveratrol ↓	resveratrol	rat primary hepatocytes	Andrieux et al., 2004
AHR binding ability of resveratrol and its derivatives ↓	resveratrol and 24 other stilbenes	47DRE reporter cell line	de Medina et al., 2005
Expression of human CYP1A1 and CYP1B1 ↓ Recruitment of the AHR complex and RNA polymerase II to the regulatory regions ↓	resveratrol	TCDD-induced human breast cancer cell line MCF-7, and human hepatocellular carcinoma cell line, HepG2	Beedanagari et al., 2009
AHR-dependent transcription of CYP1A1 and CYP1B1 ↓	resveratrol	TCDD-induced human breast cancer cells T-47D	MacPherson and Matthews, 2010
CYP1A1 and CYP1B1 expression ↓ Recruitment of AHR and ARNT to CYP1A1 and CYP1B1 enhancer regions ↓	piceatannol	TCDD-induced human breast cancer cells T-47D	MacPherson and Matthews, 2010

Table 2. AHR as a molecular target for chemopreventive action of resveratrol and its derivatives

4. Inhibitory effect of stilbene derivatives on CYP1A enzymes

4.1 *Trans*-resveratrol

The studies of the inhibitory effect of phytochemicals on cytochrome P450 dependent enzymes are mainly conducted with the use of *in vitro* techniques on cDNA-expressed enzymes. Recombinant biscistronic supersomes express particular CYP activity and cytochrome c reductase activity. It was reported that resveratrol inhibited human recombinant P450 1A1 activity in a competitive manner (Chun et al., 1999), but the IC_{50} value (the concentration that causes 50% inhibition of enzyme activity) of 23 μM was much higher than the IC_{50} value of 1.4 μM obtained for CYP1B1 inhibition (Chang et al., 2000). Interestingly, resveratrol inactivated human recombinant CYP1A2 indirectly in a mechanism-based manner (Chang et al, 2001).

Mechanism-based inhibition was not observed in rat liver microsomes; EROD (7-ethoxyresorufin-O-deethylase) activity as an indicator of both CYP1A1 and CYP1A2 was inhibited by resveratrol and piceatannol (3,3′,4,5′-tetrahydroxy-*trans*-stilbene) with K_i value of 0.4 μM for both compounds and a mixed type of inhibition (Chang et al., 2007). It was found that resveratrol is metabolized to piceatannol in the reaction of hydroxylation catalyzed by CYP1A2 (Piver et al. 2004) and CYP1B1 (Potter et al. 2002). Poor bioavailability of resveratrol caused by its fast metabolism to glucuronides and sulphates limits the use of this stilbene as a potent chemopreventive / chemotherapeutic agent (Walle et al., 2004). To explain the bioactivity of resveratrol, its accumulation to active levels in target organs or synergistic / additive effects with other food components are taken into account.

4.2 Natural resveratrol analogues

During the last decade, other naturally occurring stilbenoid compounds with potential health benefit were found and examined. Piceatannol and pterostilbene (3,5-dimethoxy-4′-hydroxy-*trans*-stilbene) occur mainly in grapes and blueberries, with their amount depending on plant variety (Rimando et al., 2004). Pterostilbene that was shown to have cancer chemopreventive activity similar to resveratrol (Rimando et al., 2002) occurs also in some medicinal plants used in traditional medicine. Beneficial bioactivity of natural resveratrol analogues have been demonstrated in numerous *in vitro* experiments and in preclinical animal models (Rimando and Suh, 2008). Resveratrol analogues exert multiple bioactivities involved in cancer chemoprevention; for example, they are efficient inhibitors of family 1 cytochromes. The inhibitory action of natural stilbenes appears to be highly selective depending on the cytochrome isoform. Moreover, the extent of CYP inhibition changes according to the stilbene structure; the types and positioning of functional groups linked to the stilbene scaffold significantly influence inhibitory activity of stilbene derivatives. Rhapontigenin (3,5,3′-trihydroxy-4′-methoxystilbene) was found to be a very selective and potent inactivator of CYP1A1 activity with IC_{50} value 0.4 μM and K_i value of 0.09 μM (Chun et al., 2001a). Pinostilbene (3,4′-dihydroxy-5-methoxy-*trans*-stilbene), pterostilbene and desoxyrhapontigenin (3,5-dihydroxy-4′-methoxy-*trans*-stilbene) were more efficient inhibitors of CYP1A1 and CYPA2 in comparison to the parent compound, while they inhibited CYP1B1 to the same extent as resveratrol (Guengerich et al., 2003; Mikstacka et al., 2006, 2007). The data on the inhibition of CYP1 enzymes by natural stilbenes are summarized in Table 3.

4.3 Resveratrol methyl ethers and other synthetic stilbenes

In the last decade, new stilbene derivatives have been designed and synthesized in order to find more potent chemopreventive agents (Szekeres et al., 2010). The additional aim of this approach was to find resveratrol derivatives demonstrating better bioavailability in comparison to the parent compound. The bioactivity of resveratrol analogues could be altered due to the presence and positioning of methoxy groups on the basic resveratrol backbone that prevent the conjugation reaction with sulphuric and glucuronic acids. Synthesized derivatives are tested with regard to their inhibitory activity toward CYP 1 enzymes in order to find more efficient and selective inhibitors. A series of *trans*-stilbene derivatives containing a 3,5-dimethoxyphenyl moiety were prepared and evaluated on human recombinant CYP1A, CYP1A2 and CYP1B1 to find a potent and selective CYP1B1 inhibitor. It was shown that substitution at the 2-position of the stilbene skeleton plays a very important role in discriminating between CYP1A1/2 and CYP1B1. Chun and his group found 3,5,2',4'-tetramethoxy-*trans*-stilbene as a new selective and very potent inhibitor of human CYP1B1 (Chun et al., 2001b). Among the whole series of compounds tested, 3,5,2',4'-tetramethoxy-*trans*-stilbene exerted the most potent inhibitory activity toward CYP1B1 with an IC_{50} value of 2 nM. 2-[2-(3,5-dimethoxyphenyl)vinyl]thiophene showed comparable inhibitory activities, but its selectivity toward CYP 1B1 was lower (Kim et al. 2002).

Another series of stilbenes with 4-methylthiophenyl moiety were synthesized and their inhibitory potency toward human recombinant CYPs: CYP1A1, CYP1A2 and CYP1B1 was evaluated. Among compounds tested, 2-methoxy-4'-methylthio-*trans*-stilbene and 3-methoxy-4'-methylthio-*trans*-stilbene demonstrated the most potent and selective inhibitory effect on CYP1A1 and CYP1B1 activities (Mikstacka et al, 2008).

Compound	CYP1A1		CYP1A2		CYP1B1	
	K_i [μM]	Mode of inhibition	K_i [μM]	Mode of inhibition	K_i [μM]	Mode of inhibition
Resveratrol	1.2[a]	mixed type	15.5[a] 5.33[c]	mixed type	0.75[a]	mixed type
Piceatannol	3.01	competitive	9.67[c]	mixed type	0.27	competitive
Desoxyrhapontigenin	0.16	competitive	1.04	mixed type	2.06	competitive
Pinostilbene	0.13	mixed type	0.94	mixed type	0.90	competitive
Pterostilbene	0.57	competitive	0.39[c]	mixed type	0.91	competitive
Rhapontigenin	0.21[b] 0.4 (IC_{50})	competitive	160 (IC_{50})	n.d.	9 (IC_{50})	n.d.

[a] Chang et al., 2001; [b] Chun et al., 2001; [c] in mouse liver microsomes (Mikstacka et al., 2006); n.d. not determined

Table 3. Effect of natural *trans*-stilbenes on human recombinant CYP1A1, CYP1A2 and CYP1B1 activities

4.4 Other natural phenols

The influence of other phenolic phytochemicals on CYP1 activities is worth presenting in the context of possible additive or synergistic effects of the micro-components of human diet. The properties of plant extracts rich in numerous bioactive substances are particularly interesting in terms of herb-drug interaction, which could be a subject of independent review. At the beginning of the last decade, Piver and collaborators (2003) discovered that non-volatile components of red wine or various Cognac beverages exert stronger inhibitory effect on CYP1A1, CYP1A2, and CYP1B1 than resveratrol and its dimer ε-viniferin. Another extract, prepared from the most widely used herbal medicine *Ginkgo biloba*, was tested for its ability to inhibit the major human cytochrome P450 enzymes (Gaudineau et al., 2004). It was demonstrated that the flavonoidic fraction of standardized extract inhibits human CYP1A2 and other cytochromes (CYP2C9, CYP2E1, and CYP3A4), wheras its terpenoidic fraction significantly inhibits only CYP2C9. *In vivo* CYP1A2 induction was observed as a result of herbal dietary supplementation (Rye et al., 2003). Effects of Cuban and Mexican herbal extracts used in traditional medicine (obtained from *Heliopsis longipes*, *Mangifera indica* L. and *Thalassia testudinum*) on CYP1A1/2 and other cytochromes involved in drug metabolism of CYP3A4 and CYP2D6 were studied with the use of human liver microsomes and compared with the pure constituents isolated from the extracts of affinin (an alkamide isolated from the *H. longipes* extract), N-*iso*-butyl-decanamide, and mangiferin. The extracts significantly inhibited CYP1A1/2 activities, which reflects the high content of flavonoids with recognized CYP1A1/2 inhibitory properties (Rodeiro et al., 2009).

Numerous natural phenols demonstrate inhibitory activity toward CYP1 enzymes. Phytochemicals that exert inhibitory effects on CYP1A enzymes comparable to natural stilbenes comprise: flavonoids, isothiocyanates, coumarin and its derivatives.

Flavonoids represent a large class of phenolic phytochemicals. They are ubiquitously present in plant-derived foods and are important microcomponents of the human diet. Humans ingest approximately 0.6-1 g of these bioactive compounds daily (Kuhnau, 1976). The effects of flavonoids on CYP1 activities have been explored since the early nineties, including the effects of flavone and five hydroxylated derivatives on the methoxyresorufin O-demethylase activity catalyzed by human recombinant CYP1A1 and CYP1A2 (Zhai et al., 1998). The authors found galangin (3,5,7-trihydroxyflavone) as the most potent inhibitor of CYP1A2 with K_i value of 8 nM. It should be mentioned that no stilbene derivative with a comparable inhibitory potency toward CYP1A2 was found. Furthermore, galangin showed almost 5-fold selectivity for CYP1A2 over CYP1A1; while, 7-hydroxyflavone exhibited 6-fold greater selectivity for CYP1A1 over CYP1A2. The other hydroxylated flavone derivatives: 3-hydroxy; 5-hydroxy; 7-hydroxy- and 3,7-dihydroxyflavone were also potent inhibitors of CYP1A1 ($IC_{50} < 0.1\ \mu M$) and CYP1A2 ($IC_{50} < 0.3\ \mu M$).

In experiments with the use of human recombinant CYPs, seven flavonoids (myricetin, apigenin, kaempferol, quercetin, amentoflavone, quercitrin, and rutin) occurring in St. John's Wort were tested. They were found to be slightly more selective for CYP1B1 activity compared to CYP1A1. Apigenin and amentoflavone were competitive inhibitors of CYP1B1, while quercetin showed a mixed type of inhibition. The most potent CYP1B1 inhibitor was apigenin with K_i of 60 nM. The same authors investigated CYP1 inhibition in cell system. Myricetin, apigenin, kaempferol and quercetin inhibited TCDD-induced EROD activity in intact 22Rv1 human prostate cancer cells. Because flavonoids were added 30 minutes prior to the EROD assay, the inhibition did not reflect down regulation of CYP1 mRNA or protein level (Chaudhary et al., 2006). The influence of flavonoid constituents of St. John's Wort were also studied by Schwarz's group. They demonstrated the differentiated inhibition of CYP1A1-catalyzed estradiol 2-hydroxylation according to CYP1A1 genotype. The variant CYP1A1.2 (Ile462Val) was significantly inhibited by quercetin, hypericin and pseudohypericin (naphthodiantrones), with IC_{50} values for 2-hydroxylation being more than two times lower than the wild-type enzyme. Additionally, the wild-type enzyme was efficiently inhibited by kaempferol, myricetin and resveratrol (Schwarz et al., 2011).

The synthesis of structures differentiated by type and positions of substituents leads to a continuation of structure and activity relationship (SAR) studies. Recently, Takemura and coworkers (2010) evaluated the structure–property relationship of 18 major flavonoids on inhibiting enzymatic activity of CYP1A1, 1A2 and 1B1 by using an ethoxyresorufin O-deethylation assay. Flavones and flavonols indicated relatively strong inhibitory effects on CYP1s compared with flavanone that does not have the double bond between C-positions 2 and 3 on the C-ring. Flavonoids used in this study selectively inhibited CYP1B1 activity.

Special attention is paid to methoxy derivatives of flavone, which have inhibitory potency exceeding that of the parent compound (Walle & Walle, 2007). In particular, methoxy types of flavones and flavonols such as chrysoeriol and isorhamnetin showed strong and selective inhibition against CYP1B1 (Takemura et al., 2010). The most potent inhibitors of CYP1 catalyzed ethoxyresorufin O-deethylation were the methoxylated flavones acacetin, diosmetin, eupatorin and the dihydroxylated flavone chrysin, indicating that the 4'-OCH₃ group at the B ring and the 5,7-dihydroxy motif at the A ring play a prominent role in EROD inhibition (Androutsopoulos et al., 2011). It was observed that high metabolic turnover of methoxylated flavonoids may result in enhanced antiproliferative activity. Several flavonoid metabolites produced in reactions catalyzed by CYP1A1 or CYP1B1 have been shown to inhibit cancer cell cycle progression. The authors observed CYP1A1-catalyzed biotransformation of acacetin to luteolin, apigenin and scutellarein. The chemopreventive ability of these metabolites was previously established. Generally, it is suggested that dietary flavonoids exhibit three distinct modes of action with CYP1 enzymes: (1) inhibitors of CYP1 enzymatic activity, (2) CYP1 substrates and (3) substrates and inhibitors of CYP1 enzymes.

Coumarin (1,2-benzopyrone) and its derivatives occur naturally in several plant families. They are components of essential oils, and are often used as fragrance ingredients in human diet. Their effect on CYP1 activities have been studied since the early nineties. The naturally occurring coumarins: bergamotin, coriandrin, isoimperatorin, imperatorin, ostruthin are potent inhibitors of the metabolic activation of benzo(a)pyrene and dimethylbenzanthracene in the cell culture model system of mouse epidermis (Cai et al., 1997). In experiments *in vitro*, mechanism-based inactivation of hepatic EROD activity by natural coumarin coriandrin was observed (Cai et al., 1996). These results demonstrate that certain coumarins to which humans are exposed in their diet are bioactivated by CYP1A1 to reactive intermediates that subsequently form covalent adducts with the apoprotein, effectively destroying enzyme activity.

Curcumin is a natural plant food additive obtained from turmeric used in spices and traditional Indian medicine. Its chemopreventive anticancer potential is well documented (Aggarwal et al., 2003). It belongs to hydroxycinnamic acid derivatives observed ubiquitously in plants. Earlier reports on the inhibition of rat liver microsomal CYPs by curcumin showed that curcumin is a strong inhibitor of CYP1A enzymes and CYP2B as well (Oetari et al., 1996; Thapliyal and Maru, 2001, 2003). However, these data were not confirmed in studies with human recombinant cytochrome P450s, where curcumin appeared to be a moderate inhibitor of CYP1A2 with IC_{50} value 40 μM (Appiah-Opong et al., 2007). Appiah-Opong and coworkers synthesized curcumin derivatives that exhibited about 10- to 40-fold greater potency towards inhibition of CYP1A2 than curcumin itself (Appiah-Opong et al., 2008).

Other natural phenols studied more recently with respect to CYP1 inhibition include **phytocannabinoids,** constituents of marijuana, and **chromene amides** from *Amyris plumieri*, a plant grown in the Caribbean, Central America and Venezuela used in folk medicine. Three major constituents in marijuana; Δ^9-tetrahydrocannabinol, cannabidiol and cannabinol inhibited activities of human recombinant CYP1s: CYP1A1, CYP1A2 and CYP1B1 in a competitive manner (Yamaori et al., 2010). One of the amides (chromene acetamide) tested appeared to inhibit potently CYP1A1 activity *in vitro* with IC_{50} and K_i values 1.547 μM and 0.37 μM, respectively (Badal et al., 2011).

Interestingly, in the studies on different natural phenols Schwarz and Roots demonstrated that the inhibitory effect depends not only on the structure of the inhibitor, but also the substrate of the reaction catalyzed by CYPs used in the assay. They found flavonoids like myricetin, apigenin, quercetin, and kaempferol, as well as tea polyphenol (-)epigallo catechin gallate, strongly inhibited the formation of benzo(a)pyrene diolepoxide, the ultimate carcinogenic product of benzo(a)pyrene activation. Furthermore, resveratrol, an inhibitor of CYP1A1-catalyzed ethoxyresorufin deethylation, exhibited only slightly inhibitory effect on CYP1A1-mediated epoxidation of 7,8-diol-B(a)P (Schwarz & Roots, 2003).

5. Docking studies – The new approach to CYPs-phytochemical interaction

Mechanistic studies of the inhibitory effect of stilbenes on enzyme activities are mainly conducted *in vitro* with the use of human recombinant cytochromes. However, the affinity of compounds to cytochromes may be determined by computational analysis of inhibitor/substrate docking in the enzyme active site. Molecular modeling is presumed to be helpful in predicting inhibitory potential of CYP regulators by characteristics of ligand-enzyme interactions. We review *in silico* research on elucidating the mechanism of inhibitory action of phytochemicals by analysis of structure and activity relationship. Potential phytochemical candidates can be selected by *in silico* virtual screening, based on natural compound libraries (www.bioscreening.com). When active chemicals are selected, they may be "docked" into the target protein by using available programs, enabling detailed protein-ligand interactions to be obtained and the best fit of a candidate compound to be identified. The main objective of molecular docking is to determine the binding interactions between protein and ligand.

Computational procedures of molecular modeling have been employed since the nineties. Studies of Lewis and coworkers (1997) on CYP1 family enzymes structure and ligand docking in enzyme cavities have been a great contribution to the development of this field. Lewis formulated the general characteristic of CYP1 ligands as planar and polar polycyclic molecules. Substituents linked to the polycyclic hydrocarbon core influence the ligand binding responsible for molecular interactions: hydrogen bonds; π-π stacking; and hydrophobic interactions. The effect of structural modification on the inhibitory selectivity of phytochemical derivatives on CYP1A1, CYP1A2, and CYP1B1 help to elucidate which interactions determine the inhibitory ability of the compounds. There are similarities between the active sites of CYP1A2 and CYP1A1 which are in accordance with the overlapping substrate specificities of the two enzymes. However, the CYP1A1 substrates are generally of higher lipophilicity than those of CYP1A2. The reason lies in the more hydrophobic character of the CYP1A1 active site region (including the access channel) in comparison to CYP1A2 active site (Lewis et al., 1999). The differences in the structure of enzyme binding sites may determine the metabolism pathways of a substrate. With the use of computational docking the mechanism of E2 2-hydroxylation and 4-hydroxylation catalyzed by CYP1A1/2 and CYP1B1, respectively, were elucidated. CYP1A1 and CYP1A2 produced 2-OH-E2 and 4-OH-E2 in a ratio of 10 : 1; whereas CYP1B1 produces 2-OH-E2 and 4-OH-E2 in a ratio of 1 : 3 (Lee et al., 2003). The docking study suggests that CYP1A1 and CYP1A2 generate 2-OH-E2 rather than 4-OH-E2, and that CYP1B1 generates both 2-OH-E2 and 4-OH-E2. Particular amino acids residues for each CYP were identified as playing an important role in estradiol recognition (Itoh et al., 2010).

Several groups of phytochemicals were tested for affinity to active sites of CYP1 members. The first studied compounds were rutaecarpine derivatives. An alkaloid rutaecarpine preferentially inhibited CYP1A2 activity with IC_{50} value of 22 nM. However, 1-methoxyrutaecarpine and 1,2-dimethoxyrutaecarpine were the most selective CYP1A2 inhibitors. Molecular modeling showed a good fitting of rutaecarpine and the active site of CYP1A2. Two hydrogen bonds between the keto- and N14-groups of rutaecarpine and the Thr[208] and Thr[473] residues of CYP1A2, respectively, were visualized with molecular modeling procedures. The C-ring moiety of rutaecarpine formed π-π stacking interaction with the aromatic ring of Phe[205] residue (Don et al., 2003).

Coumarin was shown to be a substrate of human CYPs, specifically: CYP1A1 and CYP1A2. Molecular modeling led to recognition and localization of the amino acid residues which interact with coumarin molecules resulting in the orientation of coumarin with 3,4 bond directly above the heme moiety. Coumarin 3,4-epoxide is produced and then rearranged to hydroxyphenylacetaldehyde, which can be further metabolized to toxic products. In the CYP1A1 active site, Ser[113] forms a hydrogen bond with coumarin, while Phe[205] and Phe[358] are responsible for aromatic π-π stacking. In CYP1A2, Thr[113] forms hydrogen bonds with coumarin, and Phe[205] is responsible for π-π stacking (Lewis et al., 2006). However the different key residues take part in the interactions with coumarin, they determine the same site of metabolism, and in consequence, the pathway of coumarin metabolism is the same for both CYP1A1 and CYP1A2 .

7,8-benzoflavone (α-naphthoflavone) is a prototype flavonoid which has been used to examine the mechanism of action on P450 enzymes. Molecular modeling studies revealed that 7,8-naphthoflavone is positioned in a hydrophobic cavity of CYP1A2 next to the

The Inhibitory Effect of Natural Stilbenes and Their Analogues on Catalytic Activity of Cytochromes P450
Family 1 in Comparison with Other Phenols – Structure and Activity Relationship

259

active site where it may cause a direct effect on substrate binding (Cho et al., 2003). Further studies with the use of molecular docking were aimed at methoxyflavonoids with a 2-3 double bond, which exerted strong inhibitory effect on CYP1 activities, particularly CYP1B1 (Takemura et al., 2010). The authors observed that the binding specificity of methoxyflavonoids is based on the interactions between the methoxy groups and specific CYP1s residues. For example, chrysoeriol and isorhamnetin fit well into the active site of CYP1B1, but do not fit into the active site of CYP1A2 and 1A1 because of steric collisions between the methoxy substituent of these methoxyflavonoids and Ser[122] in CYP1A1 and Thr[124] in CYP1A2. Androutsopoulos's group described molecular docking of several flavonoids with regard to their metabolism and inhibitory activity. The simulated binding orientation of the compounds tested was in accordance with the study of Takemura and coworkers (2010). Diosmetin and eupatorin are predicted to be oriented with ring-B over the prosthetic group so that 4'-methoxy group is at ~4.5 Å from the heme iron. The less substituted chrysin and acacetin also were shown to bind CYP1A1 with ring-B over the iron-heme group. However, a lower number of interactions were found within the active site of CYP1A1 (Androutsopoulos et al., 2011).

To better characterize stilbenes as ligands of CYPs, we performed molecular docking by simulation of resveratrol and pterostilbene binding in active sites of CYP1A2 and CYP1B. Resveratrol and pterostilbene molecules were docked into the cavities of CYP1A2 (PDB code: 2hi4) and CYP1B1 (PDB code: 3pm0) with the use of the CDOCKER procedure implemented in Accelrys Discovery Studio 2.5.5. CDOCKER uses a CHARMm-based molecular dynamics (MD) scheme to dock ligands into a receptor binding site. For assigning receptor and ligand atom partial charges, we applied the charging rules used in the MMFF94 forcefield. Docked poses were scored by the negative value of CDOCKER energy for the –CDOCKER_ENERGY function, which include interaction energy and internal ligand energy: the higher positive value of –CDOCKER_ENERGY, the stronger affinity of a ligand to the binding site.

Our docking experiment showed that in the CYP1A2 active site, all possible poses of resveratrol can be grouped into two sets. This observation indicated that two binding modes are possible for resveratrol molecule. In mode A, represented by the pose with highest score, a resveratrol molecule is directed with 4'-OH group toward a heme (Fig. 3a). In mode B, the second ring with 3-OH and 5-OH substituents is situated in the vicinity of a prosthetic group (Fig. 3b). In both orientations, resveratrol binding is stabilized by π–π stacking interactions, with phenyl ring of Phe[226] (mode A), and with Phe[226] and Phe[260] (mode B). Contrary to resveratrol, a pterostilbene molecule was docked in the CYP1A2 active site only in one orientation with 4'-OH group directed toward a heme (Fig. 3c). Pterostilbene binding was stabilized by π–π interaction with an aromatic ring of Phe[226]. For a resveratrol molecule docked in the active site of CYP1B1, we also distinguished two binding modes. In contrast to CYP1A2, the highest scored pose corresponded to binding mode B. In both orientations (A and B), resveratrol was stabilized by two π–π interactions between both of its rings and a phenyl ring of Phe[231], and additionally by two hydrogen bonds with Asn[265] and Asp[333] in mode B, or Asn[265] and Asn[228] in mode A (Fig. 3d and 3e).

Similar to interaction with CYP1A2, a pterostilbene molecule represented only one type of orientation in the CYP1B1 cavity (Fig. 2f). The binding conformation with 4'-OH group close to a heme was stabilized by two π–π stacking interactions with Phe[231]. In the case of

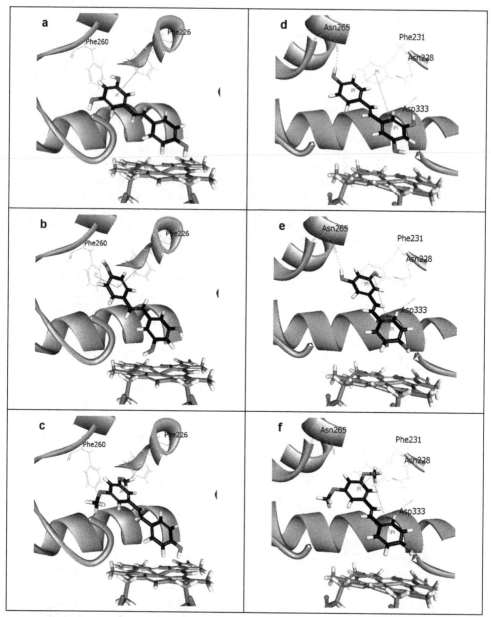

Fig. 3. Putative binding modes of resveratrol and pterostilbene in active sites of CYP1A2 (a – c) and CYP1B1 (d – f) with key residues involved in π–π stacking interactions and hydrogen bonds represented by solid blue lines and dashed blue lines, respectively. Heme molecule is at the bottom. CYP1A2 active site in complex with: (a) resveratrol in binding mode A, (b) resveratrol in mode B, (c) pterostilbene. CYP1B1 active site in complex with: (d) resveratrol in binding mode B, (e) resveratrol in mode A, (f) pterostilbene.

pterostilbene, which is a dimethoxy analogue of resveratrol, it is suggested that hydrophobic interactions might play a key role determining and stabilizing its docking orientation.

In studies of *trans*-resveratrol metabolism by human microsomal CYP1B1 enzyme (Potter et al., 2002), the authors observed formation of two metabolites, M1 and M2. The major metabolite M2 has been identified as piceatannol (3,4,3',5'-tetrahydroxystilbene), while 3,4,5,4'-tetrahydroxystilbene was proposed as the M1 product. More recent work (Piver et al., 2004) provided evidence that CYP1A2 is also engaged in the metabolism of *trans*-resveratrol to piceatannol and tetrahydroxystilbene M1. Our studies confirmed the possibility of two pathways of metabolism on the grounds of molecular docking analysis.

6. Conclusion

The finding of high affinity ligands among natural compounds for each of the CYP1 family enzymes will help to reveal more about enzyme specificity, providing a starting point for more extensive studies and improved predictive capabilities. Particularly, a selective inhibition against CYP1B1 that influences the chemopreventive properties of phytochemicals for E2 related breast cancer seems to be promising. There is a need for better characterization of potential chemopreventive/therapeutic agents in order to understand their abilities and limits to influencing numerous pathways leading to cancer development. Novel classes of anti-cancer drugs including those of plant origin are being developed that can target both drug-metabolizing enzymes and disease modifying pathways. Recently, interest in the combinatory effect of different phytochemicals is growing, with respect to the multi-targeted action of numerous components of a food matrix. Wenzel and co-workers found that metabolism of resveratrol present in beverages such as wine or grape juice is inhibited by other polyphenols due to competitive reactions with Phase -II enzymes, resulting in an increased concentration of the free form (Wenzel et al., 2005). It is suggested that an efficient chemoprevention strategy lies in the use of combinations of several chemopreventive and/or therapeutic agents which may exert multi-targeted action. In conclusion, the search for potent and selective CYP1A inhibitors appears to hold promise and should be continued with the use of novel computational techniques.

7. References

Aggarwal, B.B.; Kumar, A. & Bharti, A.C. (2003). Anticancer potential of curcumin: preclinical and clinical studies. *Anticancer Res.*, Vol. 23, No. 1A, (January-February 2003), pp. 363-398, ISSN 0250-7005

Andrieux, L.; Langouet, S.; Fautrel, A.; Ezan, F.; Krauser, J.A.; Savouret, J.F.; Guengerich, F.P.; Baffet, G. & Guillouzo, A. (2004). Aryl hydrocarbon receptor activation and cytochrome P450 1A induction by the mitogen-activated protein kinase inhibitor UO126 in hepatocytes. *Mol. Pharmacol.*, Vol. 65, No 4, (April 2004), pp. 934-943, ISSN 0026-895X

Androutsopoulos, V.P.; Papakyriakou, A.; Vourloumis, D. & Spandidos, D.A. (2011). Comparative CYP1A1 and CYP1B1 substrate and inhibitor profile of dietary flavonoids. *Bioorg. Med. Chem.*, Vol. 19, No. 9, (May 2011), pp. 2842-2849, ISSN 0968-0896

Appiah-Opong, R.; Commandeur, J.N.M.; van Vugt, B. & Vermeulen, N.P.E. (2007). Inhibition of human recombinant cytochrome P450s by curcumin and curcumin decomposition products. *Toxicology*, Vol. 235, No. 1-2, (June 2007), pp. 83-91, ISSN 0300-483X

Appiah-Opong, R.; de Esch, I.; Commandeur, J.N.; Andarini M. & Vermeulen, N.P. (2008). Structure-activity relationships for the inhibition of recombinant human cytochromes P450 by curcumin analogues. *Eur. J. Med. Chem.*, Vol. 43, No. 8, (August 2008), pp. 1621-1631, ISSN 0223-5234

Badal, S.; Williams, S.A.; Huang, G.; Francis, S.; Vendantam, P.; Dunbar, O.; Jacobs, H.; Tzeng, T.J.; Gangemi, J. & Delgoda, R. (2011). Cytochrome P450 1 enzyme inhibition and anticancer potential of chromene amides from *Amyris plumieri*. *Fitoterapia*, Vol. 82, No. 2, (March 2011), 230-236, ISSN 0367-326X

Beedanagari, S.R.; Bebenek, I.; Bui, P. & Hankinson, O. (2009). Resveratrol inhibits dioxin-induced expression of human CYP1A1 and CYP1B1 by inhibiting recruitment of the aryl hydrocarbon receptor complex and RNA polymerase II to the regulatory regions of the corresponding genes. *Toxicol. Sci.*, Vol. 110, No. 1, (July 2009), pp. 61-67, ISSN 1096-6080

Bode, A.M. & Dong, Z. (2009). Cancer prevention research - then and now. *Nature Rev. Cancer*, Vol. 9, No. 7 (June 2009), pp. 508-516, ISSN 1474-175X

Bruno, R.D. & Njar, V.C.O. (2007). Targeting cytochrome P450 enzymes: A new approach in anti-cancer drug development. *Bioorg. Med. Chem.*, Vol. 15, No. 15 (August 2007), pp. 5047-5060, ISSN 0968-0896

Cai, Y.; Baer-Dubowska, W.; Ashwood-Smith, M.J.; Ceska, O.; Tachibana, S. & DiGiovanni, J. (1996). Mechanism-based inactivation of hepatic ethoxyresorufin O-dealkylation activity by naturally occurring coumarins. *Chem. Res. Toxicol.*, Vol. 9, No. 4, (June 1996), pp. 729-736, ISSN 0893-228X

Cai, Y.; Baer-Dubowska, W.; Ashwood-Smith, M. & DiGiovanni, J. (1997). Inhibitory effects of naturally occurring coumarins on the metabolic activation of benzo[a]pyrene and 7,12-dimethylbenz[a]anthracene in cultured mouse keratinocytes. *Carcinogenesis*, Vol. 18, No. 8 (August 1997), pp. 215-222, ISSN 0143-3334

Canistro, D.; Bonamassa, B.; Pozzetti, L.; Sapone, A.; Abdel-Rahman, S.Z.; Biagi, G.L. & Paolini, M., (2009). Alteration of xenobiotic metabolizing enzymes by resveratrol in liver and lung of CD1 mice. *Food Chem. Toxicol.* Vol. 47, No. 2, (February 2009), pp. 454-461, ISSN 0278-6915

Casper, R.F.; Quesne, M.; Rogers, I.M.; Shirota, T.; Jolivel, A.; Milgrom, E. & Savouret, J.F. (1999). Resveratrol has antagonist activity on the aryl hydrocarbon receptor: implications for prevention of dioxin toxicity. *Mol. Pharmacol.* Vol. 56, No. 4, (October 1999), pp. 784-790, ISSN 0026-895X

Castro, D.J.; Baird, W.M.; Pereira, C.B.; Giovanini, J.; Lohr, C.V.; Fischer, K.A.; Yu, Z.; Gonzalez, F.J.; Krueger, S.K. & Williams, D.E. (2008). Fetal mouse Cyp1b1 and transplacental carcinogenesis from maternal exposure to dibenzo(a,1)pyrene. *Cancer Prev. Res. (Phila)*, Vol. 1, No. 2, pp. 128-134, ISSN 1940-6207

Chang, T.K.H.; Lee, W.B. & Ko, H.H. (2000). Trans-resveratrol modulates the catalytic activity and mRNA expression of the procarcinogens-activating human cytochrome P450 1B1. *Can. J. Physiol. Pharmacol.*, Vol. 78, No. 11 (November 2011), pp. 874-881, ISSN 0008-4212

Chang, T.K.H.; Chen, J. & Lee, W.B. (2001). Differential inhibition and inactivation of human CYP1 enzymes by trans-resveratrol: evidence for mechanism-based inactivation of CYP1A2. *J. Pharmacol. Exp. Ther.*, Vol. 299, No. 3, (December 2001), pp. 874-882, ISSN 0022-3565

Chang, T.K.H.; Chen, J. & Yu, C.-T. (2007). In vitro inhibition of rat CYP1A1 and CYP1A2 by piceatannol, a hydroxylated metabolite of trans-resveratrol. *Drug Metab. Lett.*, 1, 1, (January 2007), pp. 13-16, ISSN 1872-3128

Chaudhary, A. & Willett, K.L. (2006). Inhibition of human cytochrome CYP1 enzymes by flavonoids of St. John's wort. *Toxicology*, Vol. 217, No. 2-3, (January 2006), pp. 194-205, ISSN 0300-483X

Chen, Z.H.; Hurh, Y.J.; Na, H.K.; Kim, J.H.; Chun, Y.J.; Kim, D.H.; Kang, K.S.; Cho, M.H. & Surh, Y.J. (2004). Resveratrol inhibits TCDD-induced expression of CYP1A1 and CYP1B1 and catechol estrogen-mediated oxidative DNA damage in cultured human mammary epithelial cells. *Carcinogenesis*, Vol. 25, No. 10, (October 2004), pp. 2005-2013, ISSN 0143-3334

Cho, U.S.; Park, E.Y.; Dong, M.S.; Park, B.S.; Kim, K. & Kim, K.H. (2003). Tight-binding inhibition by α–naphthoflavone of human cytochrome P450 1A2. *Biochim. Biophys. Acta*, Vol. 1648, No. 1-2, (May 2003), pp. 195-202, ISSN 0006-3002

Chun, Y.J.; Kim, M.Y. & Guengerich, F.P. (1999). Resveratrol is a selective human cytochrome P450 1A1 inhibitor. *Biochem. Biophys. Res. Commun.*, Vol. 262, No. 1, (August 2999), pp. 20-24, ISSN 0006-291X

Chun, Y.J.; Ryu, S.Y.; Jeong, T.C. & Kim, M.Y. (2001a). Mechanism-based inhibition of human cytochrome P450 1A1 by rhapontigenin. *Drug Metab. Dispos.*, Vol. 29, No. 4, (April 2001), pp. 389-393, ISSN 0090-9556

Chun, Y.J.; Kim, S.; Kim, D.; Lee, S.K. & Guengerich, F.P. (2001b). A new selective and potent inhibitor of human cytochrome P450 1B1 and its application to antimutagenesis. *Cancer Res.*, Vol. 61, No. 22, (November 2001), pp. 8164-8170, ISSN 0008-5472

Ciolino, H.P. & Yeh, G.C. (1999). Inhibition of aryl hydrocarbon-induced cytochrome P-450 1A1 enzyme activity and CYP1A1 expression by resveratrol. *Mol. Pharmacol.*, Vol. 56, No. 4, (October 1999), pp. 760-767, ISSN 0026-895X

Ciolino, H.P.; Daschner, P.J. & Yeh, G.C. (1998). Resveratrol inhibits transcription of CYP1A1 in vitro by preventing activation of the aryl hydrocarbon receptor. *Cancer Res.*, Vol. 58, No. 24, (December 1998), pp. 5707-5712, ISSN 0008-5472

de Medina, P.; Casper, R.; Savouret, J.-F. & Poirot, M. (2005). Synthesis and biological properties of new stilbene derivatives of resveratrol as new selective aryl hydrocarbon modulators. *J. Med. Chem.*, Vol. 48, No. 1, (January 2005), pp. 287-291, ISSN 1520-4804

Don, M.-J.; Lewis, D.F.V.; Wang, S.-Y.; Tsai, M.-W. & Ueng, Y.F. (2003). Effect of structural modification on the inhibitory selectivity of rutaecarpine derivatives on human CYP1A1, CYP1A2, and CYP1B1. *Bioorg. Med. Chem. Lett.*, Vol. 13, No.15, (August 2003), pp. 2535-2538, ISSN 0960-894X

Gaudineau, C.; Beckerman, R.; Welbourn, S. & Auclair, K. (2004). Inhibition of human P450 enzymes by multiple constituents of the Ginkgo biloba extract. *Biochem. Biophys. Res. Commun.*, Vol. 318, No. 4, (June 2004), pp. 1072-1078, ISSN 0006-291X

Gerhauser, C.; Klimo, K.; Heiss, E.; Neumann, I.; Gamal-Eldeen, A.; Knauft, J.; Liu, G.Y.; Sitthimonchai, S. & Frank, N. (2003) Mechanism-based in vitro screening of potential cancer chemopreventive agents. *Mutat. Res.*, Vol. 523-524, (February-March 2003), pp. 163-172, ISSN 0027-5107

Gonzalez, F.J. (2002).Transgenic models in xenobiotic metabolism and toxicology. *Toxicology*, Vol. 181-182 (December 2002), pp. 237-239, ISSN 0300-483X

Goswami, S.K. & Das, D.K. (2009). Resveratrol and chemoprevention. *Cancer Lett.*, Vol. 284, No. 1, (October 2009), pp. 1-6, ISSN 0304-3835

Guengerich, F.P.; Chun, Y-J.; Kim, D.; Gillam, E.M.J. & Shimada, T. (2003). Cytochrome P450 1B1: a target for inhibition in anticarcinogenesis strategies. *Mutat. Res.*, Vol. 523-524, (February-March), pp. 173-182, ISSN 0027-5107

Itoh, T.; Takemura, H.; Shimoi, K. & Yamamoto, K. (2010). A 3D model of CYP1B1 explains the dominant 4-hydroxylation of estradiol. *J.Chem. Inf. Model.*, Vol. 50, No. 6, (June 2010), pp. 1173-1178, ISSN 1549-9596

Jang, M.; Cai, L.; Udeani, G.O.; Slowing, K.V.; Thomas, C.F.; Beecher, C.W.W.; Fong, H.H.S.; Farnsworth, N.R.; Kinghorn, A.D.; Mehta, R.G.; Moon, R.C. & Pezzuto, J.M. (1997). Cancer chemopreventive activity of resveratrol, a natural product derived from grapes, *Science*, Vol. 275, No. 5297, (January 1997), pp. 218-220, ISSN 0036-8075

Kim, S.; Ko, H.; Park, J.E.; Jung, S.; Lee, S.K. & Chun, Y.J. (2002). Design, synthesis and discovery of novel trans-stilbene analogues as potent and selective human cytochrome P450 1B1 inhibitors. *J. Med. Chem.*, Vol. 45, No. 1, (January 2002), pp. 160-164, ISSN 1520-4804

Kisselev, P.; Schunck, W.H.; Roots, I. & Schwarz, D. (2005). Association of CYP1A1 polymorphism with differential metabolic activation of 17-β-estradiol and estrone. *Cancer Res.*, Vol. 65, No. 7, (April 2005), pp. 2972-2978, ISSN 0008-5472

Kuhnau, J. (1976). A class of semiessential food components: their role in human nutrition. *World Rev. Nutr. Diet*, Vol. 24, pp. 117-191, ISSN 0084-2230

Lamb, D.C.; Waterman, M.R.; Kelly, S.L. & Guengerich, F.P. (2007). Cytochromes P450 and drug discovery. *Curr. Opin. Biotech.*, Vol. 18, No. 6, (December 2007), pp. 504-512, ISSN 0958-1669

Lee, A.J.; Cai, M.X.; Thomas, P.E.; Conney, A.H. & Zhu, B.T. (2003). Characterization of the oxidative metabolites of 17β-estradiol and estrone formed by 15 selectively expressed human cytochrome p450 isoforms. *Endocrinology*, Vol. 144, No. 8, (August 2003), pp. 3382-3398, ISSN 0013-7227

Lewis, D.F.V. (1997). Quantitative structure – activity relationships in substrates, inducers and inhibitors of cytochrome P450 (CYP1). Drug Metab. Rev., Vol. 29, No. 3, (August 1997), pp. 589-650, ISSN 0360-2532

Lewis, D.F.V.; Lake, B.G.; George, S.G.; Dickins, M.; Eddershaw, P.J.; Tarbit, M.H.; Beresford, A.P.; Goldfarb, P.S. & Guegerich, F.P. (1999). Molecular modeling of CYP1 family enzymes CYP1A1, CYP1A2, CYP1A6 and CYP1B1 based on sequence homology with CYP102. *Toxicology*, Vol. 139, No. 1-2, (November 1999), pp. 53-79, ISSN 0300-483X

Lewis, D.F.V.; Ito, Y. & Lake, B.G. (2006). Metabolism of coumarin by human P450s: A molecular modeling study. *Toxicol. in vitro*, Vol. 20, No 2, (March 2006), pp. 256-264, ISSN 0887-2333

Liehr, J.G. & Ricci, M.J. (1996). 4-Hydroxylation of estrogens as marker of human mammary tumors. *Proc. Natl. Acad. Sci. U.S.A.* , Vol. 93, No. 8, (April 1996), pp. 3294-3296, ISSN 0027-8424

MacPherson, L. & Matthews, J. (2010). Inhibition of aryl hydrocarbon receptor-dependent transcription by resveratrol or kaempferol is independent of estrogen receptor α expression in human breast cancer cells. *Cancer Lett.*, Vol. 299, No. 2, (December 2010), pp. 119-129, ISSN 0304-3835

Mc Fadyen, M.C. & Murray, G.I. (2005). Cytochrome P450 1B1: a novel anticancer therapeutic target. *Future Oncol.* 1, No. 2, (April 2005), pp. 259-263, ISSN 1479-6694

Mikstacka, R.; Przybylska, D.; Rimando, A.M. & Baer-Dubowska, W. (2007). Inhibition of human recombinant cytochromes P450 CYP1A1 and CYP1B1 by trans-resveratrol metyl ethers. *Mol. Nutr. Food Res.*, Vol. 51, No. 5, (May 2007), pp. 517-524, ISSN 1613-4125

Mikstacka, R.; Rimando, A.M.; Szalaty, K.; Stasik, K. & Baer-Dubowska, W. (2006). Effect of natural analogues of trans-resveratrol on cytochromem P450 1A2 and 2E1 catalytic activities. *Xenobiotica*, Vol. 36, No. 4, (April 2006), pp. 269-285, ISSN 0049-8254

Mikstacka, R.; Baer-Dubowska, W.; Wieczorek, M. & Sobiak, S. (2008). Thiomethylstilbenes
    as inhibitors of CYP1A1, CYP1A2 and CYP1B1 activities. *Mol. Nutr. Food Res.*, Vol.
    52, No. S1, (June 2008), pp. S77-S83, ISSN 1613-4125
Oetari, S.; Sudibyo, M.; Commandeur, J.N.M.; Samhoedi, R. & Vermeulen, N.P.E. (1996).
    Effects of curcumin on cytochrome P450 and glutathione-S-transferase activities in rat
    liver. *Biochem. Pharmacol.*, Vol. 51, No. 1, (January 1996), pp. 39-45, ISSN 0006-2952
Piver, B.; Berthou, F.; Dreano, Y. & Lucas, D. (2003). Differential inhibition of human
    cytochrome P450 enzymes by ε-viniferin, the dimer of resveratrol: comparison with
    resveratrol and polyphenols from alcoholized beverages. *Life Sci.*, Vol. 73, No. 9,
    (July 2003), pp. 1199-1213, ISSN 0024-3205
Piver, B.; Fer, M.; Vitrac, X.; Merillon, J.-M.; Dreano, Y.; Berthou, F. & Lucas, D. (2004).
    Involvment of cytochrome P450 1A2 in the biotransformation of trans-resveratrol in
    human liver microsomes. *Biochem. Pharmacol.*, Vol. 68, No. 4, (August 2004), pp.
    773-783, ISSN 0006-2952
Potter, G.A.; Patterson, L.H.; Wanogho, E.; Perry, P.J.; Butler, P.C.; Iljaz, T.; Ruparelia, K.C.; Lamb,
    J.H.; Farmer, P.B.; Stanley, L.A. & Burke, M.D. (2002). The cancer preventive agent
    resveratrol is converted to the anticancer agent piceatannol by the cytochrome P450
    enzyme CYP1B1. *Br. J. Cancer*, Vol. 86, No. 5, (March 2002), pp. 774-778, ISSN 0007-0920
Rendic, S. & Di Carlo, F.J. (1997). Human cytochromes P450 enzymes: a status report
    summarizing their reactions, substrates, inducers, and inhibitors. *Drug Metab. Rev.*,
    Vol. 29, No. 1-2, (February-May 1997), pp. 413-580, ISSN 0360-2532
Revel, A.; Raanani, H.; Younglai, E.; Xu, J.; Rogers, I.; Han, R.; Savouret, J.F. & Casper, R.F.
    (2003). Resveratrol, a natural aryl hydrocarbon receptor antagonist, protects lung
    from DNA damage and apoptosis caused by benzo[a]pyrene. *J. Appl. Toxicol.*, Vol.
    23, No. 4, (July-August 2003), pp. 255-261, ISSN 0260-437X
Rimando, A.M.; Cuendet, M.; Desmarchelier, C.; Mehta, R.G.; Pezzuto, J.M. & Duke, O.D.
    (2002). Cancer chemopreventive and antioxidant activities of pterostilbene, a
    naturally occurring analogue of resveratrol. *J. Agric. Food Chem.*, Vol. 50, No. 12,
    (June 2002), pp. 3453-3457, ISSN 0021-8561
Rimando, A.M.; Kalt, W.; Magee, J.B.; Dewey, J. & Ballington, J.R. (2004). Resveratrol,
    pterostilbene, and piceatannol in Vaccinium berries. *J. Agric. Food Chem.*, Vol. 52,
    No. 15, (July 2004), pp. 4713-4719, ISSN 0021-8561
Rimando, A.M. & Suh, N. (2008). Biological/chemopreventive activity of stilbenes and their
    effect on colon cancer. *Planta Med.*, Vol. 74, No. 13, (October 2008), pp. 1635-1643,
    ISSN 0032-0943
Rodeiro, I.; Donato, M.T.; Jimenez, N.; Garrido, G.; Molina-Torres, J.; Menendez, R.; Castell,
    J.V. & Gomez-Lechon, M.J. (2009). Inhibition of human P450 enzymes by natural
    extracts used in traditional medicine. *Phytother. Res.*, Vol. 23, No. 2, (February 2009),
    pp. 279-282, ISSN 0951-418X
Ryu, S.-D. & Chung, W.-G. (2003). Induction of the procarcinogen-activating CYP1A2 by a
    herbal dietary supplement in rats and humans. *Food Chem. Toxicol.*, Vol. 41, No. 6,
    (June 2003), pp. 861-866, ISSN 0278-6915
Schwarz, D. & Roots, I. (2003). In vitro assessment of inhibition by natural polyphenols of
    metabolic activation of procarcinogens by human CYP1A1. *Biochem. Biophys. Res.
    Commun.*, Vol. 303, No. 3, (April 2003), pp. 902-907, ISSN 0006-291X
Schwarz, D.; Kisselev, P.; Schunck, W.-H. & Roots, I. (2011). Inhibition of 17β-estradiol
    activation by CYP1A1: genotype- and regioselective inhibition by St. John's Wort

and natural polyphenols. *Biochim. Biophys. Acta*, Vol. 1814, No. 1, (January 2011), pp. 168-174, ISSN 0006-3002

Sporn, M.B. & Liby, K.T. (2005) Cancer chemoprevention: scientific promise, clinical uncertainty. *Nature Clinical Practise Oncology*, Vol. 2, No. 10, (October 2005), pp. 518-525, ISSN 1743-4254

Swanson, H.I.; Njar, W.C.O.; Yu, Z.; Castro, D.J.; Gonzalez, F.J.; Williams, D.E.; Huang, Y.; Kong, A.-N. T.; Doloff, J.C.; Ma, J.; Waxman, D.J. & Scott, E.E. (2010). Targeting drug-metabolizing enzymes for effective chemoprevention and chemotherapy. *Drug Metab. Dispos.*, Vol. 38, No. 4, (April 2010), pp. 539-544, ISSN 0090-9556

Szaefer, H.; Cichocki, M.; Brauze, D. & Baer-Dubowska, W. (2004). Alteration in phase I and II enzyme activities and polycyclic aromatic hydrocarbon-DNA adduct formation by plant phenolics in mouse epidermis. *Nutr. Cancer* Vol. 48, No. 1, (January 2004), pp. 70-77, ISSN 0163-5581

Szekeres, T.; Fritzer-Szekeres, M.; Saiko, P. & Jager, W. (2010). Resveratrol and resveratrol analogues – structure-activity relationship. *Pharm. Res.*, 27, 6, (March 2010), pp. 1042-1048, ISSN 0724-8741

Takemura, H.; Itoh, T.; Yamamoto, K.; Sakakibara, H. & Shimoi, K. (2010). Selective inhibition of methoxyflavonoids on human CYP1B1 activity. *Bioorg. Med. Chem.*, Vol. 18, No. 17, (September 2010), pp. 6310-6315, ISSN 0968-0896

Thapliyal, R. & Maru, G.B. (2001). Inhibition of cytochrome P450 isozymes by curcumins in vitro and in vivo. *Food Chem. Toxicol.*, Vol. 39, No. 6, (June 2001), pp. 541-547, ISSN 0278-6915

Walle, T.; Hsieh, F.; DeLegge, M.H.; Oatis, J.E.,Jr. & Walle, U.K. (2004). High absorption but very low bioavailability of oral resveratrol in humans. *Drug Metab. Dispos.*, Vol. 32, No. 12, (December 2004), pp. 1377-1382, ISSN 0090-9556

Walle, U.K. & Walle, T. (2007). Novel methoxylated flavone inhibitors of cytochrome P450 1B1 in SCC9 human oral cancer cells. *J. Pharm. Pharmacol.*, Vol. 59, No. 6, (June 2007), pp. 857-862, ISSN 0022-3573

Wattenberg, L.W. (1985). Chemoprevention of cancer. *Cancer Res.*, Vol. 45, No. 1, (January 1985), pp. 1-8, ISSN 0008-5472

Wenzel, E.; Soldo, T.; Erbersdobler, H. & Somoza, V. (2005). Bioactivity and metabolism of trans-resveratrol orally administered to Wistar rats. *Mol. Nutr. Food Res.*, Vol. 49, No. 5, (May 2005), pp. 482-494, ISSN 1613-4125

William, W.N., Jr.; Heymach, J.V.; Kim, E.S. & Lippman, S.M. (2009). Molecular targets for cancer chemoprevention. *Nat. Rev. Drug Discov.*, Vol. 8, No. 3, (March 2009), pp. 213-225, ISSN 1474-1776

Yamaori, S.; Kushihara, M.; Yamamoto, I. & Watanabe, K. (2010). Characterization of major phytocannabinoids, cannabidiol and cannabinol, as isoform selective and potent inhibitiors of human CYP1 enzymes. *Biochem. Pharmacol.*, Vol. 79, No. 11, (June 2010), pp. 1691-1698, ISSN 0006-2952

Zhai, S.; Dai, R.; Friedman, F.K. & Vestal, R.E. (1998). Comparative inhibition of human cytochromes P450 1A1 and 1A2 by flavonoids. *Drug Metab. Dispos.*, Vol. 26, No. 10, (October 1998), pp. 989-992, ISSN 0090-9556

Permissions

The contributors of this book come from diverse backgrounds, making this book a truly international effort. This book will bring forth new frontiers with its revolutionizing research information and detailed analysis of the nascent developments around the world.

We would like to thank Iraj Rasooli, for lending his expertise to make the book truly unique. He has played a crucial role in the development of this book. Without his invaluable contribution this book wouldn't have been possible. He has made vital efforts to compile up to date information on the varied aspects of this subject to make this book a valuable addition to the collection of many professionals and students.

This book was conceptualized with the vision of imparting up-to-date information and advanced data in this field. To ensure the same, a matchless editorial board was set up. Every individual on the board went through rigorous rounds of assessment to prove their worth. After which they invested a large part of their time researching and compiling the most relevant data for our readers. Conferences and sessions were held from time to time between the editorial board and the contributing authors to present the data in the most comprehensible form. The editorial team has worked tirelessly to provide valuable and valid information to help people across the globe.

Every chapter published in this book has been scrutinized by our experts. Their significance has been extensively debated. The topics covered herein carry significant findings which will fuel the growth of the discipline. They may even be implemented as practical applications or may be referred to as a beginning point for another development. Chapters in this book were first published by InTech; hereby published with permission under the Creative Commons Attribution License or equivalent.

The editorial board has been involved in producing this book since its inception. They have spent rigorous hours researching and exploring the diverse topics which have resulted in the successful publishing of this book. They have passed on their knowledge of decades through this book. To expedite this challenging task, the publisher supported the team at every step. A small team of assistant editors was also appointed to further simplify the editing procedure and attain best results for the readers.

Our editorial team has been hand-picked from every corner of the world. Their multi-ethnicity adds dynamic inputs to the discussions which result in innovative outcomes. These outcomes are then further discussed with the researchers and contributors who give their valuable feedback and opinion regarding the same. The feedback is then collaborated with the researches and they are edited in a comprehensive manner to aid the understanding of the subject.

Apart from the editorial board, the designing team has also invested a significant amount of their time in understanding the subject and creating the most relevant covers. They scrutinized every image to scout for the most suitable representation of the subject and create an appropriate cover for the book.

The publishing team has been involved in this book since its early stages. They were actively engaged in every process, be it collecting the data, connecting with the contributors or procuring relevant information. The team has been an ardent support to the editorial, designing and production team. Their endless efforts to recruit the best for this project, has resulted in the accomplishment of this book. They are a veteran in the field of academics and their pool of knowledge is as vast as their experience in printing. Their expertise and guidance has proved useful at every step. Their uncompromising quality standards have made this book an exceptional effort. Their encouragement from time to time has been an inspiration for everyone.

The publisher and the editorial board hope that this book will prove to be a valuable piece of knowledge for researchers, students, practitioners and scholars across the globe.

List of Contributors

Afeef S. Husni and Stephen J. Cutler
University of Mississippi, USA

Cinara V. da Silva, Fernanda M. Borges and Eudes S. Velozo
Federal University of Bahia, Brazil

João X. de Araújo-Júnior, Mariana S.G. de Oliveira, Pedro G.V. Aquino, Magna S. Alexandre-Moreira and Antônio E.G. Sant'Ana
Universidade Federal de Alagoas, Brazil

Kirley M. Canuto, Edilberto R. Silveira, Antonio Marcos E. Bezerra, Luzia Kalyne A. M. Leal and Glauce Socorro B. Viana
Empresa Brasileira de Pesquisa Agropecuária, Universidade Federal do Ceará, Brazil

Nor Hadiani Ismail, Asmah Alias and Che Puteh Osman
Universiti Teknologi MARA, Malaysia

Maha Aboul Ela, Abdalla El-Lakany and Mohamad Ali Hijazi
Dept. of Pharmacognosy, Faculty of Pharmacy, Beirut Arab University, Beirut, Lebanon

Francisco José Queiroz Monte, Telma Leda Gomes de Lemos and Edilane de Sousa Gomes
Programa de Pós-Graduação em Química Universidade Federal do Ceará, Fortaleza – Ceará, Brazil

Mônica Regina Silva de Araújo
Depatamento de Química, Universidade Federal do Piauí, Teresina - Piauí, Brazil

Young Ho Kim, Jeong Ah Kim and Nguyen Xuan Nhiem
Chungnam National University, South Korea

Indah Epriliati
Widya Mandala Catholic University, Indonesia

Irine R. Ginjom
Swinburne University of Technology, Sarawak Campus, Malaysia

L.G. Rao
Department of Medicine, St. Michael's Hospital, University of Toronto, Canada

N. Kang and A.V. Rao
Department of Nutritional Sciences, Faculty of Medicine, University of Toronto, Canada

Patricia Isabel Manzano Santana and Esther Lilia Peralta Garcìa
Laboratorio Bioproductos, Centro de Investigaciones Biotecnológicas del Ecuador, CIBE-ESPOL, Ecuador

Mario Silva Osorio
Laboratorio de Productos Naturales de la Facultad de Ciencias, Naturales y Oceanográficas de la Universidad de Concepción, Chile

Olov Sterner
Centre for Analysis and Synthesis, Lund University, Sweden

Liliana Hernández Vázquez
Universidad Autónoma Metropolitana, Unidad Xochimilco, Depto. Sistemas Biológicos, México

Javier Palazon
Laboratorio de Fisiología Vegetal, Facultat of Farmacia, Universitat de Barcelona, Spain

Arturo Navarro-Ocaña
Departamento de Alimentos y Biotecnología, Facultad de Química "E" – UNAM, México

Renata Mikstacka, Zbigniew Dutkiewicz and Stanisław Sobiak
Department of Chemical Technology of Drugs, Poznań University of Medical Sciences, Poland

Wanda Baer-Dubowska
Department of Pharmaceutical Biochemistry, Poznań University of Medical Sciences, Poland